# Care Coordination *and* Transition Management

## CORE CURRICULUM

*Editors*
Sheila A. Haas, PhD, RN, FAAN
Beth Ann Swan, PhD, CRNP, FAAN
Traci S. Haynes, MSN, RN, CEN

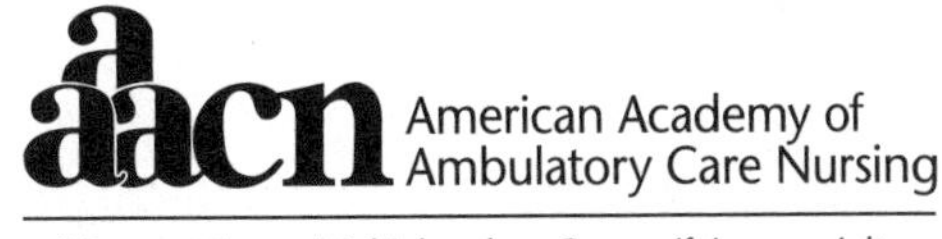

# *Care Coordination and Transition Management Core Curriculum*

**Editors**
Sheila A. Haas, PhD, RN, FAAN
Beth Ann Swan, PhD, CRNP, FAAN
Traci S. Haynes, MSN, RN, CEN

**Managing Editor:** Kenneth J. Thomas
**Managing Editor:** Katie R. Brownlow, ELS
**Director of Editorial Services:** Carol M. Ford
**Layout Design and Production:** Darin Peters
**Director of Creative Design and Production:** Jack M. Bryant

**AAACN Executive Director:** Cynthia Nowicki Hnatiuk, EdD, RN, CAE, FAAN
**AAACN Director of Association Services:** Pat Reichart
**AAACN Education Director:** Rosemarie Marmion, MSN, RN-BC, NE-BC
**AAACN Education Coordinator:** Kristina Moran

**Publication Management**
Anthony J. Jannetti, Inc.
East Holly Avenue, Box 56, Pitman, NJ 08071-0056
Phone: 856-256-2300; Fax: 856-589-7463; www.ajj.com

**FIRST EDITION**
ISBN: 978-1-940325-02-6



**DISCLAIMER**

The authors, reviewers, editors, and publishers of this book have made serious efforts to ensure that treatments, practices, and procedures are accurate and conform to standards accepted at the time of publication. Due to constant changes in information resulting from continuous research and clinical experience, reasonable differences in opinions among authorities, unique aspects of individual clinical situations, and the possibility of human error in preparing such a publication require that the reader exercise individual judgment when making a clinical decision, and if necessary, consult and compare information from other authorities, professionals, or sources.

**SUGGESTED CITATION**

Haas, S.A., Swan, B.A., & Haynes, T. S. (Eds.). (2014). *Care coordination and transition management core curriculum*. Pitman, NJ: American Academy of Ambulatory Care Nursing.

**Endorsed by the Academy of Medical-Surgical Nurses**

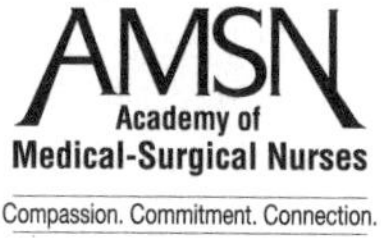




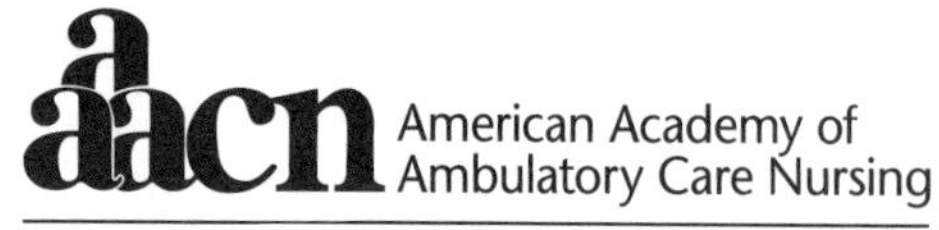


American Academy of Ambulatory Care Nursing (AAACN)
East Holly Avenue, Box 56, Pitman, NJ 08071-0056
Phone: 800-AMB-NURS; Fax: 856-589-7463
aaacn@ajj.com; www.aaacn.org

# Table of Contents

# A Message from AAACN President

## The wait is over!
## The *Care Coordination and Transition Management (CCTM) Core Curriculum* Is Here

Health care reform and the Patient Protection and Affordable Care Act (2010) challenged the American health care system to find ways to manage the complex health needs of the population by increasing access to care and managing costs while providing the highest quality of care. Interprofessional patient-centered care models like the Patient-Centered Medical Home and Accountable Care Organizations are designed to provide personalized care management with "RNs ideally positioned to serve in the care coordinator/transition manager role" (Haas, Swan, & Haynes, 2013, p. 45). Safe, efficient, and effective transitions between providers, levels of care, and various care settings will be key factors to the success of these models.

The vision for this much anticipated text grew out of the need and desire for evidence-based registered nurse (RN) competencies to provide education for and demonstrate the effectiveness of the role of the RN in care coordination and transition management (CCTM). The American Academy of Ambulatory Care Nursing (AAACN) developed an action plan in 2011 to initiate this endeavor. The project included three phases for the core curriculum development and a fourth phase to include the development of an online education course (Haas et al., 2013).

Four separate interprofessional Expert Panels were convened. The first reviewed and analyzed the literature. The second defined the nine dimensions and the core competencies and associated activities related to RN care coordination and transition management. The third built upon the work of the first two panels and created the table of evidence which includes the competencies and the knowledge, skills, and attitudes necessary to fulfill this important role. A fourth panel of nurse leaders and experts from ambulatory and acute care was enlisted to develop and create this *Core Curriculum* and the online course corresponding to the content of the text.

For our three editors – Sheila A. Haas, PhD, RN, FAAN; Beth Ann Swan, PhD, CRNP, FAAN; and Traci S. Haynes, MSN, RN, BA, CEN – this project has been a labor of love! They have worked tirelessly to facilitate the work of the Expert Panels and to champion the publication of this cutting-edge text and educational course that will serve as a CCTM resource for all registered nurses. The AAACN Board of Directors and I thank our editors, the nurses and other professional colleagues who served on the Expert Panels, and the authors and reviewers who worked so diligently to bring the vision of this *Core Curriculum* to reality. We also acknowledge the Academy of Medical-Surgical Nurses (AMSN) for their collaboration in serving on the Expert Panels; for their assistance in developing the chapter "Care Coordination and Transition Management Between Acute Care and Ambulatory Care;" and for their endorsement of the *Core Curriculum.*

I hope that you find this outstanding publication to be a valuable resource in your nursing practice wherever you coordinate care or manage patient transitions.

**Susan M. Paschke, MSN, RN-BC, NEA-BC**
*AAACN President, 2013-2014*

### References


Haas, S., Swan, B.A., & Haynes, T. (2013). Developing ambulatory care registered nurse competencies for care coordination and transition management. *Nursing Economic$, 31*(1), 44-49, 43.

Patient Protection and Affordable Care Act. (2010). Public Law 111-148, § 2702, 124 Stat. 119, 318-319.

# Foreword

## A Competency Model to Improve Quality and Safety, Care Coordination, and Transitions

Health care has been in continual change over the past few decades, implementing multiple strategies to improve outcomes. Nurses are increasingly positioned to help lead these changes through advancements in nursing education and refocusing professional practice models. Competency models are one strategy for improving care by describing standardized care objectives that address the shortcomings identified in the Institute of Medicine report *To Err is Human* (IOM, 1999), and the quality goals described in the *Crossing the Quality Chasm* report (IOM, 2001). These reports revealed startling gaps in health care and proposed a quality framework, STEEEP, to improve care outcomes: all care should be Safe, Timely, Equitable, Efficient, Effective, and Patient-centered. These goals, in addition to changes from the 2012 Affordable Care Act, are changing health care access, delivery, and reimbursement dramatically. The 2010 IOM report *Future of Nursing* called for nurses to practice to their fullest preparation and also to seek advanced educational mobility to lead changes in improving care. Thus, nurses are uniquely positioned to provide key leadership in improving care management across the myriad care delivery settings, but need guidelines for specific settings and populations that help meet new regulations and reimbursement demands.

### A Competency-Based Resource

This *Care Coordination and Transition Management Core Curriculum* is a just-in-time competency-based resource to guide nurses in the new delivery systems and payment directives. Increasing complexity of care, diverse practice settings, and payer requirements are key factors that position nurses to have a leading role in care management across providers and transitions in care. The *Core Curriculum* addresses competencies for improving care outcomes among the multiple dimensions of growing complexity of care in diverse settings, and, in particular, ambulatory populations. Most guidelines and evidence-based standards have been developed based on acute care inpatient experiences without addressing care needs across transitions in settings or multiple providers. The three editors of this text have carefully researched the competencies needed for new care management roles, both inpatient and outpatient, to coordinate and manage care effectively.

Edited by three experts in ambulatory care who have each served as president of the American Academy of Ambulatory Care Nursing, the *Core Curriculum* provides a futuristic perspective that integrates the award-winning and widely adopted Quality and Safety Education for Nurses (QSEN) competency model (American Association of Colleges of Nursing, 2012; Cronenwett et al., 2007). The goal of QSEN (www.QSEN.org) is the integration of the six competencies into all of nursing so that quality and safety are part of nurses' daily work: patient-centered care, teamwork and collaboration, evidence-based practice, quality improvement, safety, and informatics. These competencies are now part of nursing education standards and other regulatory and certification guidelines.

The *Care Coordination and Transition Management Core Curriculum* provides a critical step in improving quality and safety of care and helps nurses understand better how to incorporate the QSEN competencies in practice. Patient-centered care is at the heart of safety; the Care Coordination and Transition Management standards describe specific evidence-based principles for accurate and personalized assessment as the basis for patient-centered care. Safety awareness is even more important in considering the unique practice settings that include advanced practice nurses who may be in independent or group practice, nurses who must communicate and share care goals among interprofessional colleagues, and those who manage small care teams or supervise unlicensed personnel. Recognizing breakdowns in processes is the first step to develop quality improvement initiatives that can close gaps between ideal and actual performance measures. Competency in informatics provides a key strategy for communication, decision support, and documentation.

### Making Care Standards Accessible

The potential power of this *Core Curriculum* is in making care standards readily accessible to nurses. Standardization in care is a major component of safe care. Evidence-based standards share best practices based on the latest evidence gathered from the literature and documented experiences. Nurses are the constant patient care providers who spend the most time with patients, and as such, have key information for making care decisions. Knowing when and how to speak up is critical for improving care outcomes. Many errors occur during transitions in care, whether between providers, between settings, or unit-to-unit transfers; standardized handoff processes and communication can assure care management without interruption.

Competency objectives identifying the knowledge, skills, and attitudes for accomplishing work help to standardize care by specifying competencies for providers in a particular setting or population focus to successfully perform functions or tasks. Competencies are defined by the knowledge needed for achievement, the skills that enable application, and the attitudes that shape caregiver responses and influence decision making about care. Competency models can also provide measurement criteria for assessing competency achievement. Competency development includes developing clinical judgment, reflecting on improving one's work, and awareness of the context of practice (Tanner, 2006). Competency development is more than achieving skills or completing tasks. A competency-based practice model guides organization of tasks within a patient-centered perspective to address needs in a particular care delivery setting such as nursing in an ambulatory care center or a specific patient population. Competency statements identifying the knowledge, skills, and attitudes can be applied to developing educational curriculum or specific training, identifying licensure and certification requirements, writing position descriptions, recruiting and hiring personnel, and/or evaluating employee performance.

### Empowering Nurses and Patients

Building on the six QSEN competencies, the *Care Coordination and Transition Management Core Curriculum* culminates in care guidelines across nine evidence-based dimensions: self-management, patient and family education and engagement, communication and transition, coaching and counseling patients and families, nursing process, teamwork and collaboration, patient-centered care planning, decision support and information systems, and advocacy. The comprehensive nature of the competencies can leverage improvements across all settings and providers and be applied in multiple ways from orientation to evaluation. These competencies are about empowering nurses and empowering patients applying the change model of *Will, Ideas, and Execution.* We know nurses have the *will* to improve care when they have the *ideas* and have the resources for *execution.* The *Care Coordination and Transition Management Core Curriculum* is a vital resource for all nurses that fits the current practice arena and has the capacity to improve care for all.

**Gwen Sherwood, PhD, RN, FAAN**
*Associate Dean for Academic Affairs and Professor*
*University of North Carolina at Chapel Hill*
*School of Nursing*
*Chapel Hill, NC*

### References

American Association of Colleges of Nursing (AACN). (2012). *QSEN education consortium: Graduate-level QSEN competencies, knowledge, skills and attitudes.* Retrieved from http://www.aacn.nche.edu/faculty/qsen/competencies.pdf

Cronenwett, L., Sherwood, G., Barnsteiner, J., Disch, J., Johnson, J., Mitchell, P., Sullivan, D.T., & Warren, J. (2007). *Quality and safety education for nurses. Nursing Outlook, 55*(3), 122-131.

Institute of Medicine (IOM). (1999). *To err is human: Building a safer health system.* Washington, DC: National Academies Press.

Institute of Medicine (IOM). (2001). *Crossing the quality chasm: A new health system for the 21st century.* Washington, DC: National Academies Press.

Institute of Medicine (IOM). (2010). *The future of nursing: Leading change, advancing health.* Washington, DC: The National Academies Press.

Tanner, C. (2006). Thinking like a nurse: A research based model of clinical judgment in nursing. *Journal of Nursing Education, 45*(6), 204-211.

# Preface

The passage of the Patient Protection and Affordable Care Act (ACA) in 2010 has provisions fostering movement from a focus on acute care to care across the continuum with wellness, health promotion, and disease prevention. Settings for care, again fostered by the ACA, are the Patient-Centered Medical Home (PCMH) and Accountable Care Organizations. ACA provisions offer many opportunities for access to primary care for patients and for contributions by ambulatory care nurses as well as for nurses working in acute, subacute, and home care. The ACA also has provisions that mirror the Institute of Medicine's (IOM, 2001) *Crossing the Quality Chasm* report recommendations for health care reform, including the need for care to be safe, effective, patient centered, timely, efficient, and equitable. Other ACA provisions are focused on use of evidence-based practice to guide care provided by interprofessional teams. Again, in PCMHs and other ambulatory care settings, these expectations spelled out in health care reform legislation offer opportunities for ambulatory and acute care nurses to be major contributors. Finally, another IOM report, *The Future of Nursing: Leading Change, Advancing Health* (2010), includes recommendations, two in particular, that speak directly to opportunities for all nurses in this era of health care reform: (a) Nurses should practice to the full extent of their education and training, and (b) Nurses should be full partners, with physicians and other health care professionals, in redesigning health care in the United States (IOM, 2010).

*The Care Coordination and Transition Management Core Curriculum for Ambulatory Care Nursing* is a comprehensive, evidence-based guide designed to support the American Academy of Ambulatory Care Nursing's (AAACN) mission: "To advance the art and science of ambulatory care nursing" and provide a valid and reliable care coordination and transition management model and practice resource for nurses (AAACN, 2014). Recognizing that demand for primary and specialty care would increase with enactment of the ACA and that the numbers of patients with complex chronic illnesses were increasing, the AAACN decided to invest in a translational research project to define the dimensions of care coordination and transition management (CCTM). This foundation could provide for development of CCTM competencies for nurses and evidence-based content for professional education and continuing development of ambulatory and acute care nurses working in new models of care delivery in PCMHs and other care settings.

This *Care Coordination and Transition Management Core Curriculum* is one outcome of the CCTM project. This *Core Curriculum* text is designed for registered nurses currently working in ambulatory care and acute care settings who aspire to move into the RN in CCTM role as well as for nurses who are considering transitioning into ambulatory or other settings where they desire to develop CCTM knowledge, skills, and attitudes that are essential to the CCTM role. The *Core Curriculum* is a rich, evidence-based resource that can enhance nursing student experiences in ambulatory, acute, subacute, and home care settings. This *Core Curriculum* uses the Quality and Safety in Nursing Education (QSEN) Competency framework (Cronenwett et al., 2007) that specifies knowledge, skills, and attitudes (KSA) for each of the nine Registered Nurse Care Coordination and Transition Management dimensions. The unique KSA tables included in each chapter provide a rich resource by summarizing chapter content and enhancing understanding of the breadth and depth of each dimension. The tables categorize requisite skills and attitudes that are needed in addition to knowledge of content for each Care Coordination and Transition Management dimension.

This undertaking could not have come to fruition without the commitment and expertise of the volunteer AAACN member expert contributors who participated in one or more expert panels and were authors of chapters in this *Core Curriculum*. The AAACN Board of Directors and membership, as well as its association management firm, Anthony J. Jannetti, Inc., are to be commended for their vision, leadership, and support of this translational research project and the publication of the *Care Coordination and Transition Management Core Curriculum*. We are proud to provide this text to RNs who want to grow as care coordinators and transition managers to better serve our most vulnerable patient populations.

**Sheila A. Haas, PhD, RN, FAAN**
*Lead Editor*
**Beth Ann Swan, PhD, CRNP, FAAN**
*Co-Editor*
**Traci S. Haynes, MSN, RN, CEN**
*Co-Editor and Project Manager*

### References

American Academy of Ambulatory Care Nursing (AAACN). (2014). *Membership.* Retrieved from https://www.aaacn.org/membership

Cronenwett, L., Sherwood, G., Barnsteiner, J., Disch, J., Johnson, J., Mitchell, P., … Warren, J. (2007). Quality and safety education for nurses. *Nursing Outlook, 55*(3), 122-131.

Institute of Medicine (IOM). (2001). *Crossing the quality chasm.* Washington, DC: National Academies Press.

Institute of Medicine (IOM). (2010). *The future of nursing: Leading change, advancing health* (1st ed.). Washington, DC: National Academies Press.

Patient Protection and Affordable Care Act. (2010). Public Law 111-148, § 2702, 124 Stat. 119, 318-319.

# Contributors

**Karen Alexander, MSN, RN**
Instructor
Thomas Jefferson University
Philadelphia, PA

**Janine Allbritton, MSN, RN**
Regional Clinical Manager
USMD
Irving, TX

**Ida M. Androwich, PhD, RN, BC-NI, FAAN**
Professor and Director of Graduate HSM Programs
Loyola University Chicago
Maywood, IL

**Deborah E. Aylard, MSN, RN**
Nurse Clinical Educator
Core Physicians, LLC
Exeter, NH

**Mary Anne Bord-Hoffman, MN, RN-BC**
Nurse Manager
VA Palo Alto Healthcare System
San Jose Community Based Outpatient Clinic
San Jose, CA

**Stephanie Coffey, DNP, MBA, FNP-BC, RN-BC**
Associate Chief Nurse Executive Ambulatory Care/NP
U.S. Department of Veterans Affairs
VA Roseburg Healthcare System
Roseburg, OR

**Mary Sue Dailey, APN-CNS**
Advanced Practice Nurse, Clinical Nurse Specialist, Adult Medical-Surgical Acute Care
Advocate Good Samaritan Hospital
Downers Grove, IL

**Judy Dawson-Jones, MPH, BSN, RN**
Director of Nursing, General Care
Akron Children's Hospital
Akron, OH

**Janet Fuchs, MBA, MSN, RN, NEA-BC**
Senior Director Ambulatory Nursing
Cleveland Clinic
Cleveland, OH

**Vicki Grant, MS, RN-BC**
Professional Development Specialist
Virginia Mason Medical Center
Seattle, WA

**Kristene Grayem, MSN, CNP, RN**
Director for Clinical Systems/Performance Improvement & Nursing
Akron Children's Hospital, Department of Pediatrics
Akron, OH

**M. Elizabeth Greenberg, PhD, RN-BC, C-TNP**
Assistant Clinical Professor
Northern Arizona University
Tucson, AZ

**Sheila A. Haas, PhD, RN, FAAN**
Professor
Marcella Niehoff School of Nursing
Loyola University Chicago
Maywood, IL
Past President
American Academy of Ambulatory Care Nursing

**Denise Hannagan, MSN, MHA, RN-BC**
Education Program Coordinator
Cedars-Sinai Medical Center
Los Angeles, CA

**Traci S. Haynes, MSN, RN, CEN**
Director Clinical Services
LVM Systems
Mesa, AZ
Past President
American Academy of Ambulatory Care Nursing

**Kari J. Hite, MN, RN, CDE**
Home Telehealth RN Care Coordinator
SAVAHCS
Tucson, AZ

**Anne Talbott Jessie, MSN, RN**
Senior Director of Ambulatory Nursing Practice
Carilion Clinic
Roanoke, VA

**Sheila A. Johnson, MBA, RN**
Director, ACO Quality and Care Coordination
Dartmouth-Hitchcock
Bedford, NH

**Rosemary Kennedy, PhD, MBA, RN, FAAN**
CEO
eCare Informatics, LLC
Frazer, PA

# Contributors

**Candia Baker Laughlin, MS, RN-BC**
Director of Nursing, Ambulatory Care Services
University of Michigan Health System
Ann Arbor, MI
Past President
American Academy of Ambulatory Care Nursing

**Cheryl Lovlien, MS, RN-BC**
Nursing Education Supervisor
Mayo Clinic
Rochester, MN

**Carol Mannone, MSN, RN, CH-GC**
Educator Primary Care
Lahey Hospital & Medical Center
Beverly, MA

**Naomi Mercier, MSN, RN-BC**
Nursing Director Primary Care
Lahey Health
Burlington, MA

**Kathy Mertens, MN, MPH, RN**
Director of Clinical Care Systems
UW Medicine Harborview Medical Center
Seattle, WA

**Carol Rutenberg, MNSc, RN-BC, C-TNP**
President
Telephone Triage Consulting, Inc.
Hot Springs, AR

**Kathryn B. Scheidt, MSN, MS, BSN, RN**
Telehealth Nursing Consultant
Independent Contractor
Westminister, CO

**Kathleen T. Sheehan, MS, BSN, RN-BC, CH-GCN**
Director of Ambulatory & Transitional Case Management
Lahey Hospital & Medical Center
Burlington, MA

**Beth Ann Swan, PhD, CRNP, FAAN**
Dean and Professor
Thomas Jefferson University
Philadelphia, PA
Past President
American Academy of Ambulatory Care Nursing

**Judith M. Toth-Lewis, PhD, MSN, RN**
Clinical Quality Consultant
Kaiser Permanente
Portland, OR

**Barbara Ellis Trehearne, PhD, RN**
VP of Clinical Excellence, Quality, & Nursing Practice
VP of Primary Care
Group Health
Seattle, WA

**Mary Hines Vinson, DNP, RN-BC**
Retired
Duke University Health System
Durham, NC

**Stephanie G. Witwer, PhD, RN, NEA-BC**
Administrator Employee and Community Health
Mayo Clinic
Rochester, MN

# Reviewers

**Julie Alban, MSN, MPH, RN-BC**
RN – Patient Care Coordinator
The Villages VA Outpatient Clinic
The Villages, FL

**Carol Ann Attwood, MLS, MPH, RN, C**
Medical Librarian/Registered Nurse
Patient and Health Education Library
Mayo Clinic
Scottsdale, AZ

**Sharron D. Coffie, MSN, RN, CNS-BC, CHFN**
Manager, Nursing Practice Ambulatory Specialty Clinics
Froedtert & The Medical College of Wisconsin
Milwaukee, WI

**Sarah Creswell, BS, RN-BC**
Patient Education Specialist
Lehigh Valley Health Network
Allentown, PA

**Diane Davis, BSN, RN, DNPc**
Director, Medical Home Navigation Program
Concord Hospital
Concord, NH

**Eileen M. Esposito, DNP, RN-BC, CPHQ**
Principal & Executive Consultant
Ambulatory Expert Solutions
Jericho, NY

**Mary Anne Granger, MSN, RN**
Clinical Resource Leader, Ambulatory Services (Medical Home)
Maricopa Integrated Health Services
Phoenix, AZ

**Christine Griffel, BSN, RN-BC**
RN Care Manager
Veterans Administration Pittsburgh Healthcare System
Pittsburgh, PA

**Karla A. Hall, BSW, BSN, RN, CCM**
RN Program Coordinator, Palliative Care
PeaceHealth St. Joseph Medical Center
Bellingham, WA
Regional Coordinator, Care Transitions Program
University of Colorado Denver
Aurora, CO

**LT Dwight Hampton, MBA, BSN, RN-BC, PCMH CCE**
Deputy Director, Patient-Centered Medical Home Program Management Office
U.S. Navy Bureau of Medicine and Surgery
Falls Church, VA

**LCDR Eric J. Kulhan, MSHSA, MEd, BSN, RN-BC**
Head, Military & Staff Education
Captain James A. Lovell Federal Health Care Center
North Chicago, IL

**Cheryl Lovlien, MS, RN-BC**
Nursing Education Supervisor
Mayo Clinic
Rochester, MN

**Ann Marie Matlock, DNP, RN, NE-BC**
Service Chief, Medical-Surgical Specialties
CDR United States Public Health Service
National Institutes of Health Clinical Center
Bethesda, MD

**Cindy McConnell, MS, RN, NEA-BC**
Ambulatory Nursing Director
Children's Hospital Colorado
Aurora, CO

**Peggy Morgan-Griffin, RN-BC, MSHCA**
Supervisory Clinical Nurse, Specialty Services Clinic
Phoenix Indian Medical Center
Phoenix, AZ

**Edtrina L. Moss, MSN, RN-BC, NE-BC**
Nurse Manager
DeBakey VA Medical Center
Houston, TX

**Sue Olsson, BSN, RN-BC**
Rheumatology Nurse
University of Michigan Health System
Ann Arbor, MI

**Pamela E. Ruzic, MSN, RN-BC**
Health Coordinator – Outpatient Resident Clinic
Baylor University Medical Center
Dallas, TX

**Sandra L. Siedlecki, PhD, RN, CNS**
Senior Nurse Scientist
Office of Research & Innovation
Cleveland Clinic
Cleveland, OH

**Cynthia A. Standish, MSN, RN-BC**
Nurse Educator
Captain James A. Lovell Federal Health Care Center
North Chicago, IL

# Reviewers

**Judith M. Toth-Lewis, PhD, MSN, RN**
Clinical Quality Consultant
Kaiser Permanente
Portland, OR

**Catherine E. Vanderboom, PhD, RN**
Clinical Nurse Researcher
Mayo Clinic
Rochester, MN

**CDR Gayle L. Walker, BSN, RN-BC, PCMH CCE**
Program Manager, Navy Comprehensive Pain Management Program
U.S. Navy Bureau of Medicine and Surgery
Falls Church, VA

**Laurie Friday Walsh, MSN, RN, GNP**
Geriatric Nurse Practitioner
Kaiser Eldercare
Kaiser Sacramento
Sacramento, CA

**L. Renée Watson, MSN, RN**
Senior Director Nursing and Patient Care Coordination
St. Luke's Health System
Boise, ID

**Suzanne Wells, MSN, RN**
Manager
St. Louis Children's Hospital Answer Line
St. Louis, MO
Past President
American Academy of Ambulatory Care Nursing

**Stephanie G. Witwer, PhD, RN, NEA-BC**
Administrator Employee and Community Health
Mayo Clinic
Rochester, MN

# Expert Panels

## Phase 1 Expert Panel

Karen Alexander, MSN, RN***
Janine Allbritton, MSN, RN**
Jo Ann Appleyard, PhD, RN
Deborah E. Aylard, MSN, RN**
Jeff Bergen, MSN, RN, CIC
Deanna Blanchard, MSN, RN
Elizabeth Bradley, MSN, RN-BC
Stefanie Coffey, DNP, MBA, FNP-BC, RN-BC****
Patricia Grady, BSN, RN, CRNS, FABC
Denise Hannagan, MSN, MHA, RN-BC**
Clare Hastings, PhD, RN, FAAN
Anne Talbott Jessie, MSN, RN****
Sheila A. Johnson, MBA, RN**
CMDR. Catherine McNeal Jones, MSN, MBA, NC, USN HCM, RN-BC
Cheryl Lovlien, MS, RN-BC**
Carol Mannone, MSN, RN, CH-GC**
Sylvia McKenzie, MSN, RN, CPHQ
Shirley Morrison, PhD, RN, OCN
Janet Moye, PhD, RN, NEA-BC
Donna Parker, MA, BSN, RN-BC
Deborah Smith, DNP, RN
Erin Taylor, MSN, RN, CNOR
Debra Toney, PhD, RN, FAAN
Linda Walton, MSN, RN, CENP

## Phase 2 Expert Panel

Karen Alexander, MSN, RN***
Marc Altshuler, MD
Jill Arzouman, MS, RN, ACNS, BC, CMSRN
Stefanie Coffey, DNP, MBA, FNP-BC, RN-BC****
Sandy Fights, MS, RN, CMSRN, CNE
Janet Fuchs, MBA, MSN, RN, NEA-BC***
Jamie Green, MSN, RN
Anne Talbott Jessie, MSN, RN****
Diane Kelly, DrPH, MBA, RN
Lisa Kristosik, MSN, RN
Rosemarie Marmion, MSN, RN-BC, NE-BC***
Kathy Mertens, MN, MPH, RN***
Stephanie G. Witwer, PhD, RN, NEA-BC***

## Phase 3 Expert Panel

Stefanie Coffey, DNP, MBA, FNP-BC, RN-BC****
Janet Fuchs, MBA, MSN, RN, NEA-BC***
Anne Talbott Jessie, MSN, RN****
Rosemarie Marmion, MSN, RN-BC, NE-BC***
Nancy May, MSN, RN-C, NEA-BC
Kathy Mertens, MN, MPH, RN***
Carol Rutenberg, MNSc, RN-BC, C-TNP**
Barbara Ellis Trehearne, PhD, RN**
Stephanie G. Witwer, PhD, RN, NEA-BC***

## Phase 4 Expert Panel

Karen Alexander, MSN, RN***
Janine Allbritton, MSN, RN**
Ida M. Androwich, PhD, RN, BC-NI, FAAN
Deborah E. Aylard, MSN, RN**
Mary Anne Bord-Hoffman, MN, RN-BC
Stefanie Coffey, DNP, MBA, FNP-BC, RN-BC****
Mary Sue Dailey, APN-CNS
Judy Dawson-Jones, MPH, BSN, RN
Janet Fuchs, MBA, MSN, RN, NEA-BC***
Vicki Grant, MSN, RN-BC
Kristene Grayem, MSN, CNP, RN
M. Elizabeth Greenberg, PhD, RN-BC, C-TNP
Denise Hannagan, MSN, MHA, RN-BC**
Kari J. Hite, MN, RN, CDE
Anne Talbott Jessie, MSN, RN****
Sheila A. Johnson, MBA, RN**
Rosemary Kennedy, PhD, MBA, RN, FAAN
Candia Baker Laughlin, MS, RN-BC
Cheryl Lovlien, MS, RN-BC**
Carol Mannone, MSN, RN, CH-GC**
Rosemarie Marmion, MSN, RN-BC, NE-BC***
Naomi Mercier, MSN, RN-BC
Kathy Mertens, MN, MPH, RN***
Carol Rutenberg, MNSc, RN-BC, C-TNP**
Kathryn B. Scheidt, MSN, MS, BSN, RN
Kathleen T. Sheehan, MS, BSN, RN-BC, CH-GCN
Judith M. Toth-Lewis, PhD, MSN, RN
Barbara Ellis Trehearne, PhD, RN**
Mary Hines Vinson, DNP, RN-BC
Stephanie G. Witwer, PhD, RN, NEA-BC***

## Experts Who Performed a More Recent Review of Literature Between Phases 3 & 4

Karen Alexander, MSN, RN
Janine Allbritton, MSN, RN
Jo Ann Appleyard, PhD, RN
Stefanie Coffey, DNP, MBA, FNP-BC, RN-BC
Denise Hannagan, MSN, MHA, RN-BC
Clare Hastings, PhD, RN, FAAN
Anne Talbott Jessie, MSN, RN
Sheila A. Johnson, MBA, RN
Cheryl Lovlien, MS, RN-BC
Carol Mannone, MSN, RN, CH-GC
Debralee Quinn, MSN, RN-BC, CNN
Kathleen T. Sheehan, MS, BSN, RN-BC, CH-GCN
Linda Walton, MSN, RN, CENP

* Indicates number of Expert Panels beyond one.

# Acknowledgments

It took nurse experts from all over this nation to see the vision for the RN in CCTM role and collaborate to make it a reality. The AAACN volunteer expert panelists, writers, and reviewers have been awesome in their willingness to participate, produce, make deadlines, and bring this project to fruition on time and on budget.

None of our work as volunteers could have happened without the dedicated support of the AAACN and Anthony J. Jannetti, Inc. staff, especially Pat Reichart, Rosemarie Marmion, and Cyndee Nowicki Hnatiuk, who worked tirelessly with reams of tables and documents and innumerable requests. We made maximum use of digital files, website compendiums, online conferencing, and communication to expedite our work.

## AAACN Board Members

Susan Paschke, MSN, RN-BC, NEA-BC – President
Marianne Sherman, MS, RN-BC – President Elect
Judy Dawson-Jones, MPH, BSN, RN – Secretary
COL. (Ret) Carol A. B. Andrews, PhD, RN-BC, NE-BC, CCP – Treasurer
Debra L. Cox, MS, RN – Director
Nancy May, MSN, RN-C, NEA-BC – Director
CAPT. (Ret) Wanda C. Richards, MSM, MPA, BSN – Director
Suzanne N. Wells, MSN, RN – Immediate Past President

## AAACN and Anthony J. Jannetti, Inc. Staff

Cyndee Nowicki Hnatiuk, EdD, RN, CAE, FAAN – Executive Director
Pat Reichart – Director of Association Services
Rosemarie Marmion, MSN, RN-BC, NEA-BC – Education Director
Kristina Moran – Education Coordinator
Kenneth J. Thomas – Managing Editor
Katie R. Brownlow, ELS – Managing Editor
Darin Peters – Layout Design and Production
Carol M. Ford – Director of Editorial Services
Jack M. Bryant – Director of Creative Design and Production
Erin Fisher – PR and Association Marketing Manager
Celess Tyrell – Program Manager (Online Modules)
Stephanie McDonald – Customer Service Coordinator
Robin Maier – Customer Service Coordinator (Online Modules)

## Traci Haynes

We have never worked with a project manager as expert as Traci. She kept us on target and on time and did it with unfailing grace and tact. Traci, a million thanks!

## Personal Notes

I would like to acknowledge my husband, Eric, you are my inspiration; my daughters, Erica and Emily, who make me believe that everything is possible, including change; and my parents Elizabeth and John H. Reck, who implanted in me a voice to advocate for making the world a better place for all people.

*– Beth Ann Swan*

I would like to acknowledge my husband, Tim, for his unwavering support and encouragement and for being my sounding board. My thanks also to my children, Meg and her husband Andy, and my son John for their patience and support for my continuing work with projects in the profession that I love. Also, my four grandchildren, Nick, Grace, Madeline, and Wilson, all are respectful of my work and willing to wait at times to play when I am done. This has been one of the most enlightening projects that I have ever experienced and this has been due to the collaboration with colleagues Beth Ann and Traci, and all of our expert panelists who are not only excellent clinicians and administrators, but committed and consistently willing to go that extra mile to push the envelope to make health care better.

*– Sheila A. Haas*

I would like to thank Sheila and Beth Ann for their vision and bringing their thoughts to the AAACN Board of Directors in the fall of 2011. They knew the forthcoming changes as part of the Affordable Care Act and the Institute of Medicine's report *The Future of Nursing* would result in increased opportunities for ambulatory nursing, especially in the Care Coordination Transition Management role. They also knew that competencies were paramount in supporting this role. Their willingness to chair this initiative was driven by their passion for ambulatory nursing and AAACN. I marvel at their insight, expertise, and fortitude in making this a reality. I also want to thank all the volunteer members of the expert panels and reviewers, and the Anthony J. Jannetti, Inc. team for their knowledge, support, and diligence in meeting deadlines. Lastly, to my family – husband Greg and children Chad, Abigail, and Clint, and our grandchildren – many, many thanks to all of you for your enduring support of me and my profession throughout the years.

*– Traci S. Haynes*

# CHAPTER 1

# Introduction

*Beth Ann Swan, PhD, CRNP, FAAN*
*Sheila A. Haas, PhD, RN, FAAN*
*Traci S. Haynes, MSN, RN, CEN*

## I. Purpose

During the summer of 2011, the American Academy of Ambulatory Care Nursing (AAACN) Health Care Reform Advisory Team made a recommendation to the AAACN Board of Directors that there was a need for written competencies for the care coordination transition management (CCTM) registered nurse (RN) role. The Advisory Team worked with their Board Liaison and the Executive Team to develop a survey asking members if they had access to CCTM competencies, and if not, if they felt a need for competencies.

A nine-question survey link was sent to the AAACN membership in July 2011. Respondents were asked to complete the survey using an online survey tool. It was revealed that very few sites had access to CCTM competencies, and those that did had developed them internally. Most respondents also felt competencies needed to be evidence-based and more thorough to support the care provided to patients and their families. One member wrote, "Competency would create standardization and ensure excellence in the care we are providing." Another wrote, "They are needed because our work needs to be validated, supported, and replicated, and it needs to be evidence-based so we can provide the best quality of care." Other responses included: "I provide this type of care in a clinic setting. It is a huge part of the job and requires adequate time to do well. Yet staff is poorly oriented and trained in the skills and knowledge needed to provide this vital care. Measurable and defined competencies would support improvement in the delivery of care;" "Competencies help ensure that staff have the right level of training and knowledge which ultimately helps improve patient safety;" "From a quality perspective, competencies are always important to indicate performance and performance improvement opportunities;" "We need a system to help ensure consistency and standardization within an organization and amongst organizations;" "There is an increasing need for RN care coordination with the Medical Home initiative. This is not a skill that is taught in nursing schools or that is acquired while working in the hospital setting."

Based on feedback received from the membership, the AAACN Board of Directors made the decision to move forward in the development of the CCTM competencies. Two of AAACN's Health Care Reform Advisory Team members, Dr. Sheila Haas and Dr. Beth Ann Swan, agreed to co-chair this initiative while Ms. Traci Haynes served as the Board Liaison and Project Manager.

## II. Vision for the *Core Curriculum* as the Foundation for the Care Coordination and Transition Management (CCTM) Model

A. Vision.
1. The Care Coordination Transition Management (CCTM) Model standardizes the work of ambulatory as well as acute, subacute, and home care health care providers using evidence from interdisciplinary literature on care coordination and transition management.
2. The CCTM Model.
   a. Specifies the dimensions of care coordination and transition management and the associated competencies needed to be performed within the CCTM Model.
   b. Defines the knowledge, skills, and attitudes needed for each dimension.
   c. Meets the needs of patients with complex chronic illnesses (and their families) being cared for in Patient-Centered Medical Homes (PCMH), as well as traditional and nontraditional outpatient settings.
   d. Recommends RNs educated and prepared to work as an RN in CCTM be recognized and reimbursed by Centers for Medicare & Medicaid Services (CMS).
3. Consistent with the mission and vision of the Quality and Safety in Nursing Education (QSEN) initiative (Cronenwett et al., 2007), nurses learning about the CCTM competencies and role will develop knowledge, skills, and attitudes requisite to competent practice within the nine CCTM dimensions/competencies. Each chapter of the *Care Coordination and Transition Management Core Curriculum* will include a Knowledge, Skills, and Attitudes table that summarizes behavioral expectations for each of the nine CCTM competencies.
4. Consistent with the Institute of Medicine's Report, *The Future of Nursing: Leading Change Advancing Health* (2010), the CCTM Model:
   a. Supports RNs practicing to the full extent of their education and training.
   b. Promotes RNs achieving higher levels of education, training, and licensure through an improved education system that promotes seamless academic progression.
   c. Advocates that RNs are full partners, with physicians and other health care professionals, in redesigning health care in the United States.

   d. Highlights that effective workforce planning and policymaking require better data collection and an improved information infrastructure.
   e. Expands opportunities for nurses to lead and diffuse collaborative improvement efforts.
   f. Prepares and enables nurses to lead change to advance health.
5. Consistent with the American Nurses Association's (ANA) book, *Care Coordination: The Game Changer* (Lamb, 2014), care coordination models are vital for achieving quality and safety outcomes for patients and families (Haas & Swan, 2014).
6. Consistent with the work of national professional organizations.
   a. ANA's Position Statement on *Care Coordination and Registered Nurses' Essential Role* (2012a).
   b. ANA's white paper *The Value of Nursing Care Coordination* (2012b).
   c. ANA's *Framework for Measuring Nurses' Contributions to Care Coordination* (2013).
   d. ANA's (2013) Care Coordination Quality Measures Panel.
   e. American Academy of Nursing's (AAN) imperative for patient, family, and population-centered interprofessional approaches to care coordination and transitional care (2012).
   f. AAN's summary of the importance of health information technology in care coordination and transitional care (Cipriano et al., 2013).

## III. Definitions

A. Competence and achievement of professional practice competencies have long been expected of professionals and long assumed to be present by consumers. It is interesting, however, that consistent definitions for both are not easy to find. The American Nurses Association in 2008 issued a Position Statement on Competence. It included Definitions and Concepts in Competence that state: "An individual who demonstrates 'competence' is performing successfully at an expected level. A 'competency' is an expected level of performance that integrates knowledge, skills, abilities, and judgement. The integration of knowledge, skills, abilities and judgement occurs in formal, informal and reflective learning experiences" (ANA, 2008, p. 2).

B. Care coordination.
   1. Agency for Healthcare Research and Quality (AHRQ) definition: "Care coordination is the deliberate organization of patient care activities between two or more participants (including the patient) involved in a patient's care to facilitate the appropriate delivery of health care services. Organizing care involves the marshalling of personnel and other resources needed to carry out all required patient care activities and is often managed by the exchange of information among participants responsible for different aspects of care" (McDonald et al., 2011, p. 4; McDonald et al., 2007).
   2. National Quality Forum definition: "Care coordination is defined as an information-rich, patient-centric endeavor that seeks to deliver the right care (and only the right care) to the right patient at the right time...A function that helps ensure that the patient's needs and preferences for health services and information sharing across people, functions and sites are met over time...Care coordination maximizes the value of services delivered to patients by facilitating beneficial efficient, safe and high-quality patient experiences and improved health care outcomes" (NQF, 2010, p. 2).

C. Transition management.
   1. "Transitional care is defined as a broad range of time-limited services designed to ensure health care continuity, avoid preventable poor outcomes among at-risk populations, and promote the safe and timely transfer of patients from one level of care to another or from one type of setting to another" (Naylor, Aiken, Kurtzman, Olds, & Hirschman, 2011, p. 747).
      a. Core features of transitional care include:
         (1) Comprehensive assessment of an individual's health goals and preferences; physical, emotional, cognitive, and functional capacities and needs, and social and environmental considerations.
         (2) Implementation of an evidence-based plan of transitional care.
         (3) Care that is initiated at hospital admission, but extends beyond discharge through home and telephone visits.
         (4) Mechanisms to gather and share information across sites of care.
         (5) Engagement of patients and family caregivers in planning and executing the plan of care.
         (6) Coordinated services during and following the hospitalization by a health care professional with special preparation in the care of chronically ill people, often a master's-prepared nurse (Naylor & Sochalski, 2010, p. 2).
   2. "Care transitions refer to the movement patients make between health care practitioners and settings as their condition and care needs change during the course of a chronic or acute illness. For example, in the course of an acute exacerbation of an illness, a patient might receive care from a primary care physician or specialist in an outpatient setting, then transition to a hospital physician and nursing team during an inpatient admission before moving on to yet another care team at a skilled nursing facility. Finally, the patient might re-

turn home, where he or she would receive care from a visiting nurse. Each of these shifts from care providers and settings is defined as a care transition" (Coleman & Boult, 2003, p. 556).

3. "Transitional care is defined as a set of actions designed to ensure the coordination and continuity of health care as patients transfer between different locations or different levels of care within the same location. Representative locations include (but are not limited to) hospitals, sub-acute and post-acute nursing facilities, the patient's home, primary and specialty care offices, and long-term care facilities" (Coleman & Boult, 2003, p. 556).
   a. Transitional care is based on a comprehensive plan of care and the availability of health care practitioners who are well-trained in chronic care and have current information about the patient's goals, preferences, and clinical status.
   b. It includes logistical arrangements, education of the patient and family, and coordination among the health professionals involved in the transition.
   c. Transitional care, which encompasses both the sending and the receiving aspects of the transfer, is essential for persons with complex care needs (Coleman & Boult, 2003).
4. The authors expand on these terms and definitions of transitional care and care transitions to the term *transition management.* The authors define *transition management* as the ongoing support of patients and their families over time as they navigate care and relationships among more than one provider and/or more than one health care setting and/or more than one health care service. The need for transition management is not determined by age, time, place, or health care condition, but rather by patients' and/or families' needs for support for ongoing, longitudinal individualized plans of care and follow-up plans of care within the context of health care delivery

D. Care coordination and transition management.
   1. In the setting, care coordination and transition management are integrated functions that may occur simultaneously or separately and are not time limited as defined above. One provision of the Patient Protection and Affordable Care Act (2010) to support this expanded definition is the need for individualized plans of care and follow-up plans of care that move with patients longitudinally over time.
   2. Individualized plans of care and follow-up plans of care serve as the basis for the CCTM Model, an innovative patient-centered interprofessional collaborative practice care delivery model that integrates the RN role as care coordinator and transition manager (Swan & Haas, 2011).
   3. CCTM Model acknowledges the care coordination and transitional care activities performed by RNs and interprofessional team members in acute care, other care settings, and the community.

## IV. Background and Significance of CCTM Model

A. Rationale and need.
   1. Growing demand for care coordination and transition management.
      a. Health care spending in the United States is disproportionate; half of U.S. health care dollars are spent on 5% of the population (McDonald et al., 2011).
      b. A small percentage of individuals with complex chronic conditions consume a high proportion of health care services and account for the bulk of health care spending; chronic conditions are expensive to treat and a major driver of increased health care spending (Thorpe, 2013).
      c. Many struggle with multiple illnesses combined with social complexities such as, mental health and substance abuse, extreme medical frailty, and a host of social needs such as social isolation and homelessness (Craig, Eby, & Whittington, 2011).
      d. Individuals with multiple needs are not able to navigate the complex and fragmented health care system (Swan, 2012).
      e. Care providers recognize the need for better coordinated care that leverages community resources and aligns social determinants such as food, housing, and safe environments, but payment structures in the health care system do not allow such alignment (Kangovi et al., 2013).
      f. Patients with chronic diseases and multiple co-morbidities are a vulnerable population. Health care for these at-risk patients can be fragmented, leading to nonbeneficial or redundant testing services. Uneven quality of care for at-risk populations can lead to poor patient outcomes and increased use of limited health care resources. At-risk patients are not well served by the traditional "rescue care" approach to health care delivery, such as frequent emergency room visits and hospitalizations, and would benefit from aggressive care coordination and navigation through the health care system to ensure smooth, seamless continuity of care.
      g. The need for care coordination and transition management supports the Institute for Healthcare Improvement's Triple Aim "improving the individual experience of care, improving the health of populations, and reducing the per capita cost of care for populations" (Berwick, Nolan, & Whittington, 2008, p. 760).

B. Background for CCTM Model.
   1. March 1, 2010: Invitational conference on *Ambulatory Care Registered Nurse Performance Measurement* (Swan, Haas, & Chow, 2010).
      a. Purpose: Formulate a research agenda and develop a strategy to study the testable components of the RN role related to care coordination and care transitions, improving patient outcomes, decreasing health care costs, and promoting sustainable system change.
      b. Expert participants came from the fields of nursing, public health, managed care, research, practice, and policy.
      c. Results: *Framework for RNs' contribution to care quality and in the context of national policies.*
         (1) Recognize ambulatory as well as acute, subacute, and home care depends on an interprofessional team that significantly influences outcomes of care, and RNs are integral team members.
         (2) Build on current assets in the areas of measure endorsement, public reporting, and performance-based payment programs, and seek opportunities to "join up" with other professional organizations.
         (3) Describe and define ambulatory care RNs' contribution to "value-driven health care."
         (4) Examine new opportunities within the Patient Protection and Affordable Care Act related to the medical home and improving patient outcomes, decreasing health care costs, and promoting sustainable system change.
         (5) Explore a set of care coordination and care transition measures reflected in CMS rule-making (Swan et al., 2010).
   2. March 23, 2010: Affordable Care Act.
   3. Provisions of health care reform relate to care coordination and transition management (Swan & Haas, 2011).
   4. April 2011: AAACN Conference presentation on health care reform.
   5. Constitutionality of ACA challenged.
   6. September 2011: AHRQ grant submission – develop, implement, and evaluate a RN model for care coordination and transition management.
   7. June 2012: Supreme Court upholds ACA.
   8. *Health Affairs* article, November 2012 (Swan, 2012).
   9. *Nursing Economic$* article, January/February 2013 (Haas, Swan, & Haynes, 2013).
   10. March 23, 2013: AHRQ grant resubmitted.

C. Significance of CCTM Model in relation to Affordable Care Act.
   1. Majority of provisions are related to care coordination and care transitions, as well as health promotion and disease prevention (Naylor et al., 2011).
      a. Interventions associated with these provisions are part of RNs' independent scope of practice (ANA, 2012a).
      b. RNs have an essential role in the care coordination process (ANA, 2012a).
   2. Defined the PCMH team with RNs as team members.
   3. Focused on access to primary care versus enhanced use of specialists and acute care.
   4. Fostered care coordination for complex chronically ill persons in ambulatory settings and across the care continuum.
   5. Specified the need for individualized patient-centered care planning.
   6. Extant models of care for chronically ill in the community are staffed by RNs working with complex chronically ill patients including Boult's Guided Care Model (Boult, Karm, & Groves, 2008) and Coleman's Care Transitions Model (Coleman, Parry, Chalmers, Chugh, & Mahoney, 2007).
   7. Authorized the Accountable Care Organization program be administered by a new innovation center at CMS.
   8. In 2011, launched the *Partnerships for Patients* program to achieve two goals.
      a. Making care safer.
      b. Improving care transitions.
   9. In 2013, CMS finalized transitional care management codes. At this time these codes can be reported/billed by advanced practice nurses (APNs) but not RNs.
   10. CMS is in the process of developing care coordination codes, the current rule-making on care coordination codes includes reporting/billing by APNs but not RNs; CMS does not plan to finalize these codes until 2015.
   11. Beginning January 2015, one of the provisions of the ACA, the value modifier, will provide differential payment based on quality of care provided compared to cost during a defined performance period (CMS, 2013).

## V. Selected Extant Care Coordination Initiatives

A. Patient Aligned Care Teams (PACT) Model (True et al., 2012).
   1. In FY2010, the Veterans Health Administration (VHA) began implementation of the patient-centered medical home model, now known as PACT (Patient Aligned Care Team).
   2. Transform the VA health care delivery system to a more patient-centric model of care.

3. Primary care is the foundation of VHA health care.
4. Transformation begins with primary care and permeates other areas of the health care delivery system to include specialty care, women's health care, geriatrics, and academic training programs.
5. Long-term goals.
   a. Provide superb access to primary care (including alternatives to face-to-face care) to meet veterans' needs and expectations.
   b. Provide seamless coordination of care between VA providers and with non-VA providers.
   c. Demonstrate a patient-centered culture through the redesign of primary care practices and team roles.
6. Focus of PACT.
   a. Partnerships with veterans.
   b. Access to care using diverse methods.
   c. Coordinated care among team members.
   d. Team-based care with veterans at the center of their PACT.
7. Patient Aligned Care Team.
   a. Veterans work together with health care professionals to plan for whole-person care and lifelong health and wellness.
   b. Care team considers all aspects of patient health, with an emphasis on prevention and health promotion.
   c. Care is coordinated through collaboration.
   d. Members of the team have clearly defined roles with a focus on forging trusted personal relationships; the result is coordination of all aspects of health care.
      (1) PACT uses a team-based approach.
      (2) The patient is the center of the care team that includes family members, caregivers, and health care professionals (a primary care provider, nurse care manager, clinical associate, and administrative clerk).
      (3) When other services are needed to meet patient goals and needs, the PACT oversees and coordinates that care.

B. Guided Care Model (Boult et al., 2008).
   1. Guided care is driven by a highly skilled RN in a primary care office.
   2. The guided care nurse assists three to four physicians in providing high-quality chronic care for their patients in need of good chronic care.
   3. Those eligible for guided care are high-risk patients with several chronic conditions and complex health care needs in a primary care practice.
   4. Predictive modeling software to analyze patients' encounter data for the previous year. This "hierarchical condition category" software assigns points to each diagnosis from each encounter and computes a risk rating for each patient.

## VI. Methodology for CCTM Model for Ambulatory Care Nursing Adapted from Information Published in *Nursing Economic$* (Haas et al., 2013)

A. Developing the RN competencies for Care Coordination and Transition Management required:
   1. Expertise of ambulatory care nurse leaders.
   2. Cost-effective, expeditious approach to bring leaders together.
   3. Opportunities to dialogue and build on each individual leader's knowledge, skills, and experience.
   4. Evidentiary review completed by Expert Panel 1.
      a. Members represented practice and education, along with public, private, military, and veterans' organizations.
      b. 15 states in east, west, north, south, and central U.S. and the District of Columbia.
      c. Following a search in MEDLINE, CINAHL Plus, and PsycINFO, 82 journal articles plus white papers available online from major organizations were selected for review. Expert Panel 1 worked in dyads and reviewed four to five articles, then abstracted data to a table of evidence (TOE) concluding their work in February 2012. A second literature search was completed in the summer of 2013. An additional 58 articles were reviewed and abstracted following the same methodology by members of the Expert Panel, then added to the existing TOE.
      d. The 26-member panel worked in dyads and abstracted data to a table of TOE including:
         (1) Authors of study column.
         (2) Study title column.
         (3) Research questions column.
         (4) Research design type column.
         (5) Setting and sample, inclusion/exclusion criteria column.
         (6) Methods, intervention, and/or instruments.
         (7) Analyses column.
         (8) Key findings column.
         (9) Recommendations column.
         (10) Column listing dimension or dimensions identified with activity or activities that are supporting and/or contributing to care coordination and transition management.
   5. Use of data summary techniques to capture and share outcomes achieved by each Expert Panel.
   6. Focus group methods.
      a. Defined as a method of bringing together people from similar backgrounds or experiences to discuss a specific topic, guided by a facilitator who elicits responses from the group, but does not influence responses.

 

b. For this project, focus group method and on-line time were used to:
   (1) Clarify methods and outcome expectations.
   (2) Discuss issues with evidence evaluation such as ambiguities and contradictions in evidence.
   (3) Absence of sufficient description in evidence materials.
   (4) Sharing of concerns.
   (5) Sharing of insights and expertise.

B. Identifying dimensions of care coordination and transition management.
1. Defining dimensions.
   a. In the literature, often activities are listed that are part of care coordination such as developing a plan of care or monitoring progression of established goals.
   b. These activities fit together within a broader construct or dimension such as planning.
   c. When developing a role that reflects all of the major dimensions or constructs that make up the role, use of dimensions allows for addition or subtraction of relevant activities under each dimension as the role evolves.
2. Dimensions identified and defined by Expert Panel 2.
   a. This 16-member panel was charged with:
      (1) Defining the dimensions, identifying core competencies.
      (2) Describing the activities linked with each competency for care coordination and transition management in ambulatory and settings across the continuum.
      (3) Using focus group methods online, the expert panel identified nine patient centered-care dimensions and associated activities of care coordination and transition management.
   b. Nine evidence-based dimensions.
      (1) Support for self-management.
      (2) Education and engagement of patient and family.
      (3) Cross setting communication and transition.
      (4) Coaching and counseling of patients and families.
      (5) Nursing process including assessment, plan, implementation/intervention, and evaluation; a proxy for monitoring and intervening.
      (6) Teamwork and collaboration.
      (7) Patient-centered care planning.
      (8) Decision support and information systems.
      (9) Advocacy.
   c. The evidence-based dimensions and activities were validated using informal focus groups at the AAACN National Conference in May 2012.
3. Preliminary Competencies identified by Expert Panel 2 using the QSEN framework (Cronenwett et al., 2007).
   a. Knowledge.
   b. Skills.
   c. Attitudes.
4. Work was also guided by Wagner's Chronic Care Model (Wagner, 1998) (see Figure 1).

C. Developing Competencies for Care Coordination and Transition Management.
1. Once dimensions were discovered in the translational research project, the named dimension became the competency. Since the *CCTM Core Curriculum* is a first edition and the implementation of the RN in CCTM is a new role, the definition of each competency on the first page of each chapter offers several definitions of the competency taken from the evidence discovered in the literature. Users (organizations) are free to use the definitions offered to create a more abbreviated definition that is consonant with their setting and population served.
2. Specify education and evaluation needed for successful practice within each dimension of the role.
3. In 2003, the IOM's Health Professions Education Report recommended educators provide learning experiences so that graduates were prepared to provide patient-centered care as collaborating members of an interdisciplinary team using evidence-based practice, quality improvement methods, and informatics. This was a stimulus for development of the QSEN initiative (Cronenwett et al., 2007). The six QSEN competencies and their Knowledge, Skills, and Attitudes tables of expected behaviors have been embraced by nursing undergraduate and graduate educators. Of note is the QSEN specification of attitudes instead of abilities and judgment that were specified in the preliminary position statement (ANA, 2008). Attitudes are extremely relevant in specification of quality and safety competencies and behavior or performance expectations. It is often health care provider attitudes that override the knowledge and skills expectations of performance. A good example of this is hand hygiene. Providers have extensive knowledge of rationale for hand washing and skills to do it, but often do not practice hand hygiene, letting attitudes about emergent needs take precedence. That is why hand hygiene compliance is about 60% in health care.
4. The QSEN format (Cronenwett et al., 2007) was used to identify expected Knowledge, Skills, and Attitudes (KSA) behavior for each CCTM competency or dimension.

**Figure 1.**
**The Chronic Care Model**

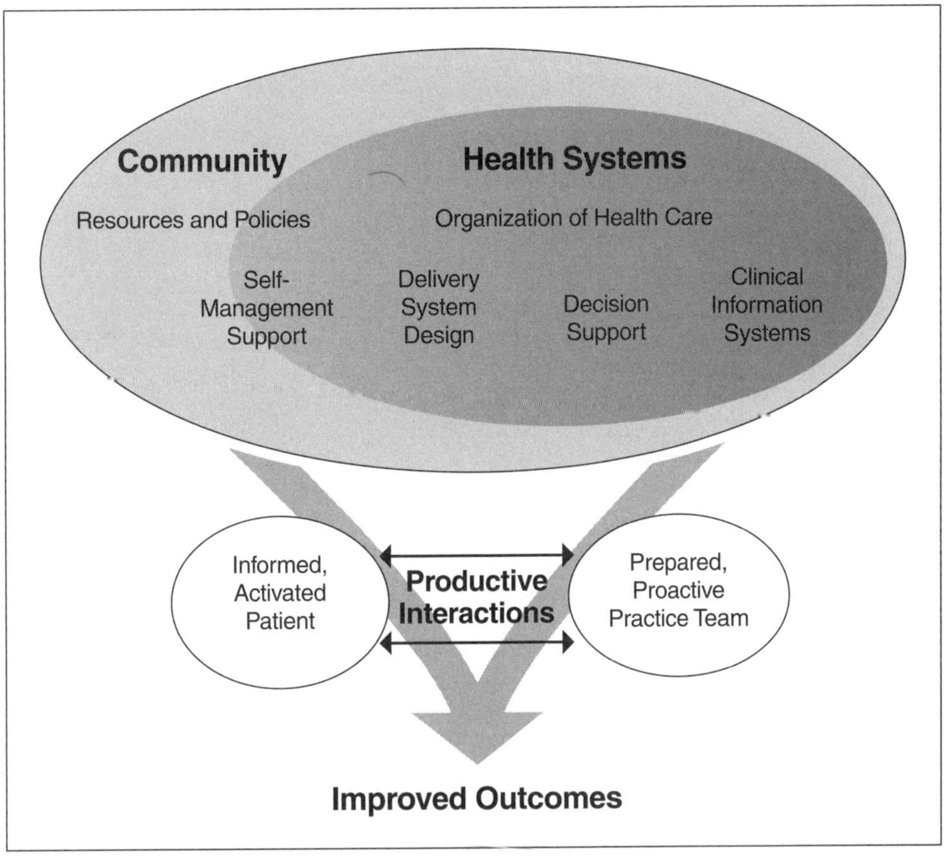

Developed by The MacColl Institute.
® ACP-ASIM Journals and Books. Reprinted with permission.

D. Verifying dimensions and competencies.
   1. In August 2012, using focus group methods online, Expert Panel 3 reviewed, confirmed, and created a table of dimensions, activities, and competencies including knowledge, skills, attitudes for ambulatory care RN care coordination, and transition management.
   2. After much discussion, Expert Panel 3 determined the original 8th dimension of decision support and information systems, as well as telehealth practice, were technologies that support all dimensions.
   3. Population health management became the new 8th dimension given the prominence it is assuming in outpatient care even though there was little discussion of it in the literature reviewed.
   4. Expert Panel 3 also determined methods to be used to enhance teamwork and interprofessional collaboration in outpatient settings.
   5. Nationally recognized core competencies for interprofessional collaborative practice QSEN competencies, and public health nursing competencies, overlap with the dimensions and competencies needed for RN care coordination and transition management (see Table 1).

E. Expert Panel 4 was convened in summer 2013. This panel was charged with writing the 13 chapters of the *CCTM Core Curriculum.* Names of panelists are in the contributor list in the beginning of this text.

## VII. Logic Model

As we prepared to work with the expert panelists who were writing chapters for the *CCTM Core Curriculum,* we developed a Logic Model to guide the organization of the chapters to identify not only activities but also processes and outcomes involved in each of the dimensions. We knew from analyzing other care coordination and transition models that the main outcomes identified were emergency room visits and hospital re-admission rates. When other quality of life outcomes were reported, there was a great variety of outcomes specified, but often there was no distinction as to whether they were short, medium, or long-term outcomes. We decided to try to plot the CCTM Model within a Logic Model as illustrated in the Appendices.

**Table 1.**
**Crosswalk of Dimensions for Care Coordination and Transition Management with Core Competencies (Haas, Swan, & Haynes, 2013)**

| Dimension RN in Care Coordination and Transition Management | Quality and Safety Education for Nurses (QSEN) Core Competencies | Interprofessional Education Collaborative Core Competencies | Public Health Nursing Competencies |
|---|---|---|---|
| Support Self-Management | Patient-Centered Care | | |
| Education and Engagement of Patient and Family | Patient-Centered Care | | |
| Cross Setting Communication and Transition | Patient-Centered Care | Interprofessional Communication | Domain #3: Communication Skills |
| Coaching and Counseling of Patients and Families | Patient-Centered Care | | Domain #4: Cultural Competency Skills |
| Nursing Process: Assessment, Plan, Intervention, Evaluation | Evidence-Based Practice Quality Improvement | Roles and Responsibilities | Domain #1: Analytic Assessment Skills |
| Teamwork and Collaboration | Teamwork and Collaboration | Teams and Teamwork | Domain #8: Leadership and System Thinking Skills |
| Patient-Centered Planning | Patient-Centered Care | Values/Ethics for Interprofessional Practice | Domain #1: Analytic Assessment Skills |
| Population Health Management | Quality Improvement Informatics | | Domain #5: Community Dimensions of Practice Skills Domain #6: Basic Public Health Sciences Skills |
| Advocacy | Patient-Centered Care Safety | | Domain #2: Policy Development/Program Planning Skills |

## VIII. Mechanics

A. The content in the *CCTM Core Curriculum* is presented in outline format for easy review and reference. Key terms that are defined in the text are captured in the Glossary. Resources and published references are identified throughout the text and at the end of chapters for further information. It is important to realize that this content captured the best evidence and information available at a point in time, and the reader is encouraged to seek current sources of information as new research and evidence on care coordination and transition management are being published.
B. Organization of each chapter.
   1. Definition of the dimension for the chapter using evidence from literature reviewed and enhanced where necessary by expert opinion.
   2. Purpose of chapter: Broad outcome statement or goal that summarizes the specific topic and aim of the chapter.
   3. Learning objectives: Brief, clear statements that describe what the reader is expected to achieve as a result of reading the chapter.
   4. Brief introduction to the competency.
   5. Content outline for the competency.
   6. Competencies: Sets of knowledge, skills, and attitudes that enable a nurse to perform in a specific role such as the registered nurse in care coordination and transition management.
   7. Finalized list of knowledge, skills, and attitudes for each competency modeled after the QSEN (Cronenwett et al., 2007) entry/pre-licensure competencies.
   8. Nationally recognized core competencies for interprofessional collaborative practice (American Association of Colleges of Nursing, 2011), QSEN competencies (Cronenwett et al., 2007), and public health nursing competencies (Quad Council of the Public Health Nursing Organizations, 2011), overlap with the dimensions and competencies needed for RN care coordination and transition management.
   9. Suggested process and outcome indicators for competencies where available.
   10. References.

## IX. Contents

A. The majority of the book is composed of nine chapters listed below, one for each evidence-based dimension, written by nurse experts. This compilation is the work of a large number of ambulatory care and acute care nurse leaders representing practice, education, and research. The authors would like to acknowledge the collaboration with the leadership from the Academy of Medical-Surgical Nurses (AMSN) on the four Expert Panels.
   1. Advocacy.
   2. Education and Engagement of Patients and Families.
   3. Coaching and Counseling of Patients and Families.
   4. Patient-Centered Care Planning.
   5. Support for Self-Management.
   6. Nursing Process (Proxy for Monitoring and Evaluation).
   7. Teamwork and Collaboration.
   8. Cross Setting Communications and Care Transitions.
   9. Population Health Management.

B. One chapter is dedicated to the transition from acute care to ambulatory care and the critical nature of handoffs in ensuring patient safety and quality of care.

C. Two chapters are devoted to technologies that provide decision support and information systems for all dimensions of care coordination and transition management.
   1. Informatics Nursing Practice.
   2. Telehealth Nursing Practice.

## X. Who Will Benefit From This Book?

This text is written for you, the registered nurse – whether you are a nurse working in ambulatory care, in a hospital, an extended care facility, a patient's home, a community setting; a student nurse; a nurse educator; or a nurse who functions in any of the other diverse places where nurses are coordinating care and managing transitions. Whatever your role, you will find this groundbreaking new reference an indispensable guide to the state of research evidence for care coordination and transition management.

## XI. How Can I Use This Book?

This core resource on care coordination and transition management is ideal for:

A. Orienting nurses transitioning into ambulatory care settings as well as acute, subacute, and home care across the continuum about care coordination and transition management.

B. Orienting existing nursing staff in acute care settings and ambulatory care settings about care coordination and transition management.

C. Orienting nurses' transition into the RN care coordination and transition management role.

D. Developing competencies, standards, policies, and procedures.

E. Revising performance appraisal instruments for ambulatory care nurses and nurses in other settings doing CCTM.

F. Enhancing educational materials/programs for nurses in CCTM.

G. Identifying nurses' structure and process contributions to patient outcomes.

H. Enhancing high-risk patient outcomes in a pay-for-performance environment.

I. Delineating the value proposition of the RN in the context of interprofessional team-based care.

J. Expanding/enhancing the use of longitudinal care planning for patients across providers of care and settings of care.

K. Developing, implementing, and evaluating quality improvement projects in your organizations around the dimensions.

L. Developing and implementing evidence-based projects and research projects guided by the dimensions.

M. Planning and implementing action plans to meet the new Magnet® standards related to ambulatory care.

## References

American Academy of Nursing (AAN). (2012). *The imperative of patient, family, and population centered interprofessional approaches to care coordination and transitional care: Policy brief.* Washington, DC: Author.

American Association of Colleges of Nursing. (2011). Health educators and foundations release competencies and action strategies for interprofessional education. *Journal of Professional Nursing, 27*(4), 195-196.

American Nurses Association (ANA). (2008). *Position statement on competence and competency.* Silver Spring, MD: Author.

American Nurses Association (ANA). (2012a). *Care coordination and registered nurses' essential role: Position statement.* Silver Spring, MD: Author.

American Nurses Association (ANA). (2012b). *The value of nursing care coordination: White paper.* Silver Spring, MD: Author.

American Nurses Association (ANA). (2013). *Framework for measuring nurses' contributions to care coordination.* Silver Spring, MD: Author.

Berwick, D., Nolan, T., & Whittington, J. (2008). The triple aim: Care, health, and cost. *Health Affairs, 27*(3), 759-769.

Boult, C., Karm, L., & Groves, C. (2008). Improving chronic care: The "Guided Care" model. *The Permanente Journal, 12*(1), 50-54.

Centers for Medicare & Medicaid Services (CMS). (2013). *Summary of 2015 physicians' value-based payment modifier policies.* Baltimore, MD: Author. Retrieved from http://www.cms.gov/Medicare/Medicare-Fee-for-ServicePayment/PhysicianFeedbackProgram/Downloads/CY2015ValueModifierPolicies.pdf

Cipriano, P., Bowles, K., Dailey, M., Dykes, P., Lamb, G., & Naylor, M. (2013). The importance of health information technology in care coordination and transitional care. *Nursing Outlook, 61,* 475-489.

Coleman, E., & Boult, C. (2003). Improving the quality of transitional care for persons with complex care needs. *Journal of the American Geriatrics Society, 51*(4), 556-557.

Coleman, E.A., Parry, C., Chalmers, S.A., Chugh, A., & Mahoney, E. (2007). The central role of performance measurement in improving the quality of transitional care. *Home Health Care Services Quarterly, 26*(4), 93-104.

*continued on page 12*

## Appendix 1.
## Program: CCTM Depicted within a Logic Model

**Situation:** The Care Coordination and Transition Management (CCTM) Model evolved to standardize work of ambulatory care nurses using evidence from interdisciplinary literature on care coordination and transition management. The vision is the CCTM Model would specify dimensions of CCTM and competencies needed to perform CCTM and make possible development of knowledge, skills, and attitudes needed for each competency so the registered nurse (RN) will meet needs of patients with complex chronic illnesses (and their families) being cared for in Patient-Centered Medical Homes (PCMH), as well as traditional and nontraditional outpatient settings, and acute, subacute, and home care settings, and their preparation so work as an RN in CCTM would be recognized and reimbursed by the Centers for Medicare & Medicaid Services.

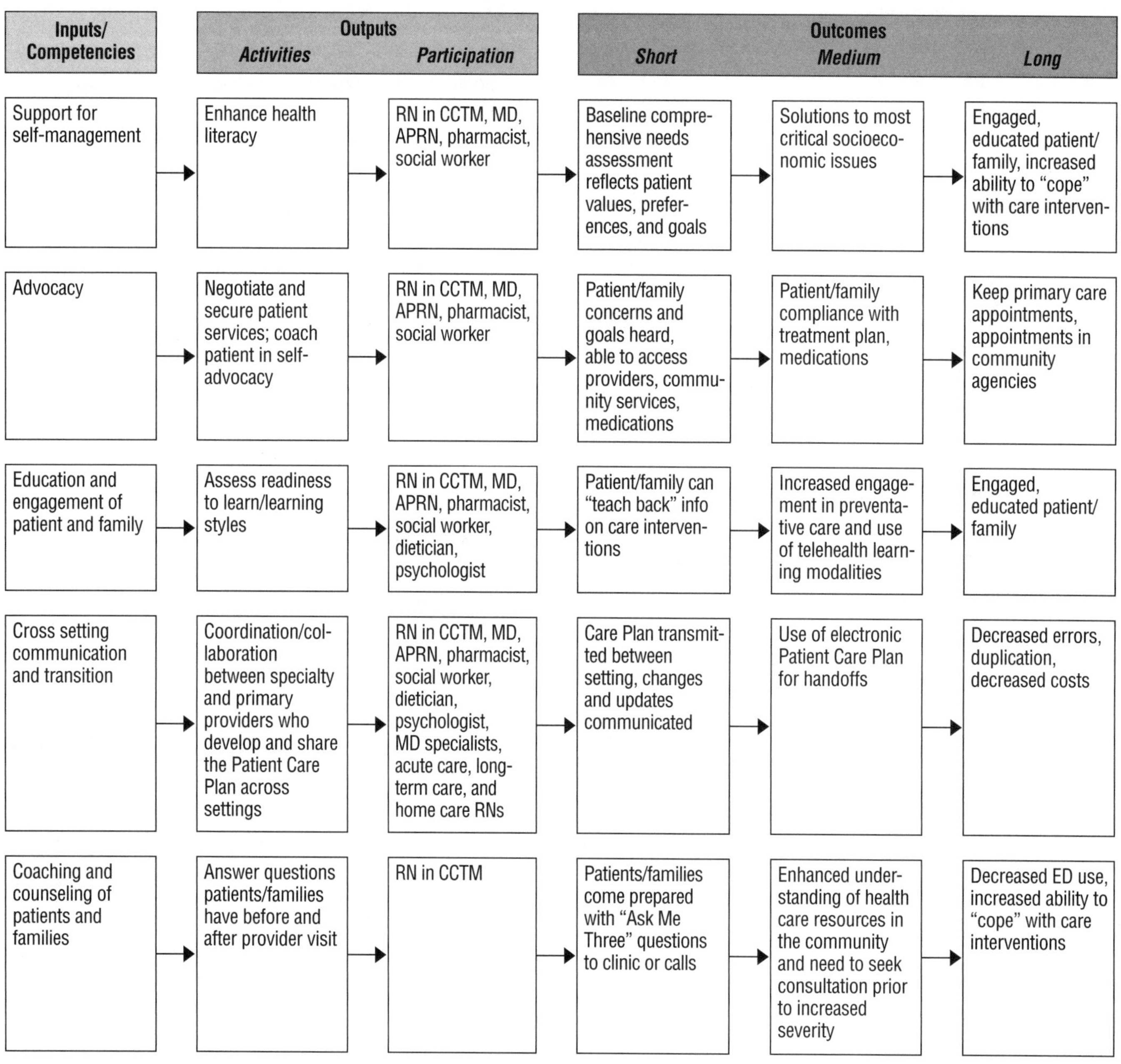

| Inputs/ Competencies | Outputs: Activities | Outputs: Participation | Outcomes: Short | Outcomes: Medium | Outcomes: Long |
|---|---|---|---|---|---|
| Support for self-management | Enhance health literacy | RN in CCTM, MD, APRN, pharmacist, social worker | Baseline comprehensive needs assessment reflects patient values, preferences, and goals | Solutions to most critical socioeconomic issues | Engaged, educated patient/ family, increased ability to "cope" with care interventions |
| Advocacy | Negotiate and secure patient services; coach patient in self-advocacy | RN in CCTM, MD, APRN, pharmacist, social worker | Patient/family concerns and goals heard, able to access providers, community services, medications | Patient/family compliance with treatment plan, medications | Keep primary care appointments, appointments in community agencies |
| Education and engagement of patient and family | Assess readiness to learn/learning styles | RN in CCTM, MD, APRN, pharmacist, social worker, dietician, psychologist | Patient/family can "teach back" info on care interventions | Increased engagement in preventative care and use of telehealth learning modalities | Engaged, educated patient/ family |
| Cross setting communication and transition | Coordination/collaboration between specialty and primary providers who develop and share the Patient Care Plan across settings | RN in CCTM, MD, APRN, pharmacist, social worker, dietician, psychologist, MD specialists, acute care, long-term care, and home care RNs | Care Plan transmitted between setting, changes and updates communicated | Use of electronic Patient Care Plan for handoffs | Decreased errors, duplication, decreased costs |
| Coaching and counseling of patients and families | Answer questions patients/families have before and after provider visit | RN in CCTM | Patients/families come prepared with "Ask Me Three" questions to clinic or calls | Enhanced understanding of health care resources in the community and need to seek consultation prior to increased severity | Decreased ED use, increased ability to "cope" with care interventions |



*continued on next page*

## Appendix 1. (continued)
## Program: CCTM Depicted within a Logic Model

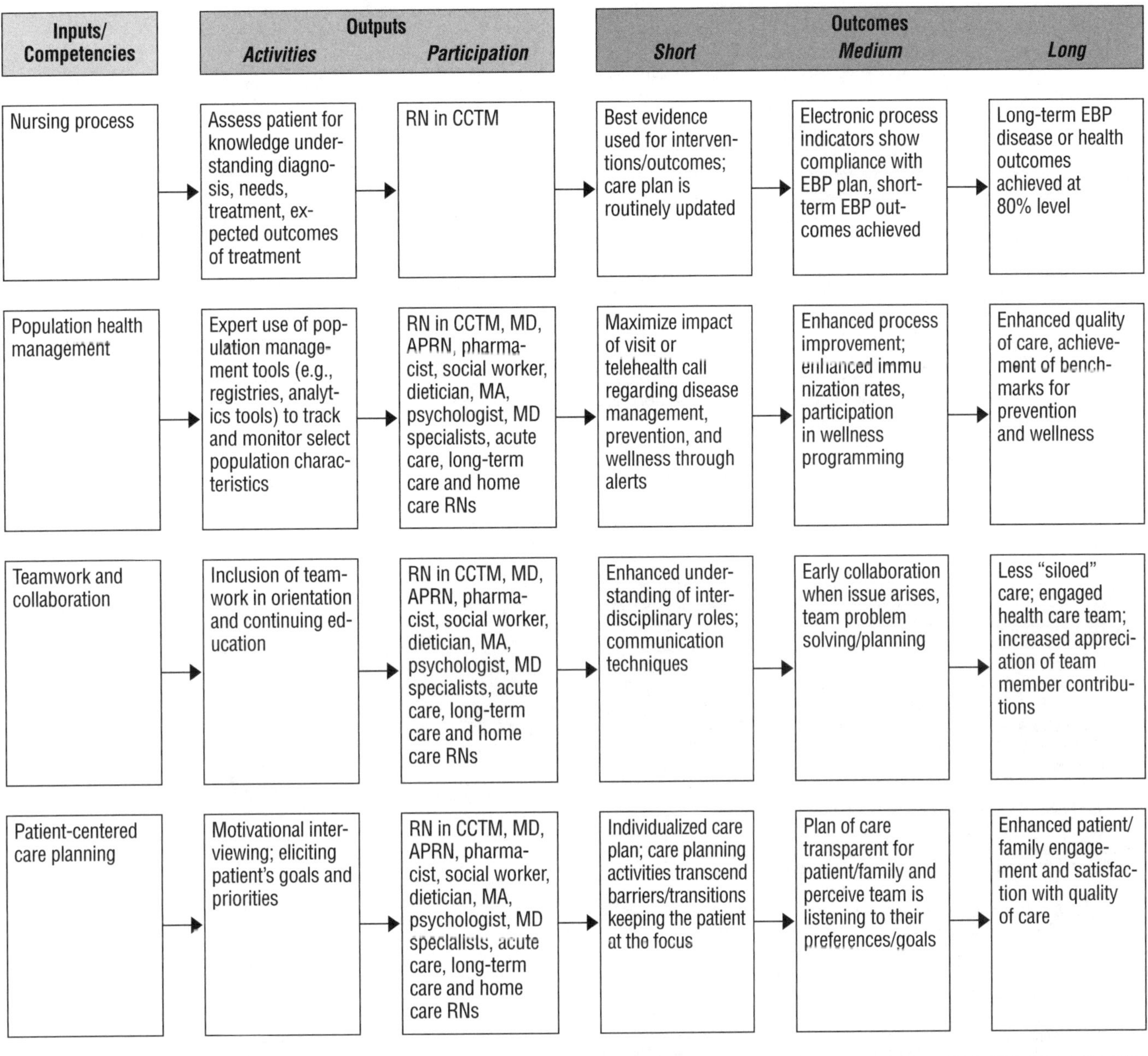

| Inputs/ Competencies | Outputs: *Activities* | Outputs: *Participation* | Outcomes: *Short* | Outcomes: *Medium* | Outcomes: *Long* |
|---|---|---|---|---|---|
| Nursing process | Assess patient for knowledge understanding diagnosis, needs, treatment, expected outcomes of treatment | RN in CCTM | Best evidence used for interventions/outcomes; care plan is routinely updated | Electronic process indicators show compliance with EBP plan, short-term EBP outcomes achieved | Long-term EBP disease or health outcomes achieved at 80% level |
| Population health management | Expert use of population management tools (e.g., registries, analytics tools) to track and monitor select population characteristics | RN in CCTM, MD, APRN, pharmacist, social worker, dietician, MA, psychologist, MD specialists, acute care, long-term care and home care RNs | Maximize impact of visit or telehealth call regarding disease management, prevention, and wellness through alerts | Enhanced process improvement; enhanced immu nization rates, participation in wellness programming | Enhanced quality of care, achievement of benchmarks for prevention and wellness |
| Teamwork and collaboration | Inclusion of teamwork in orientation and continuing education | RN in CCTM, MD, APRN, pharmacist, social worker, dietician, MA, psychologist, MD specialists, acute care, long-term care and home care RNs | Enhanced understanding of interdisciplinary roles; communication techniques | Early collaboration when issue arises, team problem solving/planning | Less "siloed" care; engaged health care team; increased appreciation of team member contributions |
| Patient-centered care planning | Motivational interviewing; eliciting patient's goals and priorities | RN in CCTM, MD, APRN, pharmacist, social worker, dietician, MA, psychologist, MD specialists, acute care, long-term care and home care RNs | Individualized care plan; care planning activities transcend barriers/transitions keeping the patient at the focus | Plan of care transparent for patient/family and perceive team is listening to their preferences/goals | Enhanced patient/family engagement and satisfaction with quality of care |

**Assumptions:** Patients will use primary care settings; patients will access CCTM providers; patients will be engaged in care processes; providers will collaborate, work in teams, develop and use patient-centered care plans; organization will have EHRs that operate across settings; outcomes are shared by team, not discipline specific.

**External Factors:** Slow development of interdisciplinary team education and practice. Changes in reimbursement and penalties for "never events" are decreasing revenues, slow implementation of EMRs that are operable across settings, and slow development of model of care plan that moves between settings.

## References

continued from page 9

Craig, C., Eby, D., & Whittington, J. (2011). *Care coordination model: Better care at lower costs for people with multiple health and social needs.* Cambridge, MA: Institute for Healthcare Improvement. Retrieved from http://www.ihi.org/knowledge/Pages/IHIWhitePapers/ IHICareCoordinationModelWhitePaper.aspx

Cronenwett, L., Sherwood, G., Barnsteiner, J., Disch, J., Johnson, J., Mitchell, P., … Warren, J. (2007). Quality and safety education for nurses. *Nursing Outlook, 55*(3), 122-131.

Haas, S., & Swan, B.A. (2014). Care coordination models for achieving quality and safety outcomes for patients and families. In G. Lamb (Ed.), *Care coordination: The game changer – How nursing is revolutionizing quality care.* Silver Spring, MD: American Nurses Association.

Haas, S., Swan, B.A., & Haynes, T. (2013). Developing ambulatory care registered nurse competencies for care coordination and transition management. *Nursing Economic$, 31*(1), 44-49, 43.

Institute of Medicine (IOM). (2003). *Health professions education: A bridge to quality.* Washinton, DC: National Acadamies Press.

Institute of Medicine. (IOM). (2010). *The future of nursing: Leading change, advancing health* (1st ed.). Washington, DC: National Academies Press.

Kangovi, S., Barg, F., Carter, T., Long, J., Shannon, R., & Grande, D. (2013). Understanding why patients of low socioeconomic status prefer hospitals over ambulatory care. *Health Affairs, 32*(7), 1196-1203.

Lamb, G. (Ed.) (2014). *Care coordination: The game changer – How nursing is revolutionizing quality care.* Silver Spring, MD: American Nurses Association.

McDonald, K.M., Schultz, E.S., Albin, L., Pineda, N., Lonhart, J., Sundaram, V., … Malcolm, E. (2011). *Care coordination measures atlas* (AHRQ Publication No.11-0023-EF). Rockville, MD: Agency for Healthcare Research and Quality.

McDonald, K., Sundaram, V., Bravata, D., Lewis, R., Lin, N., Kraft, S.A. … Owens, D.K. (2007). Care coordination. In K. Shojania, K. McDonald, R. Wachter, & D. Owens (Eds.), *Closing the quality gap: A critical analysis of quality improvement strategies* (AHRQ Publication No. 04(07)-0051-7). Technical Review 9 (Prepared by Stanford-UCSF Evidence-Based Practice Center under contract No. 290-02-0017). Vol. 7. Rockville, MD: Agency for Healthcare Research and Quality.

National Quality Forum. (2010). *Preferred practices and performance measures for measuring and reporting care coordination: A consensus report.* Washington, DC: Author.

Naylor, M., Aiken, L., Kurtzman, E., Olds, D., & Hirschman, K. (2011). The CARE SPAN: The importance of transitional care in achieving health reform. *Health Affairs, 30*(4), 746-754.

Naylor, M., & Sochalski, J. (2010). Scaling up: Bringing the transitional care model into the mainstream. *Commonwealth Fund Issue Brief, 1453*(103), 1-11.

Patient Protection and Affordable Care Act. (2010). Public Law 111-1148, §2702, 124 Stat. 119, 318-319.

Quad Council of Public Health Nursing Organizations. (2011). *Quad Council competencies for public health nurses.* Retrieved from http://www.achne.org/files/Quad%20Council/QuadCouncilCompetenciesforPublicHealthNurses.pdf

Swan, B.A. (2012). A nurse learns firsthand that you may fend for yourself after a hospital stay. *Health Affairs, 31*(11), 2579-2582.

Swan, B.A., & Haas, S. (2011). Health care reform: Current updates and future initiatives for ambulatory care nursing. *Nursing Economic$, 29*(6), 331-334.

Swan, B.A., Haas, S., & Chow, M. (2010). Ambulatory care registered nurse performance measurement. *Nursing Economic$, 28*(5), 337-339, 342.

Thorpe, K. (2013). Treated disease prevalence and spending per treated case drove most of the growth in health care spending in 1987-2009. *Health Affairs, 32*(5), 851-858.

True, G., Butler, A., Lamparska, B., Lempa, M., Shea, J., Asch, D., & Werner, R. (2012). Open access in the patient-centered medical home: Lessons learned from the Veterans Health Administration. *Journal of General Internal Medicine, 28*(4), 539-545.

Wagner, E.H. (1998). Chronic disease management: What will it take to improve care for chronic illness? *Effective Clinical Practice, 1*(1), 2-4.

## Additional Reading

Naylor, M. (2000). A decade of transitional care research with vulnerable elders. *Journal of Cardiovascular Nursing, 14*(3), 1-14.

# CHAPTER 2

# Advocacy

*Mary Hines Vinson, DNP, RN-BC*
*Judith M. Toth-Lewis, PhD, MSN, RN*
*Vicki Grant, MS, RN-BC*

## Learning Outcome Statement

The purpose of this chapter is to enable the reader to integrate professional standards of nursing related to advocacy into the Care Coordination and Transition Management (CCTM) role for the registered nurse (RN).

## Learning Objectives

After reading the chapter, the RN working in the CCTM role will be able to:

- Demonstrate patient advocacy in all CCTM activities.
- Describe the application of professional practice standards to the CCTM role in ambulatory care.
- Discuss the concept of patient advocacy as it relates to ethical principles.
- Apply the ethical principles of autonomy, beneficence, fidelity, and justice to the CCTM role of patient advocate.
- Develop and implement a plan of care in collaboration with the patient that reflects advocacy needs, interventions, and outcomes.
- Identify provisions in the Patient Protection and Affordable Care Act (PPACA) that require health care providers advocate for patient needs, goals, and preferences.
- Recognize the importance of CCTM participation in organizational and public policy formation that facilitates advocacy for patients in ambulatory care as well as other settings across the care continuum.
- Describe ways in which ambulatory care nurses can influence policy development focused on advocacy on behalf of patients, families, and nursing.
- Demonstrate the knowledge, skills, and attitudes required for the advocacy dimension (see Table 1).

## Competency Definition

Patient *advocacy* is the support and empowerment of patients to make informed decisions, navigate the health care system to access appropriate care, and build strong partnerships with providers, while working toward system improvement to support patient-centered care. Patient advocates are dedicated first and foremost to the well-being of the patients and populations they serve (Gilkey & Earp, 2009). System-level *advocacy* includes policy development and change at the organizational, local, state, and national levels to effect health care delivery and design (French, Gilkey, & Earp, 2009; Johnson, 2013).

Nursing as a profession is dynamic, not static, and includes the evolving role of advocacy as an essential element of professional practice. Professional nursing practice is based on social responsibility, which has its roots in long-standing core values and ethics of the profession (Neuman, 2012). The current definition of nursing (American Nurses Association [ANA], 2010a) states: "Nursing is the protection, promotion and optimization of health and abilities; prevention of illness and injury; alleviation of suffering through the diagnosis and treatment of human response; and advocacy in the care of individuals, families, communities and populations" (p. 8). Transformation of the U.S. health care system will require that nurses recognize and commit to patient advocacy as an important element of care coordination and transition management. The nurse in the ambulatory setting is, and will continue to be, the voice of the patient in navigating an increasingly complex system of care. Ambulatory care nurses work to assure the patient "maintains control of the encounter and treatment plan, with the nurse acting in a consultative role" (American Academy of Ambulatory Care Nursing [AAACN], 2010, p. 6). The clinical role of ambulatory care nurses includes advocating for patients, assuring care that is culturally competent and age appropriate (AAACN, 2010).

Health care reform, as described by the Patient Protection and Affordable Care Act (PPACA) of 2010, introduces changes related to health insurance coverage, access to services, quality of care, costs of health care, and overall population health (Silberman, 2013). Political and social tensions related to these changes have increased the need for advocacy and support for patients in making decisions. In a recent poll, the majority of respondents indicated they lack adequate information regarding the new health care law and how it will affect them. Although many knew of upcoming insurance mandates, few understood proposed expansion of Medicaid, the creation of health insurance marketplaces, or the availability of subsidies to provide financial support (The Henry J. Kaiser Family Foundation, 2013). As patient advocates, nurses provide guidance for patients and families in identifying and accessing appropriate resources, making prudent health care decisions, and adapting to new administrative processes related to insurance coverage.

Our responsibility as professional nurses to the *Nursing Code of Ethics* (ANA, 2001) should lead us to dialogue with administrators, medical staff, and other health professionals on matters of patient rights. Our understanding of patients' needs as they relate to the organization of services and appropriate staffing models should lead us to advocate for appropriate organizational policies that are patient centered. Our expertise in caring for patients at both individual and population levels should guide us in advocating at the community, state, and federal levels for policies which protect, support, and respect the needs and rights of patients and families. Professional nursing practice takes nurses "beyond the bedside" as advocates with the knowledge, skills, and attitudes to understand the connectivity of complex systems in this age of complexity (Zimmerman & Ng, 2008) (see Table 1).

Advocacy as a dimension of Care Coordination and Transition Management (CCTM) for ambulatory care nurses is broad in scope. Specialized knowledge and skills which include relationship building, effective written and verbal communication, negotiation, and critical analysis (Case Management Society of America [CMSA], 2010) must be integrated with clinical expertise to provide a foundation for advocacy in nursing. As stated by French and colleagues (2009), "The role of a patient advocate calls on the skills of the diplomat, the inquisitiveness of the educator and problem solver, and the courage of the activist to speak up in difficult situations" (p. 117).

## I. Advocacy and Professional Practice Standards

The definition of professional ambulatory care nursing charges the nurse with responsibility for patient advocacy and describes the patient as the one who maintains "control of the encounter and treatment with the nurse acting in a consultative role" (AAACN, 2010, p. 6).

A. Application of Professional Standards to the CCTM Model, specifically the dimension of advocacy.
   1. Standard 5b: Health Teaching and Promotion (AAACN, 2010).
      a. Utilize strategies that promote individual and community wellness.
      b. Orient to health care delivery system, services, access to care, and available resources.
      c. Support development of self-efficacy skills.
      d. Tailor teaching methods to the individual.
      e. Create environments promoting positive collegial staff and patient-staff interactions.
   2. Standard 11: Collaboration (AAACN, 2010).
      a. Collaborate with patients, family members, caregivers, and other health professionals.
      b. Communicate openly about patient care and the nurse's role in that care.
      c. Partner with patients, caregivers, and other health care providers to create, implement, and revise a plan of care focused on outcomes and decisions related to delivery of services.
      d. Partner with colleagues to promote changes that will improve patient outcomes.
      e. Use effective communication skills.
   3. Standard 12: Ethics (AAACN, 2010).
      a. Apply principles of professional codes of ethics to ensure individual rights.
      b. Actively participate in identification and resolution of ethical issues and concerns.
      c. Preserve patients' rights to confidentiality, privacy, and self-determination within legal, regulatory, and ethical parameters.
      d. Ensure care reflects cultural and age-appropriate differences.
      e. Advocate for informed decision making by the patient or legally designated representative.
      f. Educate and support patients in developing skills for self-efficacy.
   4. Standard 15: Resource Utilization (AAACN, 2010).
      a. Consider the effectiveness, cost, and impact on practice and the organization in the planning and delivery of services.
      b. Consider availability, effectiveness, efficiency, cost, and benefits of proposed care for the patient.
      c. Assist in obtaining appropriate and available services to meet health care needs and concerns with the aim of attaining positive health status over the lifespan.
      d. Support patients in becoming informed consumers regarding options, costs, risks, and benefits of health services.

## II. The Influence of Ethics on the Nurse as Patient Advocate

A. Ethics is a philosophical framework for examining values as they relate to human behaviors; how behaviors are viewed as right or wrong, good or bad, concerned with both the motives and the outcomes of actions (Steinmetz as cited in Johnson, 2013).
   1. Ethics provides a conceptual framework within which advocacy presents an opportunity to act (Johnson, 2013).
   2. Nursing's professional code of ethics states the nurse's primary commitment is to the patient (ANA, 2001).

a. Commitment is directly to the patient and to collegial interactions in the course of advocacy.
   (1) "We all have a moral obligation to work together to improve care for patients" (Pronovost & Vohr as cited in Interprofessional Education Collaborative Expert Panel [IPEC], 2011).

3. According to Fowler (as cited in Johnson, 2013), patient advocacy requires the nurse to balance ethical principles and learned professional values promoting health, well-being, and independence in care of the patient.
   a. "The registered nurse practices ethically" (ANA, 2010b, p. 47).

B. Ethical principles related to advocacy.
1. Autonomy: the right to self-determine a course of action; support of independent decision making (ANA, 2011).
   a. Concept of person-centered care found to be pivotal to coordinated care delivery (Ehrlich, Kendall, Muenchberger, & Armstrong, 2009; IPEC, 2011).
   b. Empowerment of the person, ensuring control over own care (Ehrlich et al., 2009).
   c. Customizing plan of care to be consistent with the values and needs of the patient (Schifalacqua as cited in Ehrlich et al., 2009).
   d. Helping individuals assume more of their own health-promoting activities (Craig, Eby, & Whittington, 2011).
2. Beneficence: compassion; taking positive action to help others; desire to do good; the core principle of our patient advocacy (ANA, 2011).
   a. Nonjudgmental listening, planning, and evaluation of care (Craig et al., 2011).
   b. Involving other professions in care as appropriate (IPEC, 2011).
   c. Understanding the vulnerability of the patient (Olsson, Larsson, Flennsner, & Back-Peterson, 2012).
3. Fidelity: the concept of keeping a commitment, based upon the virtue of caring (ANA, 2011).
   a. Protecting confidentiality and upholding individual's rights (Schifalacqua as cited in Ehrlich et al., 2009).
   b. Protecting the health, safety, and rights of the patient (ANA, 2001).
   c. Nurse's primary commitment to patient (ANA, 2001).
4. Justice: refers to equal and fair distribution of resources. Justice implies all citizens have an equal right to resources, regardless of what they have contributed or who they are (ANA, 2011).
   a. Proactive leveraging of services (Ehrlich et al., 2009).
   b. Providing opportunities for patients to participate in planning care (ANA, 2001).

C. Moral courage as an essential skill for nurses as advocates (Lachman as cited in Johnson, 2013).
1. Ability to overcome fear and stand up for core values and ethical obligations.
2. Knowledge of professional ethical obligations.
3. Required in individual and in organizational advocacy.
4. The preservation of integrity is viewed as "an aspect of wholeness of character" in nursing's professional code of ethics (ANA, 2001).

## III. The Nurse as Advocate in the CCTM Model

The primary care ambulatory nurse must demonstrate an understanding of the dimension of advocacy in the following areas in order to optimize the care coordination and transition management needs of the patient and family.

A. Nursing assessment.
1. Encompasses the total patient, including medical, psychosocial, behavioral, socioeconomic, and spiritual needs.
2. Document using standardized or electronic tools when available to ensure portability of care.

B. Plan of care: development of the plan of care is a collaborative process.
1. Acting as patient advocate, the RN in CCTM provides information about treatment options and plans, assesses the patient's abilities, evaluates care and treatment, and communicates with other health care providers (Olsson et al., 2012).
2. The primary purpose of care planning in the ambulatory environment is to provide continuity of care, ensuring the patient's needs are met on a long-term basis as well as to prevent unplanned hospital admissions (Olsson et al., 2012).
3. The RN in CCTM understands the unique situation of the patient, which allows the nurse to evaluate the effectiveness of the plan of care in meeting the patient's individual needs over time.

C. Negotiate patient services with patient and family; the goal of negotiating services is to maintain flexibility, moving the patient to optimal levels of health based on his or her current situation.
1. Practice cultural competence with awareness and respect diversity.
2. Comprehensive assessment to identify actual or potential barriers.
   a. Financial.
   b. Transportation.
   c. Psychosocial.
   d. Health literacy.
3. Promote evidence-based care.
   a. Provide preventive care.
4. Provide optimal patient safety.
5. Utilize behavioral change science.
   a. Motivational interviewing.

6. Link with community resources.
7. Assist with navigating the health care system.

D. Support and assistance with access to appropriate type and level of services.
   1. Facilitate patient access to necessary and appropriate services while educating the patient, family, or caregiver regarding available resources.
   2. Basic needs such as housing, food, transportation, and medical equipment.
   3. Medications.
      a. Available pharmacy services.
      b. Medication review and reconciliation to assure the patient's understanding of medications, including schedule, actions, and precautions.

E. Recognition, prevention, and elimination of disparities.
   1. Culture, race, ethnicity, national origin, migration background.
   2. Gender, gender identity or gender expression, sexual orientation, marital status.
   3. Religious, political beliefs.
   4. Mental or cognitive disability.

F. Serve as voice of the patient across settings and disciplines.
   1. Empower the patient to problem-solve by exploring options of care when available and alternative plans of care when necessary.
   2. Promote patient's self-determination.
      a. Informed and shared decision making.
      b. Autonomy.
      c. Growth.
      d. Self-advocacy.
   3. Education of other health care providers in recognizing and respecting the patient's needs, strengths, preferences, and goals.

G. Communication and patient education: communication, education, and decision making regarding choices in treatment plan, disease management, community resources, insurance benefits, and psychosocial concerns to facilitate timely and informed decisions (CMSA, 2010).
   1. Establish relationships: identify patient and family/caregiver goals.
      a. Development and maintenance of proactive, patient-centered relationships and communication with the patient and other necessary stakeholders to maximize outcomes.
      b. Mediation and negotiation to improve communication and relationships.
      c. Utilize problem-solving skills and techniques to reconcile differing points of view between patient and family and/or patient, family, and provider, or between providers.
   2. Collaborative efforts to optimize patient outcomes.
      a. Work with community, local, and state resources.
      b. Collaborate with primary care provider, other members of the health care team, the payer, and other relevant stakeholders, such as social worker for transportation needs or pharmacist for medication needs.
      c. Advocate for process and outcome indicators that can be embedded in standardized nursing documentation tools using standardized coding which enables processes and outcomes of care to be tracked.
   3. Telephone follow up and surveillance for high-risk patients and populations.

H. Provide support to achieve desired outcomes: maximize the patient's health, wellness, safety, adaptation, and self-care through quality case management, patient satisfaction, and cost efficacy (CMSA, 2010).
   1. Evaluation of effectiveness of interventions/processes of care, and achievement of goals in the plan of care.
   2. Demonstration of the efficacy, quality, and cost-effectiveness of interventions in achieving the goals documented in the plan of care.
   3. Utilization of and adherence to evidence-based guidelines, standardized tools, and evidence-based processes to measure the patient's preference for and understanding of:
      a. Proposed plan of care.
      b. Willingness to change.
      c. Support to maintain health behavioral change.

I. Enhance patient satisfaction: reflects patient's perception of care delivered and outcomes achieved, including:
   1. Concerns heard.
   2. Ability to access community services.
   3. Able to obtain medications and other therapies.
   4. Patient/family satisfaction and compliance with treatment plan.
   5. Long-term ability to keep appointments.
   6. Competent in self-management of health.

## IV. Advocacy Role in the Care of Underserved and Vulnerable Populations

Understanding the connection between health and poverty, mental illness, and homelessness is an important element of effective practice for the RN in CCTM involved in coordinating the care of impoverished, underserved, and vulnerable populations.

A. Understand contributing factors leading to health care disparities that continue to worsen for lower income people.
   1. Children in impoverished households are at increased risk of experiencing profound health problems and unmet medical needs.

2. The functionally impaired, low income, frail, and elderly represent a population with the least access to high-quality health care and the worst health outcomes (Allen et al., 2011).
3. Approximately 4.5 million people in the United States with intellectual and developmental disabilities (I/DD) require community-based services (Lind & Archibald, 2013).

B. Increase awareness of association between health disparities and hospital re-admissions.
   1. The urban underserved compose a disproportionate share of hospital re-admissions at many academic medical centers (Long, Genao, & Horwitz, 2013).

C. Understand barriers to access for underserved and vulnerable populations.
   1. Lack of housing.
      a. Refer to social worker or directly to community resources for supportive housing.
   2. Lack of health insurance.
      a. Extending health insurance coverage is a necessary step in improving access to quality health care services (Berenson, Doty, Abrams, & Shih, 2012).
      b. Assist or refer patient/family to resources for enrollment in public programs.
         (1) Medicaid – barriers to enrollment.
            (a) Restrictive eligibility and complex enrollment process.
            (b) Shortage of Medicaid providers poses challenges to families with limited resources.
   3. Lack of transportation.
      a. Collaborate with social worker to identify options and available services.
   4. Lack of child care.
      a. Collaborate with social worker or community services to explore family dynamics and options for support.
   5. Lack of established primary care provider (PCP) or medical home.
      a. Referral to PCP.
   6. Lack of care delivery models to address complex service needs of I/DD population.
      a. Promote patient-centered medical home with multidisciplinary care team.

D. Emergency departments and walk-in clinics are often first choice for homeless, underserved, and frail elderly individuals requiring medical attention.
   1. Assist in navigating patient to appropriate level of care and services.
   2. The RN in CCTM in emergency departments or community walk-in clinics should manage referral to appropriate resources for access to primary care services.
   3. The RN in CCTM should consistently offer education, encouragement, and advice to patients regarding advantages of seeking majority of care from primary care medical home.

E. Publicly financed programs pay for many I/DD services.
   1. Refer to medical home which supports care needs and access to behavioral health and long-term services.

## V. The Role of Advocacy in Organizational Policy Development

Policies and procedures provide blueprints for the behavior of an organization and a framework that guides organizational consistency. Policies describing nursing practice serve as the basis for action and decisions (Kerfoot & Chafee, 2007). Once established, such policies will lead to further development of consistent and measureable nursing outcomes for patients and families.

A. Advocacy involvement for the CCTM includes developing and updating organizational policies that define process and outcome indicators related to care coordination.
   1. Clinical practice committees (CPC): Membership on a health system, hospital, service line, or departmental CPC provides opportunities for nurses to introduce or contribute to nursing policies related to care coordination and transition management.
      a. Nursing policies, procedures, and standards provide evidence-based rationale for the practice of nursing.
      b. Nursing process standards define nursing practice and provide consistency in the delivery of care.
   2. Appointment of CCTM ambulatory care nurses to multidisciplinary committees at the organizational level contributes to effective care coordination and transition management across the continuum of care.
      a. Ambulatory CCTM perspective and voice needed on:
         (1) Medication safety committees.
         (2) Patient safety and quality assurance committees.
         (3) Executive-level oversight committees.
   3. Magnet® designation.
      a. Ambulatory nursing perspective is essential in describing care coordination activities contributing to nursing excellence in organizations with or seeking Magnet® designation.
      b. Ambulatory nurses must continue to advocate for National Database of Nursing Quality Indicators outcome measures, which reflect ambulatory nurse contributions to care coordination and transition management.

## VI. Advocacy, Public Policy Development, and Health Care Reform

Improvements in care coordination and transition management are essential to achieve desired changes in health care as described in the PPACA. The time has arrived to assure that the importance of CCTM activities by ambulatory nurses as well as nurses in CCTM in other settings across the continuum is inherently reflected in public policy.

A. Social and political priorities for nursing include addressing the cost and quality of services (Neuman, 2012).
   1. As the most trusted professionals in health care, nurses have a potentially powerful voice.
   2. To achieve concrete system-wide change, nurses must engage in broad partnerships with physicians, pharmacists, and other health care professionals to influence transformation on behalf of patients and families.
      a. Multidisciplinary coalitions are effective political strategies for influencing health policy (Bowers-Lanier, 2007).
      b. Individual responsibility and interprofessional involvement are essential (Neuman, 2012).

B. Care delivery models.
   1. In the transformed health system envisioned by the PPACA, building a more robust primary care model will mitigate the need for more expensive acute care services.
   2. Nurses must assume roles essential to meeting the rapidly expanding demand for these services.

C. Long-term solutions related to patient access must be built into public policy.
   1. Participate in state and national-level policy work through involvement in professional nursing organizations.

D. Engage in coalition partnerships.
   1. Join multidisciplinary community, state, and national coalitions whose collective voice can influence positive change.

**Table 1.**
**Advocacy: Knowledge, Skills, and Attitudes for Competency**

Advocacy is the support and empowerment of patients to make informed decisions, navigate the health care system to access appropriate care and build strong partnerships with providers, while working towards system improvement to support patient-centered care.

| Knowledge | Skills | Attitudes | Sources |
|---|---|---|---|
| Discuss principles of effective communication. | Communicate patient values, preferences, and expressed needs to other members of the health care team. | Value active partnership with patients or designated surrogates in planning, implementation, and evaluation of care. | Craig et al., 2011<br>Cronenwett et al., 2007 |
| Examine common barriers to active involvement of patients in their own health care processes. | Remove barriers in presence of families and other designated surrogates based on patient preferences. | Value the patient's expertise with own health and symptoms. | Cronenwett et al., 2007 |
| | "Act with honesty and integrity in relationships with patients, families, and team members." | "Embrace the cultural diversity and individual differences that characterize patients, populations, and the health care team." | Interprofessional Education Collaborative Expert Panel, 2011, p.19 |
| Identify resources available to support patient needs. | Provide access to resources across settings and providers. | | Ehrlich etal., 2009 |
| | | Respect patient's right to access to personal health records. | Cronenwett et al., 2007 |
| Recognize system barriers to patient access specific to the underserved populations. | Participate in advocacy efforts to improve quality of health care services for low-income and vulnerable populations. | | Berenson et al., 2012 |
| | | Value the influence of activism and organizational leadership for nurses. | Bowers-Lanier, 2007 |
| Understand individual and interprofessional advocacy as essential elements of nursing's responsibility to society. | | | Neuman, 2012 |
| | Participate in public debate and activism on behalf of an improved system of health care delivery for patients and families. | Value active participation by nurses in policy formation. | Bowers-Lanier, 2007 |
| Describe how diverse cultural, ethnic, and social backgrounds function as sources of patient, family, and community values. | | Recognize personally held attitudes about working with patients from different ethnic, cultural, and social backgrounds.<br>Willingly support patient-centered care for individuals and groups whose values differ from our own. | Cronenwett et al., 2007 |

*continued on next page*

**Source Note:** Cronenwett et al. (2007) reprinted from *Nursing Outlook,* 55(3), 122-131, with permission from Elsevier.

### Table 1. (continued)
### Advocacy: Knowledge, Skills, and Attitudes for Competency

Advocacy is the support and empowerment of patients to make informed decisions, navigate the health care system to access appropriate care and build strong partnerships with providers, while working towards system improvement to support patient-centered care.

| Knowledge | Skills | Attitudes | Sources |
|---|---|---|---|
| "Understand principles of change management." | "Apply change management principles by using data to improve patient and systems outcomes." | "Demonstrate leadership in affecting necessary change." | QSEN Education Consortium, 2012, p. 6 |
| Analyze moral problems in the practice of moral courage.<br>Recognize cultural differences that influence the practice of moral courage | Participate in open dialogue and deliberation regarding ethical issues. | "Accept values of the profession of nursing" (p. 3).<br>"Support ethical responsibilities essential to professional values" (p. 2).<br>Act on ethical beliefs despite potential risks. | Murray, 2010 |
| | Use communication skills including assertiveness, negotiation, and conflict resolution. | Develop capacity to overcome fear.<br>Demonstrate courage by speaking up against unethical, unlawful, or outdated practices. | Lachman, 2010 |

## References


Allen, K.R., Hazelett, S.E., Jarjoura, D., Wright, K., Fosnight, S.M., Kropp, D.J., ... Pfister, E.W. (2011). The after discharge care management of low income frail elderly (AD-LIFE) randomized trial: Theoretical framework and study design. *Population Health Management, 14*(3), 137-142. doi:10.1089/pop.2010.0016

American Academy of Ambulatory Care Nursing (AAACN). (2010). *Scope and standards of practice for professional ambulatory care nursing* (8th ed.). Pitman, NJ: Author.

American Nurses Association (ANA). (2001). *ANA's code of ethics with interpretive statements.* Silver Spring, MD: Author.

American Nurses Association (ANA). (2010a). *Nursing's social policy statement: The essence of the profession.* Silver Spring, MD: Author.

American Nurses Association (ANA). (2010b). *Nursing: Scope and standards of practice.* Silver Spring, MD: Author.

American Nurses Association (ANA). (2011). *Short definitions of ethical principles and theories – Familiar words, what do they mean?* Silver Spring, MD: Author. Retrieved from http://www.nursingworld.org/MainMenuCategories/EthicsStandards/Resources/Ethics-Definitionc.pdf

Berenson, J., Doty, M.M., Abrams, M.K., & Shih, A. (2012). *Achieving better quality of care for low income populations: The role of health insurance and the medical home for reducing health inequities* (Commonwealth Fund pub 1600, vol. 11). Washington, DC: The Commonwealth Fund. Retrieved from http://www.commonwealthfund.org/~/media/Files/Publications/Issue%20Brief/2012/May/1600_Berenson_achieving_better_quality_care_low_income_v2.pdf

Bowers-Lanier, R. (2007). Coalitions: A powerful political strategy. In D.J. Mason, J.K. Leavitt, & M.W. Chaffee (Eds.), *Policy and politics in nursing and health care* (5th ed., pp. 135-144). St. Louis, MO: Saunders Elsevier, Inc.

Case Management Society of America (CMSA). (2010). *Standards of practice for case management.* Little Rock, AR: Author.

Craig, C., Eby, D., & Whittington, J. (2011). *Care coordination model: Better care at lower cost for people with multiple health and social needs.* IHI Innovation Series white paper. Cambridge, MA: Institute for Healthcare Improvement.

Cronenwett, L., Sherwood, G., Barnsterner, J., Disch, J., Johnson, J., Mitchell, P., ... Warren, J. (2007). Quality and safety education for nurses. *Nursing Outlook, 55*(3), 122-131.

Ehrlich, C., Kendall, E., Muenchberger, H., & Armstrong, K. (2009). Coordinated care: What does that really mean? *Health and Social Care in the Community, 17*(6), 619-627.

French, E.A., Gilkey, M.B., & Earp, J.L. (2009). Patient advocacy: Putting the vocabulary of patient centered care in action. *North Carolina Medical Journal, 70*(2), 114-119.

Gilkey, M.B., & Earp, J.L. (2009). Defining patient advocacy in the post-quality chasm era. *North Carolina Medical Journal, 70*(2), 120-124.

Henry J. Kaiser Family Foundation, The. (2013). *Kaiser health tracking poll.* Retrieved from http://kaiserfamilyfoundation.files.wordpress.com/2013/03/8425-t1.pdf

Interprofessional Education Collaborative Expert Panel (IPEC). (2011). *Core competencies for interprofessional collaborative practice: Report of an expert panel.* Washington, DC: Interprofessional Education Collaborative.

Johnson, E.M. (2013). Patient advocacy and use of community resources. In C. Laughlin (Ed.), *Core curriculum for ambulatory care nursing* (3rd ed., pp. 113-124). Pitman, NJ: American Academy of Ambulatory Care Nursing.

Kerfoot, K., & Chafee, M. (2007). Ten keys to unlocking policy change in the workplace. In D.J. Mason, J.K. Leavitt, & M.W. Chaffee (Eds.), *Policy and politics in nursing and health care* (5th ed., pp. 482-485). St. Louis, MO: Saunders Elsevier, Inc.

Lachman, V.D. (2010). Strategies necessary for moral courage. *OJIN: Online Journal of Issues in Nursing, 15*(3). Retrieved from http://nursingworld.org/MainMenuCategories/EthicsStandards/Courage-and-Distress/Strategies-and-Moral-Courage.html

Lind, A., & Archibald, N. (2013). *Structuring new service delivery models for individuals with intellectual and developmental disabilities.* (CHCS Policy Brief). Retrieved from http://www.chcs.org/usr_doc/New_Service_Delivery_Models_for_IDD_020413.pdf

Long, T., Genao, I., & Horwitz, L.I. (2013). Reasons for readmission in an underserved high-risk population: A qualitative analysis of a series of inpatient interviews. *BMJ Open, 3*(9), 1-6. doi:10.1136/bmjopen-2013-003212

Murray, J.S. (2010). Moral courage in healthcare: Acting ethically even in the presence of risk. *OJIN: The Online Journal of Issues in Nursing, 15*(3). Retrieved from http://www.nursingworld.org/MainMenuCategories/EthicsStandards/Courage-and-Distress/Moral-Courage-and-Risk.html

Neuman, C.E. (2012). Nursing's social policy statement. In K.N. White & A. O'Sullivan (Eds.), *The essential guide to nursing practice.* Silver Spring, MD: American Nurses Assocation. Retrieved from http://essentialguidetonursingpractice.files.wordpress.com/2012/07/pages-from-essential-guide-to-nursing-practice-chapter-1.pdf

Olsson, M., Larsson, L.G., Flennsner, G., & Back-Peterson, S. (2012). The impact of concordant communication in outpatient care planning – Nurses' perspective. *Journal of Nursing, 20*(6), 748-757. doi: 10.1111/j.1365-2834.2012.01479.x

QSEN Education Consortium. (2012). *Graduate-level QSEN competencies: Knowledge, skills and attitudes.* Washington, DC: American Association of Colleges of Nursing. Retrieved from http://www.aacn.nche.edu/faculty/qsen/competencies.pdf

Silberman, P. (2013). Implementing the Affordable Care Act in North Carolina: The rubber hits the road. *North Carolina Medical Journal, 74*(4), 298-307.

Zimmerman, B., & Ng, S. (2008). Beyond the beside: Nursing as policymaking. In C. Lindberg, S. Nash, & C. Lindberg (Eds.), *On the edge: Nursing in the age of complexity.* Bordentown, NJ: PlexusPress.

# CHAPTER 3

# Education and Engagement of Patients and Families

*Cheryl Lovlien, MS, RN-BC*

## Learning Outcome Statement

The purpose of this chapter is to enable the reader to identify methods to assess patient and family learning needs, create learning opportunities, and promote an open learning environment in which the learner work toward self-management and optimal health.

## Learning Objectives

After reading this chapter, the registered nurse (RN) working in the Care Coordination and Transition Management (CCTM) role will be able to:

- Identify patient and family education needs, goals, and expected behavioral outcomes.
- Discuss steps to assess learning needs, readiness to learn, health literacy needed to plan, implement, and evaluate education and learning across the lifespan for patients and family members.
- Employ methods to engage patients/families and caregivers in health care.
- Review educational principles and theories of learning.
- Apply methods of teaching and learning that focus on special populations and how they best learn, assimilate information, and improve outcomes.
- Employ methods such as "teach back" to assess learning and health literacy.
- Demonstrate the knowledge, skills, and attitudes required for the education and engagement of patients and families dimension (see Table 1).

## Competency Definitions

*Patient education* is the process of influencing patient behavior and producing the changes in knowledge, attitudes, and skills necessary to maintain or improve health (American Academy of Family Physicians, 2004). Bastable (2011) further identifies patient education as a process of assisting people to learn health-related behaviors they can incorporate into everyday life with the goal of optimal health and independence in self-care.

*Health education* is "any combination of planned learning experiences based on sound theories that provide individuals, groups, and communities the opportunity to acquire the information and skills needed to make quality health decisions" (Wurzbach, 2004, p. 219).

*Engagement* in health care is "actions individuals must take to obtain the greatest benefit from the health care services available to them" (Rovner et al., 2010). According to Lorig and Holman (2003), the nature of having health or illness requires that the individual manage his or her disease. People have shifting perspectives of their disease due to changes in perception of the illness and their psychological state. The tasks the patient needs to take on for self-management and engagement in health care include medical tasks, knowledge and behaviors related to the disease or condition, and the role of the individual and family in "managing" health or illness (Lorig & Holman, 2003). Self-management is based on the individual needs and not on the provisions of the health care provider or educator. The ability of the patient to have control over his or her health and plans for improvement improve the outcome of health status.

*Patient activation* is defined as "understanding one's own role in the care process and having the knowledge, skills, and confidence to take on that role" (Hibbard, Greene, & Overton, 2013, p. 216) and is a four-stage process for the patient in development of the patient's role in self-care. These stages include a belief by the patient he or she serves a role in his or her health, the development of patient confidence and knowledge related to his or her health, initiation of healthy activities, and maintenance of health activities over the long term (Hibbard, Stockard, Mahoney, & Tusler, 2004).

Health care education has long incorporated a tradition of "telling." Telling the patient and family what they will do and how they will do it. The information flow has traditionally been a one-way communication between a member of the care team and the receiver, either patient/family or caregiver, with little time or effort placed in identifying if the education was clear, meaningful, or able to be accomplished. Cognitive theory identifies the need for the learner to gain attention, receive the information, and identify how that information is used. Learners need to process information in order to demonstrate understanding (Bastable, 2014).

Education of patients and families is a major dimension of the role of the registered nurse (RN) in Care Coordination and Transition Management (CCTM), with the expectation patients and families will adapt and apply health practices to improve health care outcomes. Once the provider and/or RN in CCTM have completed the provision of care and the patient leaves the clinic or hospital, it is up to the patient and family to implement the continuing care plans and activities to promote or improve health. The success of the educational efforts will hinge upon the ability of the patient/family to understand the disease process and treatment plan, and to understand and incorporate that knowledge into actionable behaviors that will promote lifestyle changes (Peikes, Genevro, Scholle, & Torda, 2011). To achieve this goal, the patient needs to understand health, illness, and influencing factors through communication that meet his or her level of understanding in a manner that is respectful and engaging. The patient should be able to use this information to implement self-care and/or make a change in lifestyle to meet health goals. In addition, the RN in CCTM must be aware of the patient's and family's level of health literacy and find resources that best help him or her to learn new concepts, to integrate and internalize those concepts, and to have the ability to change behaviors with reinforcement of those concepts from members of the health care team. This is a collaborative relationship between the RN in CCTM and patient/caregiver and a relationship that must be constantly nurtured.

Engaging patients in their health care improves outcomes (Scholle, Torda, Peikes, Han, & Genevro, 2010). Patients within the context of the Patient-Centered Medical Home should receive patient-centered care focused on the needs of the person, and within the context of his or her culture, values, and preferences (Agency for Healthcare Research and Quality, 2011). Patients should receive support for self-care efforts and involvement with the health care plan. Providing education and information to patients and families is a core dimension in the RN Care Coordination and Transition Management Model. Expectations and tools necessary for that role are identified.

## I. Assess Readiness for Learning

A. Identify the audience.
   1. Identify who will participate in learning and assure timing of education meets scheduling needs.
   2. Establish relationships with patients and families that are open to conversation and discussion. Patients/families/caregivers are the experts of their health experience and will identify what they want to know. "Honor the patient's experience" (Osborne, 2013, p. 30).
   3. Considerations of health concerns that may interfere or inhibit learning.
      a. Hearing loss may affect one in three over the age of 60 and one-half of those over 85 (U.S. Department of Health and Human Services [DHHS], 2014).
      b. Learning disabilities (e.g., dyslexia): learning disabilities (LD) are a group of varying disorders that have a negative impact on learning. They may affect one's ability to speak, listen, think, read, write, spell, or compute. The most prevalent LD is in the area of reading, known as dyslexia (National Center for Learning Disabilities, 2013).
      c. Depression and other mental health illnesses influence the ability of the patient to concentrate on learning (Wolf, Gazmararian, & Baker, 2005).
      d. Cognitive impairment: failing of short and long-term recall and general thinking logic skills (Federman, Sano, Wolf, Siu, & Halm, 2009).

B. Create an environment of learning (London, 2009).
   1. Identify the "right" time for the discussion: provide education when the patient/family is ready.
   2. Decrease distractions such as environmental noise (e.g., TV, radio, other conversations).
   3. Arrange furniture that allows discussion.
   4. Prepare patient learning materials: reading materials that are at the appropriate reading level, note taking, graphics, pictures, videos, computers, etc.

C. Alternate learning environments.
   1. Convene shared medical appointments.
   2. Initiate telephone calls to patient/family/caregiver to engage in self-care and lifestyle counseling.
   3. Initiate programs such as grocery shopping with dietician, cooking demos, and providing recipes.
   4. Provide small group informational seminars.
   5. Prepare and provide simple exercises that can be done at home; no gym required (Cesta, 2011).

## II. Assessment of Knowledge and Abilities

A. Health literacy.
   1. "Represents the cognitive and social skills which determine the motivation and ability of individuals to gain access to and understand and use information in ways which promote and maintain good health" (Nutbeam, 2000, p. 264).

2. Individuals who have the ability to understand, recognize, and choose to act on information provided in a way to achieve health (Osborne, 2013). This includes participating in health care decisions, interpreting information, and making changes to achieve a healthy lifestyle.

B. Literary assessment.
   1. Language: one-third to one-half of all adults cannot comprehend the written word and 24%-59% of people are in the lowest categories of health literacy (Cibulskis, Giardino, & Moyer, 2011).
   2. Nine out of ten people may lack essential skills to handle their health (National Center for Education Statistics, 2006).
      a. Identify and determine the best way for the learner to understand information provided and his or her role in managing the information.
      b. Choose the method or modality that patient and family members identify as an effective method for learning in the past.

C. Culture affects how people communicate, understand, and respond to health information (DHHS, n.d.). The ability to work with people in other cultures related to their health literacy requires cultural competence. This means sensitivity to and valuing of the individual's cultural beliefs, values, attitudes, traditions, language, and health practices. Using the knowledge of culture to work toward a positive health outcome (DHHS, 2001).
   1. Use interpreters.
      a. Help patients feel welcome by greeting in their native language.
      b. Allow sufficient time for interactions.
      c. Look at the patient not the interpreter.
      d. Use language tools available.
      e. Communicate with drawings such as:
         (1) Anatomical models.
         (2) Rating scales.
      f. Appreciate differences in body language.
      g. Notice signs of difficulty.
      h. Verify understanding asking the patient/family to explain in their own words or describe through an interpreter.

D. Social groups: generations are social groups bound by a shared life experience usually grouped into 20-year spans of time. The Centers for Disease Control and Prevention (CDC, 2012) provides information on the perspective of several generations accessing health care such as "Moms," "Tweens" (age 9-12), "Teens" (age 12-17), "Boomers" (born 1946-1962), and the "Responsible Generation" (age 64-84).

E. Assess styles in which people learn.
   1. Visual: seeing/watching.
   2. Auditory: listening.
   3. Kinesthetic: hands-on learning (using touch and manipulatives).
   4. One or more of the above.

F. Assess patient/caregiver knowledge of health/disease.
   1. What does the learner know or not know about the following relating to his or her health/disease.
      a. Risk factors for disease.
      b. Symptoms.
      c. Infection control practices.
      d. Communication of errors and omissions.
      e. Resources for care for disease, health, and wellness.

## III. Methods to Provide Education

Teach to meet needs of health literacy: patients and caregivers have poor recall with only 50% retention (Cibulskis et al., 2011).

A. Teach using a "universal precautions" approach, so that all communications are clear, assuming that all patients have trouble understanding (DHHS, 2010).
   1. Design written materials, format, and information delivery to match learning needs.
   2. For those unable to process written materials, other techniques and modalities must be used including illustrations, DVDs or CDs, streaming media, podcasts, etc.
   3. Use plain language to make written and oral information easier to understand for all people.
      a. Provide most important information first.
      b. Break content into smaller, understandable "chunks" of information.
      c. Use simple words and define technical terms.
      d. Use active voice (National Institutes of Health, 2013).
   4. Picture-based instructions/illustrations: show patient and family members illustrative diagrams or pictures of anatomical representations of organs (e.g., show normal heart and then heart with signs of valvular issues).
   5. Graphs to illustrate health risk: utilize graphs on disease morbidity and quantitative health risks in specific age groups, ethnic populations, etc. (Ancker, Senathirajah, Kukafka, & Starren, 2006).

B. Use active listening.
   1. Recognize words used and body language, eye contact, voice intonation.
   2. Listen for what is not said.
   3. Reinforce with positive comments when patients learn well.
   4. Reiterate content that is missed and supplement with written instructions and illustrations.
   5. Break teaching into short manageable sections.
   6. Reinforce previously learned content prior to moving on to other areas of information.

C. Utilize "teach back:" a method of teaching patients providing clear information for patients and families (Always Use Teach-back!, 2014).

 

1. Patients and families are encouraged to discuss their health care concerns in their own words and to re-explain or reiterate information to the health care provider. This process can improve patient health outcomes and provider communication (Schillinger et al., 2003).
    a. Assist patients to ask questions.
        (1) Offer a notepad.
        (2) Allow time to write answers.
        (3) Provide a writing surface.
    b. Acknowledge what patients have already heard or read.
    c. Confirm they heard what you said.
    d. Confirm you heard what they said.
    e. Provide ways for patients to learn more, offering pamphlets, websites, videos, and reliable sources of medical information.
    f. Ask questions that require more than a "yes/no" answer: ask open-ended questions and examples of what the patient is most concerned about (e.g., "What concerns you most about this diagnosis?" or "Tell me about how you see your life changing").
    g. Encourage the patient to:
        (1) Take note of symptoms: timing, intensity, characteristics.
        (2) Invite patients to bring the family/advocate to learning sessions.
        (3) Use devices such as hearing aids/eyeglasses.
        (4) Learn only as much as they want to know.
        (5) Create personal medical record (Osborne, 2013).
    h. Simplify language for translation (avoid using multisyllabic words such as hypertension, replace with "high blood pressure").
    i. Inform patients about availability of translations into their native language.
    j. Use culturally appropriate/age appropriate examples.
    k. Avoid jargon, abbreviations (write it out), acronyms, homonyms (gait, stool), idioms ("heads up" or "feeling blue") (Plain Language Action and Information Network, n.d.).
    l. Talk about topics one at a time, gain an understanding, and then move on.
    m. Build on the familiar: ask patients what they are currently doing to manage their condition and offer suggestions of ways to optimize what they are doing or to support problem solving.
    n. Explain in plain language (make it real: 5 lb. bag of flour).
    o. Prioritize information based on needs for survival.
        (1) Actions for survival.
        (2) Actions easy to do.
        (3) Resources needed to get to actions (Osborne, 2013).
    p. Watch for cues the discussion is moving too fast or slow such as wandering eyes, shifting positions, looking to family members for support, etc.

D. Pediatrics.
    1. Talk to the child based upon his or her developmental level and perceived understanding.
    2. Prepare for the procedure using models, visuals, and objects.
    3. Encourage and use laughter.
    4. Avoid teaching when there are obvious signs of pain, anxiety, confusion, medications, sleep deprivation, and frequent changes in regimen.
    5. Encourage "active" learning using dolls, toys, models, or other items that can be manipulated.

E. Use "Ask Me 3" (National Patient Safety Foundation, 2013).
    1. What is my main problem?
    2. What do I need to do?
    3. Why is it important for me to do this?

F. Use of acronyms: acronyms help learning by allowing the learner to attach words or mnemonics in order of actions to identify steps of a process for easier recall and retention. For example:
    1. PREPARED (Cibulskis et al., 2011)
        a. **P**resenting history.
        b. **R**eceived therapies.
        c. **E**xisting baseline.
        d. **P**ending test for follow-up.
        e. **A**nticipated needs.
        f. **R**ecords to be sent.
        g. **E**nd-of-life preferences.
        h. **D**iscussion with family and provider.

## IV. Collaboration and Teamwork (IPEC, 2011)

A. Set tone with the patient and family as a partnership: identify that health care provider is working collaboratively with the learners. Incorporate both interdisciplinary and interprofessional relationships which are demonstrated by two or more departments, individuals, and groups that work together symbiotically toward a common goal.

B. Utilize appropriate resources within the health care interprofessional teams to engage patients in meaningful behavioral changes.

C. Use collective knowledge of the health care team to assess, plan, implement, and evaluate information shared and alter plans as needs change along the continuum of care.
    1. Coordinate with care team so all members are targeting the same health literacy level.

2. Information needs: ask patient/family opinion and assess when it is enough and continually reassess needs and evaluation of the understanding of information already given.
    a. Tailor the message to fit understanding.
    b. Reframe the message based on the patient's experience.

D. Encourage best practices for all disciplines to benefit the patient and family members.

E. Move fluidly within the organization's culture to build partnerships as a basis for collaboration.

F. Demonstrate and promulgate linkages between services and goals to be achieved that results in improved patient safety.

G. Identify and use appropriate community resources to supplement the patient's understanding and utilization of support measures provided (social services, support groups, etc.).

H. Use team huddles and care conferences to bring all of the members of the health care team together to optimize needs identification, plan of action, and outcome evaluation.

## V. Evaluation of Learning

A. Confirm understanding by asking an application question.
1. What will you do?
2. What is your greatest concern?
3. How can I help you to better understand what to do?

B. Consider reasons for not understanding and assist to seek resources to support the patient/family with:
1. Learning disabilities.
2. Hearing loss.
3. Cognitive impairment.
4. Depression.
5. Limited literacy (cognitive decline, developmental disabilities, autism, etc.).
6. Language skills.
7. Cultural.
8. Readiness to learn and adapt to change that is needed to optimize outcomes.

C. Utilize "teach back" to validate understanding.
1. Confirm understanding by having the patient "teach back" in his or her own words.

D. Communicate teaching that has been done with patient and family through documentation in the medical record so subsequent interactions can start from the information already known and move onward to new information that is needed.

## VI. Accessing and Evaluating Reliable Health Information

A. Improves the patient and family members' level of knowledge, skills, and attitude to effectively adopt/reinforce healthy behaviors.

B. Evaluate effectiveness of mediums of learning.
1. Printed: books, leaflets, magazines, newspaper.
2. Electronica media (CD, DVD, online or web-based).
3. Mobile applications and social media websites (e.g., YouTube videos, Facebook, podcasts, webcasts, news, blogs, and Twitter).

C. How to evaluate health information (Medical Library Association, 2013).
1. Look for authorship/sponsorship of material.
    a. Government: identified as a part of federal or state-based organization (e.g., Agency for Healthcare Research & Quality, Centers for Disease Control and Prevention, National Institutes of Health. See http://health.nih.gov for a list of government health sites; web-based sites end in .gov = government agency or .mil = military agency).
    b. Education: institutions of higher education may provide educational resources for patients and families (e.g., created and sustained by the work of the educational institution such as http://goaskalice.columbia.edu).
        (1) Websites end in .edu = educational institution.
    c. Nonprofit organization: health care, professional organization, or volunteer institutions (e.g., companies that serve the public to provide health services or to support disease-specific research and education).
        (1) Websites end in .org = nonprofit organization.
    d. For-profit organization: commercial or enterprise or business. Examples may be any company creating health-related products and services such as drugs, medical equipment, insurance, health equipment, and supplies.
        (1) Websites end in .com or .net.
2. Currency: look for updates and the date of posted information.
    a. Look at the back of a brochure or at the bottom of a website for the date published.

3. Fact-based information: look for clues that information is based on evidence or research; look for an authoritative source such as a professional organization or government agency. There should be references citing the source of the information. If links to research articles are included, ensure links are intact. If links are broken, information may not be current.
4. Intent: provided for the learner to receive accurate nonbiased information. The intention should be clear to provide health information to the learner. Information should be provided without bias to a particular service or product.
5. Website reliability.
   a. Medical Library Association (2013) published recommendations for searching websites and top ten lists for reliable health information.
   b. Health on the Net Foundation (2013) provides identification of reliable health information on the Internet.

## VII. Engagement

A. Identify the roles of care team, patient/family/caregiver in:
   1. Information and communication.
      a. RN in CCTM identifies how the medical system works and offers written and/or visual directions on how to navigate the system.
      b. RN in CCTM describes roles of the team members and offers examples of how different members can address different needs.
      c. RN in CCTM and patient/family/caregiver assist to organize patient information.
   2. Self-care.
      a. Patients learn to care for themselves, participate in collaborative goal setting and decision making (Bodenheimer, 2005).
      b. Patients/families/caregivers work with providers to identify and monitor treatment and self-care goals.
      c. Patients/families/caregivers identify the need to receive help related to chronic illness.
      d. Patients/families/caregivers work toward decreasing health risks.
      e. Patients/families/caregivers engage in support groups or group visits.
      f. Patients/families/caregivers implement self-management tactics to contribute to success of management of health care over time (Erlich, Kendall, Muenchberger, & Armstrong, 2009).

B. Identify decision-making role of RN in CCTM and patient/family/caregiver.
   1. Formal.
      a. RN in CCTM reviews evidence-based information and methods to determine plan of care.
      b. RN in CCTM discusses risks, benefits, and options.
      c. Patient/family/caregiver makes decisions about treatment and includes providers in discussion of values and preferences.
   2. Informal (not created in the context of the formal provider/patient relationship).
      a. Patient/family/caregiver and/or RN in CCTM find and review options.
      b. Patient/family/caregiver, RN in CCTM, and provider create an environment of open discussion (conversational) and identify the meaning of the health care situation with the patient/family/caregiver.
      c. All roles discussed as an open review of interventions as a basis of conversation with no expectation of a formal decision.

C. Safety.
   1. Patients and families work with the health care team to review treatment and results.
   2. Patients/families discuss treatments and medications.
   3. Patients/families report events and potential safety problems, such as medication events or infection control concerns.

## VIII. Five Core Self-Management Skills (Lorig & Holman, 2003)

A. Problem solving: defining problems, generating solutions and gaining support, and knowledge from health care professionals and friends.
B. Decision making: making daily decisions based on what they know about their disease/wellness, how they will react based on their role, knowledge, and psychological involvement in the decision.
C. Utilization of resources: the ability of the individual to gain knowledge and access to resources available to assist in decision making or in support of achieving health or wellness. Successful access of resources may rely on persistence of the individual to continue to seek access to resources.
D. Partnerships with health care providers: the ability of the individual to gain access to health care team members and attain an open communication loop between the health care provider, patient, and family.
E. Taking action: patients need to be able to achieve health goals by performing activities and tasks required to achieve wellness or stability in the disease process.

**Table 1.**
**Education and Engagement of Patients and Families: Knowledge, Skills, and Attitudes for Competency**

| Knowledge | Skills | Attitudes | Sources |
|---|---|---|---|
| **Patient-Centered Planning** | | | |
| Identify care centered on the patient. | | | Boult et al., 2008 |
| Seek to understand patient/family/community preferences and values regarding health and illness. | Elicit patient values, preferences, and expressed needs as part of clinical interview, implementation of care plan, and evaluation of care. | Value seeing health care situations through patients' eyes.<br><br>Respect and encourage individual expression of patient values, preferences, and expressed needs. | Cronenwett et al., 2007 |
| Define assessment of physical, psychological, emotional, social, and cultural barriers to learning. | | Support patient-centered care for individuals and groups whose values differ from own.<br><br>Believe patients/families are able to follow a plan of care.<br><br>Flexible, seek to solve problems, with a commitment to patient and family. | Laughlin & Beisel, 2010 |
| Identify components of a coordinated, integrated plan of care.<br><br>Create an evidence-based plan of care including promotion of patient engagement, self-management and monitoring of health condition, coaching on healthy behaviors, and recognition of emergent signs and symptoms. | | | Boult et al., 2008 |
| | Use evidence-based clinical care plan and evaluate effectiveness. | | Epping-Jordan et al., 2004 |
| | | Value patient/family involvement in planning health care changes and activities.<br><br>Seek learning opportunities with patients who represent all aspects of human diversity.<br><br>Recognize personally held attitudes about working with patients from different ethnic, cultural, and social backgrounds. | Hibbard et al., 2004 |

*continued on next page*

**Source Note:** Cronenwett et al. (2007) reprinted from *Nursing Outlook, 55*(3), 122-131, with permission from Elsevier.

**Table 1. (continued)**
**Education and Engagement of Patients and Families: Knowledge, Skills, and Attitudes for Competency**

| Knowledge | Skills | Attitudes | Sources |
|---|---|---|---|
| **Patient-Centered Planning** | | | |
| Identify patient/family/caregiver need for physical comfort and emotional support. | Provide patient-centered care with sensitivity and respect for the diversity of human experience. | Willingly support patient-centered care for individuals and groups whose values differ from own.<br><br>Value the patient's expertise with own health and symptoms. | Cronenwett et al., 2007 |
| Identify the support found through involvement of family and friends.<br><br>Identify transition and continuity. | | | Wennberg et al., 2010 |
| | Use motivational interviewing. | Interpersonal mutual respect and trust that supports patient learning.<br><br>Accept changes in the plan and maintain flexibility in planning educational activities. | Coleman et al., 2006 |
| Integrate multiple dimensions of the patient/family to provide information, communication, and transition care. | | Respect and encourage expression of values.<br><br>Create relationships where evaluation of progress is open and nonthreatening. | Counsell et al., 2007 |
| **Knowledge** | **Skills** | **Attitudes** | **Sources** |
| **Collaborative Teamwork** | | | |
| Discuss principles of effective communication.<br><br>Describe basic principles of consensus building and conflict resolution. | Assess own level of communication skill in encounters with patients and families.<br><br>Participate in building consensus or resolving conflict in the context of patient care.<br><br>Communicate care provided and needed at each transition in care. | Appreciate shared decision making with empowered patients and families, even when conflicts occur.<br><br>Value continuous improvement of own communication and conflict resolution skills. | Cronenwett et al., 2007 |
| | | Act with honesty and integrity in relationships with patient, family, and caregivers. | Interprofessional Education Collaborative Expert Panel (IPEC), 2011 |
| Understand scope of practice in order to effectively highlight members of the team who are best prepared to handle the issue and delegate to appropriate team member. | Establish collaborative relationships with patient/family by explanations of care coordination-collaborative care to meet patient's needs. | Identify one's own attitude concerning support of family members and expectations). | Dennison & Hughes, 2009 |
| | Use active listening and encourage ideas and opinions from members of the team. | | IPEC, 2011 |

*continued on next page*

**Table 1. (continued)**
**Education and Engagement of Patients and Families: Knowledge, Skills, and Attitudes for Competency**

| Knowledge | Skills | Attitudes | Sources |
|---|---|---|---|
| **Collaborative Teamwork** | | | |
| | Communicate patient values, preferences, and expressed needs to other members of health care team. | Value active partnership with patients or designated surrogates in planning, implementing, and evaluating care.<br><br>Respect patient preferences for degree of active engagement in care process. | Cronenwett et al., 2007 |
| | Facilitate patient support groups for shared learning and coping. | | Dennison & Hughes, 2009 |
| Explain the role and responsibilities of care providers and how members of the team work together to provide care. | | | IPEC, 2011 |
| Reach out to each provider to inform them of your role to assist in meeting the health care needs of patients with specific interventions. | | | Katon et al., 2010 |
| | | Allow family members to determine their ability to provide support. | Wennberg et al., 2010 |
| Knowledge of patient education, coaching process to support self-management. | Demonstrate coaching methods to engage and motivate patients.<br><br>Use motivational interviewing or other techniques. | Belief that patients and families are able to manage their chronic conditions. | Leff et al., 2009 |
| | Teach self-care actions, how to manage symptoms, how to manage care, and how to adapt to changes brought on by changing health. | | Riegel & Carlson, 2002 |
| | | Accept patient self-management as important component of care management. | Wennberg et al., 2010 |

*continued on next page*

 

**Table 1. (continued)**
**Education and Engagement of Patients and Families: Knowledge, Skills, and Attitudes for Competency**

| Knowledge | Skills | Attitudes | Sources |
|---|---|---|---|
| **Education and Engagement of Patients and Families** | | | |
| Define information, communication, and education.<br><br>Coordinate the provision of patient education and learning reinforcement across the team and inform and update the care team as the plan evolves to meet the needs of the patient. | | Creatively plan experiences for patient and family learning.<br><br>Value creativity in adapting learning to meet the need of the patient/family.<br><br>Respect patient/family values, allowing space for discussion and common understanding. | Boult et al., 2008 |
| | Assess patient and family readiness, which is dependent on psychological readiness (aware of condition and implications, level of anxiety and/or depression), physiological readiness (level of pain, sedation), and social readiness (able to share with family and/or caregivers). | | Cesta, 2011 |
| | | Create an environment of communication and questioning that empowers patient/ family to engage in planning care. | Coleman et al., 2006 |
| | Identify primary support person/persons at first encounter.<br><br>Assess cognition and aptitude and readiness to learn. | | Epping-Jordan et al., 2004 |
| | | Organize and communicate with patients, families, and health care team in a way that is understandable, avoiding discipline-specific terminology when possible. | IPEC, 2011 |
| Identify appropriate approach to convey teaching after evaluation of health literacy. | | | Naylor et al., 2011 |
| Examine common barriers to active involvement of patients in their own health care processes. | Develop patient/family/ caregiver ability to engage in decision making. | Value active partnerships with patients or designated surrogates in planning, implementating, and evaluating care. Respect patient preferences for degree of active engagement in care process. | Cronenwett et al., 2007 |
| Demonstrate knowledge of engaging patients and families in health care. | Assess and teach to meet the learner's need. | Belief that knowledge and education make a difference in health care outcomes. | Manderson et al., 2011 |

*continued on next page*

**Table 1. (continued)**
**Education and Engagement of Patients and Families: Knowledge, Skills, and Attitudes for Competency**

| Knowledge | Skills | Attitudes | Sources |
|---|---|---|---|
| **Education and Engagement of Patients and Families** | | | |
| Identify questions to ask and cues for physical, psychological, and social readiness.<br><br>Identify ways to ask open-ended questions and seek to understand patient/family needs. | Address need for self-care.<br><br>Engage and invite patient and others in learning.<br><br>Create trusting relationships.<br><br>Enable patients and families from multiple generations to cope and adapt to patient health stages, encouraging and engaging them in self-management. | | Boult et al., 2008 |
| Implement teaching. | Use teach back.<br><br>Able to impart skills to patient/family.<br><br>Develop and use content that is appropriate to the age of the learner.<br><br>Teach and coach self-management skills.<br><br>Engage patients or designated surrogates in active partnerships that promote health, safety and well-being, and self-care management.<br><br>List resources available to meet patient/family needs.<br><br>Identify priorities in education:<br>• Provide critical information.<br>• Provide printed documents and communicate during transitions in care.<br>• Identify when information exceeds ability of patient to absorb. | Flexible and creative in understanding that all patients learn differently.<br><br>Acknowledge differences in learning abilities.<br><br>Adapt a creative and engaging atmosphere for education. | Boult et al., 2008<br><br>Cronenwett et al., 2007<br><br>Peter et al., 2011 |
| | Identify patient/family level of knowledge related to medication management.<br><br>Recognize the boundaries of therapeutic relationships. | Belief that patients are able to manage their medications. | Laughlin & Beisel, 2010 |

*continued on next page*

**Table 1. (continued)**
**Education and Engagement of Patients and Families: Knowledge, Skills, and Attitudes for Competency**

| Knowledge | Skills | Attitudes | Sources |
|---|---|---|---|
| **Education and Engagement of Patients and Families (continued)** | | | |
| Identify reliable resources.<br><br>Describe reliable sources for locating evidence reports and clinical practice guidelines. | Read original research and evidence reports related to area of practice.<br><br>Locate evidence reports related to clinical practice topics and guidelines.<br><br>Question rationale for routine approaches to care that result in less-than desired outcomes or adverse events. | Appreciate the importance of reading relevant professional journals regularly. | Cronenwett et al., 2007 |
| Evaluate undestanding. | Participate in structuring the work environment to facilitate integration of new evidence into standards of practice.<br><br>Identify the ability of the family member to comprehend the level of information given.<br><br>Assess learning and retention through evaluation of key topics and how to implement self-care measures. | Value the need for continuous improvement in clinical practice based on new knowledge. | Cronenwett et al., 2007<br><br>Laughlin & Beisel, 2010 |
| **Advocacy** | | | |
| Explore ethical and legal implications of patient-centered care.<br><br>Describe the limits and boundaries of therapeutic patient-centered care. | Recognize the boundaries of therapeutic relationships. | Acknowledge the tension that may exist between patient rights and the organizational responsibility for professional, ethical care.<br><br>Appreciate shared decision making with empowered patients and families, even when conflicts occur.<br><br>Examine nursing roles in assuring coordination, integration, and continuity of care. | Cronenwett et al., 2007 |

*continued on next page*

**Table 1. (continued)**
**Education and Engagement of Patients and Families: Knowledge, Skills, and Attitudes for Competency**

| Knowledge | Skills | Attitudes | Sources |
|---|---|---|---|
| **Coaching and Counseling of Patients and Families** | | | |
| Identify the informed, motivated, and prepared patient and family. | Coach patients and caregivers in resolving problems, writing down resources and providing support during transitions. | | Cronenwett et al., 2007 |
| | | Value active partnership in patient/family/caregiver in health care process. | Laughlin & Beisel, 2010 |
| | Assess the role of the family members in patient care and support.<br>Encourage patient and family communication of concerns and reinforce independent decision making in their care | | Wennberg et al., 2010 |

## References


Agency for Healthcare Research and Quality. (2011). *Patient-centered medical home: Strategies to put patients at the center of primary care.* Publication No. AHRQ 11-0029. Rockville, MD: Author.

Always Use Teach-back! (2014). *Using the teach-back toolkit.* Retrieved from http://www.teachbacktraining.com/using-the-teach-back-toolkit

American Academy of Family Physicians. (2004). *Education, patient.* Retrieved from http://www.aafp.org/about/policies/all/patient-education.html

Ancker, J.S., Senathirajah, Y., Kukafka, R., & Starren, J.B. (2006). Design features of graphs in health risk communication: A systematic review. *Journal of the American Medical Informatics Association, 13*(6), 608-618. doi:10:1197/jamia M2115

Bastable, S.B. (2011). *Health professional as educator: Principles of teaching and learning.* Sudbury, MA: Jones & Bartlett Learning.

Bastable, S.B. (2014). *Nurse as educator: Principles of teaching and learning for nursing practice.* Sudbury, MA: Jones & Bartlett Learning.

Bodenheimer, T. (2005). Helping patients to improve their health-related behaviors: What system changes do we need? *Disease Management, 8*(5), 319-330.

Boult, C., Reider, L., Frey, K., Leff, B., Boyd, C.M., Wolff, J.L., … Scharfstein, D. (2008). Early effects of "guided care" on the quality of health care for multimorbid older person: A cluster-randomized controlled trial. *Journal of Gerontology, 63*(3), 321-327.

Centers for Disease Control and Prevention (CDC). (2012). *Gateway to health communication & social marketing practice: Audience.* Retrieved from http://www.cdc.gov/healthcommunication/Audience/

Cesta, T. (2011). Reducing readmissions: Case management's critical role. *Hospital Case Management, 19*(3), 39-42.

Cibulskis, C.C., Giardino, A.P., & Moyer, V.A. (2011). Care transitions from inpatient to outpatient settings: Ongoing challenges and emerging best practices. *Hospital Practice, 39*(3), 128-139.

Coleman, E.A, Parry, C., Chalmers, S., & Min, S.J. (2006). The care transitions intervention: Results of a randomized control trial. *Archives of Internal Medicine, 166*(17), 1822-1828.

Counsell, S.R., Callahan, C.M., Clark, D.O., Tu., W., Buttar, A.B., Stump, T.E., & Ricketts, G.D. (2007). Geriatric care management for low income seniors: A randomized controlled trial. *JAMA, 298,* 2623-2633.

Cronenwett, L., Sherwood, G., Barnsteiner, J., Disch, J., Johnson, J., Mitchell, P., … Warren, J. (2007). Quality and safety education for nurses. *Nursing Outlook, 55*(3), 122-131.

Dennison, C.R., & Hughes, S. (2009). Progress in prevention: Imperative to improve care transitions for cardiovascular care. *Journal of Cardiovascular Nursing, 24*(3), 249-251.

Epping-Jordan, J.E., Pruitt, S.D., Bengoa, R., & Wagner, E.H. (2004). Improving the quality of health care for chronic conditions. *Quality and Safety in Health Care, 13*(4), 299-305.

Erlich, C., Kendall, E., Muenchberger, H., & Armstrong, K. (2009). Coordinated care: What does that really mean? *Health and Social Care in the Community, 17*(6), 619-627.

Federman, A.D., Sano, M., Wolf, M.S., Siu, A.L., & Halm, E.A. (2009). Health literacy and cognitive performance among older adults. *Journal of American Geriatric Society, 57*(8), 1475-1480.

Health on the Net Foundation. (2013). *Looking for reliable health information?* Retrieved from http://www.hon.ch/HONcode/Patients/visitor_safeUse2.html

Hibbard, J.H., Greene, J., & Overton, V. (2013). Patients with lower activation associated with higher costs. *Health Affairs, 32*(2), 216-222.

Hibbard, J.H., Stockard, J., Mahoney, E.R., & Tusler, M. (2004). Development of the patient activation measure (PAM): Conceptualizing and measuring activation in patients and consumers. *HSR: Health Services Research,* 39(4 pt. 1), 1005-1026.

Interprofessional Education Collaborative Expert Panel (IPEC). (2011). *Core competencies for interprofessional collaborative practice.* Washington, DC: Interprofessional Education Collaborative.

Katon, W.J., Lin, E.H., Von Korff, M., Ciechanowski, P., Ludman, E.J., Young, B., & McCulloch, D. (2010). Collaborative care for patients with depression and chronic illnesses. *New England Journal of Medicine, 363*(27), 2611-2620.

Laughlin, C.B., & Beisel, M. (2010). Evolution of the chronic care role of the registered nurse in primary care. *Nursing Economic$, 28*(6), 409-414.

Leff, B., Reider, L., Frick, K.D., Scharfstein, D.O., Boyd, C., Frey, K., … Boult, C. (2009). Guided care and the cost of complex healthcare: A preliminary report. *The American Journal of Managed Care, 15*(8), 555-559.


 

London, F. (2009). *No time to teach.* Atlanta, GA: Prichett & Hull Associates, Inc.

Lorig, K.R., & Holman, H.R. (2003). Self-management education: History, definition, outcomes and mechanisms. *Annals of Behavioral Medicine, 26*(1), 1-7.

Manderson, B., McMurray, J., Piraino, E., & Stolee, P. (2012). Navigation roles support chronically ill older adults through healthcare transitions: A systematic review of the literature. *Health and Social Care in the Community, 20*(2), 113-127. doi:10.1111/j.1365-2524.2011. 01032.x

Medical Library Association. (2013). *A user's guide to finding and evaluating health information on the web.* Retrieved from http://www.mlanet.org/resources/userguide.html

National Center for Education Statistics. (2006). *The health literacy of America's adults: Results from a national assessment of adult literacy.* Washington, DC: U.S. Department of Education.

National Center for Learning Disabilities. (2013). *Learning disabilities fast facts.* Retrieved from: http://www.ncld.org/types-learning-disabilities/what-is-ld/learning-disability-fast-facts

National Institutes of Health. (2013). *Quick guide to health literacy.* Retrieved from http://www.health.gov/communication/literacy/quickguide/

National Patient Safety Foundation. (2013). *Ask me 3.* Retrieved from http://www.npsf.org/for-healthcare-professionals/programs/ask-me-3/

Naylor, M.D., Aiken, L.H., Kurtzman, E.T., Olds, D.M., & Hirschman, K.B. (2011). The importance of transitional care in achieving health reform. *Health Affairs, 30*(4), 746-754.

Nutbeam, D. (2000). Health literacy as a public health goal: A challenge for contemporary health education and communication strategies into the 21[st] century. Health literacy as a public goal. *Health Promotion International.* Retrieved from http://heapro.oxfordjournals.org/content/15/3/259.abstract

Osborne, H. (2013). *Health literacy from A to Z: Practical ways to communicate your health message.* Burlington, MA: Jones and Bartlett Learning.

Peikes, D., Genevro, J., Scholle, S.H., & Torda, P. (2011). *The patient-centered medical home: Strategies to put patients at the center of primary care.* AHRQ Publication No. 11-0029. Rockville, MD: Agency for Healthcare Research and Quality.

Peter, S., Chaney, C., Zappia, T., Van Veldhuisen, C., Pereira, S., & Santamaria, N. (2011). Care coordination for children with complex care needs significantly reduces hospital utilization. *Journal for Specialists in Pediatric Nursing, 16,* 305-312.

Plain Language Action and Information Network (n.d.). Retrieved from www.plainlanguage.gov

Riegel, B., & Carlson, B. (2002). Facilitators and barriers to heart failure self-care. *Patient Education and Counseling, 46*(4), 287-295.

Rovner, M.H., French, M., Sofaer, S., Shaller, D., Prager, D., & Kanouse, D. (2010). *A new definition of patient engagement: What is engagement and why is it important?* Washington, DC: Center for Advancing Health. Retrieved from http://www.cfah.org/pdfs/CFAH_Engagement_Behavior_Framework_current.pdf

Schillinger, D., Piette, J., Grumbach, K., Wang, F., Wilson, C., Daher, C., … Bindman, A.B. (2003). Closing the loop: Physician communication with diabetic patients who have low health literacy. *Archives of Internal Medicine, 163*(1), 83-90. Retrieved from http://archinte.ama-assn.org/cgi/content/full/163/1/83

Scholle, S.H., Torda, P., Peikes, D., Han, E., & Genevro, H.E. (2010). *Engaging patient's and families in the medical home.* AHRQ Publication No. 10-0083-EF. Rockville, MD: Agency for Healthcare Research and Quality.

U.S. Department of Health and Human Services (DHHS). (n.d). *Quick guide to health literacy.* Retrieved from http://www.health.gov/communication/literacy/quickguide/Quickguide.pdf

U.S. Department of Health and Human Services (DHHS). (2001). *National standards for culturally and linguistically appropriate services in health care.* Washington, DC: Office of Minority Health. Retrieved from http://minorityhealth.hhs.gov/assets/pdf/checked/finalreport.pdf

U.S. Department of Health and Human Services (DHHS). (2014). *Quick guide to health literacy and older adults.* Retrieved from http://www.health.gov/communication/literacy/olderadults/hearing.htm

U.S. Department of Health and Human Services, Office of Disease Prevention and Health Promotion. (2010). *National action plan to improve health literacy.* Washington, DC: Author.

Wennberg, D.E., Marr, A., Lang, L., & O'Malley, S.G. (2010). A randomized trial of a telephone care-management strategy. *New England Journal of Medicine, 363,* 1245-1255.

Wolf, M.S., Gazmararian, J.A., & Baker, D.W. (2005). Health literacy and functional health status among older adults. *Archives of Internal Medicine, 165,* 1946-1952.

Wurzbach, M.E. (2004). *Community health education and promotion: A guide to program design and* evaluation (2nd ed.) Boston, MA: Jones and Bartlett.

## Additional Reading

Nash, D.B., Reifsnyder, J., Fabius, R.J., & Pracilio, V.P. (2010). *Population health management: Creating a culture of wellness.* Sudbury, MA: Jones & Bartlett Learning.

# CHAPTER 4

# Coaching and Counseling of Patients and Families

*Karen Alexander, MSN, RN*
*Judy Dawson-Jones, MPH, BSN, RN*
*Kristene Grayem, MSN, CNP, RN*

## Learning Outcome Statement

The purpose of this chapter is to enable the reader to utilize the existing strengths of the care team to create innovative ways to engage patients and families in the care plan.

## Learning Objectives

After reading this chapter, the registered nurse (RN) working in the Care Coordination and Transition Management (CCTM) role will be able to:

- Discuss methods of developing a relationship with the patients and families in order to capitalize on their strengths and identify the barriers to fulfilling care plan goals.
- Demonstrate respect and valuing of patients and families preferences, interaction styles, and goals.
- Describe strategies to empower patients and families in all aspects of the health care process (Cronenwett et al., 2007).
- Explain how to equip patients and families with the tools needed to fulfill their responsibilities.
- Discuss ways to maintain a relationship with patients and families in order to guide and reinforce the care plan.
- Demonstrate competence by positive patient outcomes as evidenced by increased care team communication, decreased emergency department visits, and reduced hospital re-admissions.
- Demonstrate the knowledge, skills, and attitudes required for the coaching and counseling of patients and families dimension (see Table 1).

## Competency Definition

*Coaching and counseling* of patients and their families involves developing a relationship that emphasizes communication, teamwork, and skill development (Schenk & Hartley, 2002). In some instances, patients' caregivers may not be family members. For the remainder of this chapter these caregivers will be termed *families.* The registered nurse coaches by guiding patients to set goals, providing them with health information, and directing them and their families toward resources (Butterworth, Linden, & McClay, 2007). The registered nurse gives feedback on successes and constructive counseling to empower patients in all aspects of their care so they can actively participate and positively influence their health outcomes.

To achieve effective implementation of the registered nurse (RN) in Care Coordination and Transition Management (CCTM) Model in ambulatory care, the nurse (RN) will coach and counsel the patients and families as they work to understand and cope with chronic disease demands and multiple dimensions of care as well as socioeconomic issues in their lives. Patients should be empowered in all aspects of their care so they can actively participate with the care team and positively influence their care plan goals. In this dimension, the registered nurse (RN) will learn the knowledge, skills, and attitudes necessary to prepare the patients and families to confidently carry out their responsibilities within the care plan (see Table 1).

### I. Develop a Relationship with the Patients and Families

A. Need to acknowledge and utilize the strengths of patients' existing support structure at home.
   1. Inclusion of family members and community partners in the care team is key to success (Dennison & Hughes, 2009), but this cannot occur until shared goals, resources, and limitations are known.
      a. "Value seeing health care situations through the patient's eyes" (Cronenwett et al., 2007, p. 123).
      b. Communicate regarding limitations of each team member and have defined responsibilities for the family members.
      c. Acknowledge the limitations of the RN in CCTM and set availability boundaries.

 

2. Families bring familiarity with local, culturally competent resources in their neighborhood.
   a. Recognize personally held attitudes about working with patients from different ethnic, cultural, and social backgrounds (Cronenwett et al., 2007).
   b. Willingly support patient-centered care for individuals and groups whose values differ from own (Cronenwett et al., 2007).

B. Barriers to coping and participating in the care plan include patient readiness to change; limited resources; and physical, mental, and educational limitations to include low health literacy.
1. Readiness to change may not be present in the patients or families.
   a. Nurses can guide a patient through the stages of change as patients identify their own health goals and create autonomous control over their choices (Miller, 2010).
   b. Assess level of patient's decisional conflict and provide access to resources (Cronenwett et al., 2007).
2. DiClemente and Prochaska (1998) created and tested the transtheoretical model to describe behavioral change which takes into account the patient's desire to change.
   a. Pre-contemplation: the time when the individual is not aware of a need to change behavior.
   b. Contemplation: the intention to take action is in the next 6 months.
   c. Preparation: the intention to take action in the next month with some new behaviors tried in the last 12 months.
   d. Action: initiation of behavioral modification.
   e. Maintenance: continuation of the behavior for more than 6 months.
3. Identify what stage of readiness the patient is in before initiating interventions as a nurse coach (Schenk & Hartley, 2002).
   a. Understanding that not all patients will be prepared for action, allow a relationship to build based on trust and not coercion.
   b. Health outcomes desired by the patient may not mesh with the outcomes the medical team desires; however, reflecting on best care may help the team come to a shared goal (Howard & Ceci, 2013).
4. Educational level of the patient and family needs to be determined before a care plan can be best carried out.
   a. Medical jargon and low health literacy contribute to patients not hearing the messages we are trying to deliver (Dennison & Hughes, 2009).
   b. Education will be individualized to the patient's chronic disease management needs, and reading and health literacy levels.

C. Activities and skills that will develop a relationship with the patient and family.
1. Motivational interviewing is a proven technique which was first established within addiction therapy and has translated well into all types of health coaching.
   a. Motivational interviewing is an effective behavior change tool where patients are guided towards talking about change in their own words (Miller, 2010).
   b. The RN in CCTM can guide patients through the stages of change as they identify their own health goals and create autonomous control over their choices (Miller, 2010).
2. Empathy and listening must be at the heart of the interview process (Miller, 2010).
3. Communication, whether face to face, via telephone, or email is at the core of a coaching relationship.
   a. Respect the dignity and privacy of patients while maintaining confidentiality in the delivery of team-based care (Interprofessional Education Collaborative [IPEC], 2011).
   b. Participate in building consensus or resolving conflict in the context of patient care (Cronenwett et al., 2007).

## II. Encourage Patients and Families to Be Active Members of the Team

A. The RN in CCTM is the day-to-day communicator in an outpatient setting and therefore can strive to include the patient and family in the team (Butterworth et al., 2007).

B. Place interdisciplinary team collaboration in high importance with the patient as a valued member.
1. Patient is a co-laborer in the health goals, not an observer or a recipient.
2. Patient-centered practice means care will look different for different patients.

C. Activities that demonstrate the value of a patient on the team:
1. If patient-centered goals and participation are valued as team outcomes, then nurses will be able to communicate these goals with all members of the interdisciplinary team (Schenk & Hartley, 2002).
   a. Communicate patient values, preferences, and expressed needs to other members of health care team (Cronenwett et al., 2007).
   b. Promote individualized self-management goals (Huffman, 2007).
2. Frequently incorporate reflective practice after initiating goals.
   a. Benner (1985) initially identified coaching as a nursing skill, emphasizing relational support and the art of caring.
   b. Recognize one's limitations in skills, knowledge, and abilities (IPEC, 2011).

3. In-person nurse-only visits as well as telephone and email communication can facilitate this interaction effectively (Parry, Coleman, Smith, Frank, & Kramer, 2003).

## III. Strategies in Identifying the Best Family Members to Support the Patient in the Health Care Plan

A. It is important for the care team to identify which family member can most effectively provide the necessary level of support required by the patient.
   1. Value active partnership with patients or designated surrogates in planning, implementation, and evaluation of care (Cronenwett et al., 2007).
   2. Respect patient preferences for degree of active engagement in care process (Cronenwett et al., 2007).

B. Motivational interviewing promotes trust between the care team, patient, and family, promoting an atmosphere of safety and acceptance for individuals to explore and modify health-related behaviors (Miller, 2010).
   1. Developing trust builds a collaborative team between the nurse, patient, and family.
   2. Motivational interviewing relies on patients' self-efficacy and families' understanding and desire to improve patients' health outcomes.

C. Refined listening skills are essential for clinicians to identify the family member who is best suited to support the patient's recovery plan.

D. The Fundamental Guidelines for Motivational Interviewing include (Miller, 2010):
   1. Encourage and promote confidence in the patients' and families' ability to achieve positive health outcomes.
   2. Resist the reflex to direct rather than guide the recovery plan. Encourage patient input and respect the patient's perspective.
   3. Understand a patient's motivation and desired health outcome.
   4. Listen to patients and family members to understand their interpersonal dynamics as it relates to the practical support and care during the patient's recovery process.
   5. Empower patients to control their own personal health outcomes.
   6. Encourage and celebrate participation and contributions to wellness by patients and families.
   7. Initiate and promote collaborative conversation with patients and families.
   8. Identify and discuss all available resources with patients and families.
   9. Respect a person's autonomy and privacy.

E. When utilizing motivational interviewing, consider four general principles in your approach to collaborating with the family.
   1. Use honesty regarding matters of health and be empathetic to the patient's challenges relative to recovery (Miller, 2010).
      a. Engaging in honest discussions regarding patients' medical conditions along with a structured path to recovery fosters realistic expectations by the patients and their families.
      b. Managing expectations and expanding patients' understanding regarding their condition is essential to positive behavioral change.
      c. Consistent feedback and recognition of patient progress is indispensable to patient stability and positive outcomes.
      d. Acknowledging the role of the family caregivers in progress discussions is invaluable to continued support and progress.
      e. Recognizing that ambivalence is normal and often inherent in longer recoveries (Miller, 2012).
   2. Discuss potential discrepancies in desired outcomes and behaviors that are inconsistent with the recovery plan (Miller, 2010).
      a. The relationship between the clinician, patients, families, and caregivers should address the benefits of changing behaviors that will facilitate desired outcomes.
      b. It is important to help patients recognize contradictions between what they want and what they are doing.
   3. Acknowledge resistance and frustration by the patient and caregivers (Miller, 2010).
      a. Confront the problem, not the person. Resistance is a signal to reinforce goals and refresh the care plan (Miller, 2010).
      b. Care and recovery plans must include alternative care options that will accomplish the same goals and outcomes. Resistance often stems from fear of change and fear of failure.
      c. Encouragement and recognition of patient efforts and family contributions by the clinicians is critical to maintaining the patient's progress, recovery, and positive outcomes.
   4. Support self-efficacy (Miller, 2010).
      a. Patients and families must understand the value of changed behavior and have a solid belief in their ability to accomplish the desired change.
      b. Appreciate shared decision making with empowered patients and families, even when conflicts occur (Cronenwett et al., 2007).

## IV. Equip the Patient and Family

A. Health coaching has been defined by a variety of experts as a practice that educates patients while promoting self-management of individualized health goals (Huffman, 2007).

1. A self-management model can engage patients in activities that promote health.
2. The use of a self-management model is critical in equipping patients and families with tools needed to fulfill their responsibilities.
3. A self-management model is a set of tools used collaboratively by both the patients and their health care providers.
   a. It is a systematic approach to assessing the patient's self-management beliefs, behavior, and knowledge.
   b. Use of a self-management model improves partnerships with patient's health care team, aids in sustaining behavior changes, collaboratively identifies goals, and targets interventions to reduce barriers.

B. The 5 A's Behavior Change Model Adapted for Self-Management Support Improvement (Glasgow, 2002) is an interactive closed loop model for implementing self-management strategies (see Figure 1).

C. The 5 A's are Assess, Advise, Agree, Assist, and Arrange. Each of the 5 A's feed into the patient's personal action plan (Glasgow, 2002).
1. Assess: beliefs, behavior, and knowledge (Glasgow, 2002).
   a. Assess patient's knowledge about his or her health status.
   b. Elicit patient values, preferences, and expressed needs (Cronenwett et al., 2013).
   c. Assess levels of physical and emotional comfort (Cronenwett et al., 2013).
   d. Assess patient's confidence in dealing with his or her health goals and barriers.
   e. Assess patient's knowledge, skills, and beliefs related to perceived health status.
2. Advise: provide specific information about health risks and benefits of change (Glasgow, 2002).
   a. Provide patient-centric recommendations to promote health.
   b. Relate all health information to healthy behaviors.
   c. Stress the importance of behavior changes.
3. Agree: collaboratively set goals based on patients' interests and confidence in their ability to change behaviors (Glasgow, 2002).
   a. Set collaborative goals.
   b. Make SMART goals: Specific, Measurable, Attainable, Realistic, and Timely (Meyer, 2003).
   c. Incorporate family into plan to support and accomplish goals.
   d. Communicate goals to all team members.
   e. Consider both short and long-term goals.
   f. Discuss risks and benefits of proposed behavior changes.
4. Assist: identify personal barriers, strategies, problem-solving techniques, and social/environmental support (Glasgow, 2002).
   a. Promote creative strategies to lead to planned change.
   b. Collaboratively design patient-centric plans to address patient concerns.
   c. Provide evidence-based care strategies.
   d. Develop strategies and self-monitoring skills to address barriers to change.
5. Arrange: specify plan for follow-up (Glasgow, 2002).
   a. Continually monitor and follow-up action plans that facilitate open communication.
   b. Utilize strategies to monitor progress (email, phone calls, visits) as outlined in plan.
6. Personal action plan (Glasgow, 2002).
   a. Identify specific goals.
   b. List anticipated barriers.
   c. Create strategies to minimize barriers.
   d. Develop follow-up plan.
   e. Communicate plan to patient/family and entire health care team.

D. Benefits to use of Self-Management Model.
1. Shared decision making.
2. Prompts behavior changes.
3. Relevant strategies and interventions.
4. Knowledge of treatment.
5. Patient partnership with health care team.

E. Awareness of patient support structure within the health care team.
1. Telephone (and texting) contact.
2. Nurse only visits.
3. Home visits.
4. Technology (Internet-based interventions).

## V. Maintain a Relationship with the Patients and Families

A. Building a trusting relationship between clinicians, patients, and families is a key component of successful coaching.
1. Establishing strong nurse-patient relationships can determine the quality of patient outcomes as well as the length of recovery (Halldorsdottir, 2008).
2. Development of a nurse-patient relationship theory delineates conditions under which essential connections can be nurtured to attain the desired health outcomes (Halldorsdottir, 2008).
3. The prerequisite for patient trust is the sense that the nurse is genuinely caring, compassionate, competent, and a knowledgeable expert regarding the patient's health care needs.

B. Halldorsdottir's (2008) theory was derived from an analysis of patient/family perceptions of the nurse-patient relationship. Building a relationship of trust between the nurse and patient can be categorized in six phases.

1. “Reaching out” (Halldorsdottir, 2008, p. 647).
   a. Either the nurse or the patient reaching out to the other can accomplish a connection; however, the other party needs to respond positively.
   b. If the patient reaches out to the nurse, the nurse needs to take the time to employ good listening skills to demonstrate a sense of genuine care.
   c. This initial communication can lay the foundation for building an effective bridge between nurse and patient/family members (Halldorsdottir, 2008).
2. “Removing the mask of anonymity” (Halldorsdottir, 2008, p. 647).
   a. Begin the development of removing the stereotypes of the patient and nurse.
   b. The nurse and patient acknowledge that each is essential to the patient’s recovery program.
   c. Open discussion is an opportunity for the nurse to express interest and understanding of the broader dimension of the patient’s life (Halldorsdottir, 2008).
3. “Acknowledgment of connection” (Halldorsdottir, 2008, p. 647).
   a. At this juncture, the patient recognizes the connection because the nurse is responding to him or her as a whole person.
   b. Verbal, nonverbal, and body language are strong indicators of genuine caring.
   c. The nurse provides consistent eye-to-eye contact with the patient using dialogue assuring the patient the nurse is listening and focused on his or her care and concerns (Halldorsdottir, 2008).
4. “Reaching a level of truthfulness” (Halldorsdottir, 2008, p. 647).
   a. In this progressive phase of connection, the patient has developed the feeling of being safe in the nurse’s care.
   b. The patient will honestly share inner feelings, concerns, and level of knowledge and skill.
   c. The nurse acknowledges the patient’s concerns, vulnerabilities, and feelings of uncertainty (Halldorsdottir, 2008).
5. “Reaching a level of solidarity” (Halldorsdottir, 2008, p. 647).
   a. The patient becomes more confident the nurse is on his or her side and they are equal in the partnership.
   b. Feelings of mistrust disappear because the nurse has demonstrated genuine care about the patient and understands the patient’s personal life situation, goals, and expectations for recovery.
6. “True negotiation of care” (Halldorsdottir, 2008, p. 647).
   a. The nurse and patient work equally to develop the plan of care and goals.
   b. The nurse is able to be supportive while not creating a dependency. The nurse better understands the patient’s world and the patient has an increased sense of well-being (Halldorsdottir, 2008).

C. Careful, thoughtful navigation through these phases can influence an atmosphere that promotes a sense of support and well-being for patients.

## VI. Evaluation and Outcomes

A. Patients utilize the accessibility of the RN in CCTM with increased phone, email, home, and office visits.
B. Patients demonstrate increased understanding of resources available to meeting their self-management goals.
C. The patient demonstrates ability to seek help prior to escalation of symptoms.
D. The patient demonstrates increased self-efficacy and ability to cope.

**Figure 1.**
**5 A's Behavior Change Model**
**Adapted for Self-Management Support Improvement**

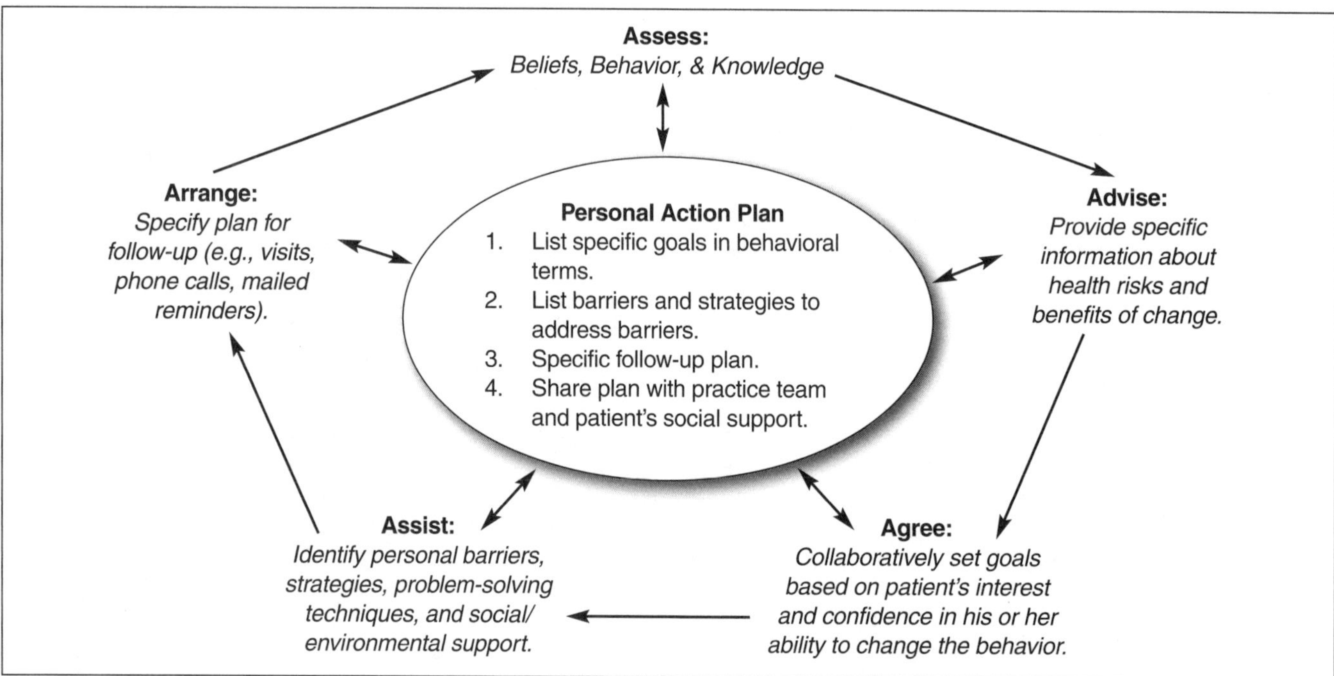


**Source:** Reprinted from Glasgow (2002) with permission from Springer Science and Business Media.

| Five A's Change Concept | Patient Level (patient-provider interaction) | Office Environment (standard operating procedure) | Community/Policy (community org. and both internal system and external community policy) |
|---|---|---|---|
| **Assess**<br>*CCM element:*<br>Have patient periodically complete valid health behavior surveys and provide him or her with feedback. | - Try brief behavior survey in (a) waiting room, (b) on computer.<br>- Assess patient knowledge about his or her chronic condition.<br>- Ask patient, "What about Self-Management (SM) is most important to talk about today?"<br>- Ask patient, "What are your most challenging barriers?," recognizing physical, social, and economic barriers.<br>- Provide patient with personalized feedback and results.<br>- Assess conviction and confidence regarding target behaviors. | - Select or develop HRA survey.<br>- Employ conviction and confidence rulers.<br>- Revise self-care surveys to make appropriate.<br>- Add fields to the medical record to record behavior status for smoking, weight, exercise.<br>- Add behaviors to the problem list for patient.<br>- Prompt staff to collect or update key behaviors status at each visit.<br>- Have computer in waiting room for HRA assessment with printouts for providers and/or patients.<br>- Employ outreach and population-based approach to assess all patients across multiple chronic illnesses.<br>- Pilot approaches to providing feedback to patients; check for understanding. | *Community:*<br>- Conduct needs assessment in partnership with community groups (e.g., include formative eval with potential users and non-users, small-scale recruitment studies to enhance methods).<br>- Work on state health dept or other coalition to develop community health behavior survey or assess barriers to change.<br>- Share data on BRFSS (Behavioral Risk Factor Surveillance System) items or other behaviors with other organizations.<br><br>*Internal system policy:*<br>- Employ longitudinal patient assessment system (e.g., using interactive computer technology).<br>- Make screening on all four health behaviors a vital sign; and require reporting on all patients at some frequency. |

*continued on next page*

**Figure 1. (continued)**
**5 A's Behavior Change Model**
**Adapted for Self-Management Support Improvement**

| Five A's Change Concept | Patient Level (patient-provider interaction) | Office Environment (standard operating procedure) | Community/Policy (community org. and both internal system and external community policy) |
|---|---|---|---|
| **Advise**<br>*CCM element:*<br>Provide personally relevant, specific recommendations for behavior change. | - Relate patient symptoms or lab results to patient behavior, recognizing patient's culture or personal illness model.<br>- Inform patient that behavioral issues are as important as taking medications.<br>- Provide specific, documented behavior change advice in the form of a prescription.<br>- Share evidence-based guidelines with patients to encourage their participation. | - Develop list of benefits of behavior change/risk reduction.<br>- Develop list of common symptoms that exercise, losing weight, or stopping smoking can improve.<br>- Arrange prompt system to remind physicians to advise behavior change.<br>- Provide prompt to have physician advise on importance of calling if any trouble taking medication as prescribed. | *Internal system policy:*<br>- Reinforce/Recognize/Reward staff for documented advice to change behavior.<br><br>*External policy:*<br>- Recommend or lobby purchasers, health plan, and government to reimburse five A's/SM Action Planning. |
| **Agree**<br>*CCM element:*<br>Use shared decision-making strategies that include collaborative goal setting. | - Have patient develop specific, measurable, feasible SM goal for behavior change.<br>- Provide options and choices among possible SM goals.<br>- Do above with input from family or spouse, and with support/assistance from caregiver.<br>- Share perspectives with patient on what is most important short-term goal; agree on a specific target.<br>- Present evidence on benefits and harms to patient and let him or her decide on course. | - Make sure patient SM goals are in chart and all team members refer to them.<br>- Provide staff with training in patient-centered counseling or empowerment training, which may include videos on motivational interviewing or goal setting.<br>- Have in-service from expert on shared decision making.<br>- Incorporate videos on patient role or choice into practice, and have patients see prior to consultation.<br>- Develop multi-modal intervention to promote practice change rather than one utilizing single strategy. | *Community:*<br>- Meet with organizations to identify agreed upon self-management support (patient education) priorities for coming year.<br><br>*Internal system policy:*<br>- Create field or permanent space in medical record for behavioral goals.<br>- Develop assessment method to determine that goals were set in a collaborative fashion.<br>- Require peer observation and feedback on real or simulated patients at a minimum of every 4 months.<br><br>*External policy:*<br>- Require or reimburse documentation of collaboratively set goals in medical records.<br>- Recognize providers who have completed training in motivational interviewing; Bayer course on collaboration; etc. |

*continued on next page*

**Figure 1. (continued)**
**5 A's Behavior Change Model**
**Adapted for Self-Management Support Improvement**

| Five A's Change Concept | Patient Level (patient-provider interaction) | Office Environment (standard operating procedure) | Community/Policy (community org. and both internal system and external community policy) |
|---|---|---|---|
| **Assist**<br>*CCM element:*<br>Use effective self-management support strategies that include action planning and problem solving. Help patients create specific strategies to address issues of concern to them. | - Help patient develop strategies to address barriers to change (write on Action Plan form).<br>- Implement patient discussion of SM Action Plan (a) during PCP visit, (b) immediately before or after with nurse.<br>- Refer patient to evidence-based education or behavioral counseling (individual or group).<br>- Elicit patient's views and plans regarding potential resources and support within family and community.<br>- Use planned interactions to support evidence-based care.<br>- Give care that patient understands and that fits with his or her cultural background.<br>- During follow-up visits, review progress, experience, concerns; renegotiate goals and revise action plan. | - Select/develop SM Action Plan form.<br>- Adapt SM Action.<br>- Plan for your setting, specifically focusing on the four S's (size, scope, scalability, and sustainability) in planning any office restructuring.<br>- Develop specific plan to enhance SM resources, by addressing the REAIM dimensions, to make sure you are addressing all key issues for panel wide or community impact.<br>- Make sure blank Action Plan forms are in each exam room. | *Community:*<br>- Work with community groups and referrals to develop Action Plans and communication avenues.<br>- Get list of your patients who have used resources; get their feedback.<br>*Internal system policy:*<br>- Compile list of recommended quality resources that can be shared with staff and patients.<br>- Evaluate adverse outcomes and quality of life for program revision and cost-benefit analysis.<br>- Recognize/reward teams that have higher levels of documented action plans.<br>*External policy:*<br>- Add behavior change counseling to HEDIS criteria for each behavior for adult patients who receive such counseling.<br>- Also, make problem solving, shared decision making, or approved SM support programs a HEDIS criterion. |
| **Arrange**<br>*CCM elements:*<br>Follow-up on action plans.<br>Follow-up on referrals.<br>Establish two-way communication and partner with community groups to improve services and linkages. | - Give patient copy of SM Action Plan.<br>- Follow-up call to patient within a week after visit as "booster shot" for SM Action Plan.<br>- E-mail follow-up or brief letter restating plan and inviting questions.<br>- Arrange for patient to contact specific community resources that could support his or her goals.<br>- Follow-up with goals set in action plan at each nonacute visit. | - Develop collaborative process that can facilitate communications and support with other practices.<br>- Develop follow-up checklist/prompt to make sure follow-up is provided.<br>- Include blank on Action Plan form for follow-up date. | *Community:*<br>- Invite community program representatives to present at patient group visit, diabetes class, or health fair.<br>- Follow-up with community programs to see how many patients attended and to get information on their progress.<br>*Internal system policy:*<br>- Employ longitudinal patient monitoring and feedback systems related to SM goals.<br>- Provide time or incentives for follow-up contacts.<br>*External policy:*<br>- Recognize/reward social and economic environment in which these health systems interventions occur.<br>- Reimburse follow-up phone calls, email contacts, etc., outside of face-to-face visit. |

**Source:** Reprinted from Glasgow (2002) with permission from Springer Science and Business Media.

**Table 1.**
**Coaching and Counseling of Patients and Families: Knowledge, Skills, and Attitudes for Competency**

| Knowledge | Skills | Attitudes | Sources |
|---|---|---|---|
| Describe the benefit of the coaching relationship to the patient.<br>Describe the benefit of the coaching relationship to the health care team. | Teaches and supports patients and families skills for self-management.<br>Elicit patient values, preferences, and expressed needs as part of clinical interview. | Respect and encourage patient expression of values and preferences.<br>Value the patient's expertise with own health and symptoms.<br>Belief that patients' and families' perspectives and participation are important in developing effective care plan. | Cronenwett et al., 2007 |
| Describe motivational techniques. | Assessment of life stressors motivating patients towards self-care. | Values involvement of patients and families in shared decision making. | Cronenwett et al., 2007 |
| Understand SMART goals. | Provide patient-centered care with sensitivity and respect of health care team. | Patient as partner. | Meyer, 2003 |
| Integrate understanding of multiple dimensions of patient-centered care. | Motivational interviewing may illicit shared, patient-centered goals. | Empathy and listening.<br>Implement reflective practice and awareness of one's own limitations. | Miller, 2010 |
| Community resources and how to access services.<br>Examine common barriers to active involvement of patients in their own health care processes. | Assessment of family's strengths.<br>Assessment of needs and barriers to health care goals. | Open and accepting attitude toward patients and families.<br>Family-centered care. | Cronenwett et al., 2007 |
| Demonstrate comprehension of self-management model. | Initiate 5 A's of Behavior Change. | Values involvement of patients and families in self-management to prevent rehospitalization. | Glasgow, 2002 |

**Source Note:** Cronenwett et al. (2007) reprinted from *Nursing Outlook, 55*(3), 122-131, with permission from Elsevier.

## References


Benner, P. (1985). Quality of life: A phenomenological perspective on explanation, prediction, and understanding in nursing science. *Advances in Nursing Science, 8*(1), 1.

Butterworth, S.W., Linden, A., & McClay, W. (2007). Health coaching as an intervention in health management programs. *Disease Management & Health Outcomes, 15*(5), 299-307.

Cronenwett L., Sherwood G., Barnsteiner J., Disch J., Johnson J., Mitchell P., … Warren J. (2007). Quality and safety education for nurses (QSEN). *Nursing Outlook, 55*(3), 122-131.

Dennison, C., & Hughes, S. (2009). Imperative to improve care transitions for cardiovascular patients. *Journal of Cardiovascular Nursing, 24*(3), 249-251.

DiClemente, C.C., & Prochaska, J.O. (1998). *Towards a comprehensive, transtheoretical model of change: Stages of change and addictive behaviors.* New York, NY: Plenum Press.

Glasgow, R.E. (2002). *Self-management aspects of the improving chronic illness care breakthrough series: Implementation with diabetes and heart failure teams.* New York, NY: Springer Science + Business Media.

Halldorsdottir, S. (2008). The dynamics of the nurse-patient relationship: Introduction of a synthesized theory from the patient's perspective. *Scandinavian Journal of Caring Sciences, 22*(4), 643-652. doi:10.1111/j.1471-6712.2007.00568x

Howard, L.M., & Ceci, C. (2013). Problematizing health coaching for chronic illness self-management. *Nursing Inquiry, 20*(3), 223-231. doi:10.1111/nin.12004

Huffman, M. (2007). Health coaching: A new and exciting technique to enhance patient self-management and improve outcomes. *Home Healthcare Nurse, 25*(4), 271-274.

Interprofessional Education Collaborative (IPEC). (2011). *Core competencies for interprofessional collaborative practice.* Retrieved from http://www.aacn.nche.edu/education-resources/ipecreport.pdf

Meyer, P.J. (2003). *Attitude is everything: If you want to succeed above and beyond.* Waco, TX: Meyer Resource Group.

Miller, N.H. (2010). Motivational interviewing as a prelude to coaching in healthcare settings. *Journal of Cardiovascular Nursing, 25*(3), 247-251.

Parry, C., Coleman, E.A., Smith, J.D., Frank, J., & Kramer, A.M. (2003). The care transitions intervention: A patient-centered approach to ensuring effective transfers between sites of geriatric care. *Home Health Care Services Quarterly, 22*(3), 1-17.

Schenk, S., & Hartley, K. (2002). Nurse coach: Healthcare resource for this millennium. *Nursing Forum, 37*(3), 14-20. doi:10.1111/j.1744-6198.2002.tb01006.x

## Additional Readings


Agency for Healthcare Research and Quality. (2008). *Integrating chronic care and business strategies in the safety net* (Prepared by Group Health's MacColl Institute for Healthcare Innovation, in partnership with RAND and the California Health Care Safety Net Institute, under Contract No./Assignment No: HHSA2902006000171). AHRQ Publication No. 08-0104-EF. Rockville, MD: Author. Retrieved from http://acc.rmhp.org/Files/tools/qi_teams/AHRQ_Integrating_Chronic_Care_and_Business_Strategies_in_the_Safety_Net.pdf

Leveille, S.G., Huang, A., Tsai, S.B., Allen, M., Weingart, S.N., & Lezzoni, L.I. (2009). Health coaching via an Internet portal for primary care patients with chronic conditions: A randomized controlled trial. *Medical Care, 47*(1), 41-47.

Martins, R.K., & McNeil, D.W. (2009). Review of motivational interviewing in promoting health behaviors. *Clinical Psychology Review, 29*(4), 283-293. doi:http://dx.doi.org/10.1016/j.cpr.2009.02.001

Noordman, J., de Vet, E., van der Weijden, T., & van Dulmen, S. (2013). Motivational interviewing within the different stages of change: An analysis of practice nurse-patient consultations aimed at promoting a healthier lifestyle. *Social Science & Medicine, 87*(0), 60-67. doi:http://dx.doi.org/10.1016/j.socscimed.2013.03.019

# CHAPTER 5

# Patient-Centered Care Planning

*Judith M. Toth-Lewis, PhD, MSN, RN*
*Kathleen T. Sheehan, MS, BSN, RN-BC, CH-GCN*
*Anne Talbott Jessie, MSN, RN*

## Learning Outcome Statement

The purpose of this chapter is to enable the reader to demonstrate the ability to develop, implement, and provide ongoing management of a comprehensive plan of care – based upon the individual patient's values, preferences, and needs – in partnership with the primary care provider and larger interdisciplinary care team.

## Learning Objectives

After reading this chapter, the registered nurse (RN) working in the Care Coordination and Transition Management (CCTM) role will be able to:

- Perform a comprehensive needs assessment on the patient focusing on the overall needs so interventions can be planned and implemented accurately.
- Identify gaps in care and individualize the plan focus through a pre-visit chart review and visit planning.
- Describe the process for identification of high-risk populations and determine appropriate risk.
- Utilize motivational interviewing as a communication style to guide the patient and family planning to make positive behavior changes to improve health.
- Develop a plan of care utilizing input from patient, family, and multidisciplinary team members.
- Design interventions founded in evidence-based clinical guidelines.
- Demonstrate the knowledge, skills, and attitudes required for the patient-centered care planning dimension (see Table 1).

## Competency Definition

"Patient- and family-centered care is an approach to the planning, delivery, and evaluation of health care that is grounded in mutually beneficial partnerships among health care providers, patients, and families" (Institute for Patient- and Family-Centered Care, 2014, para. 1).

In designing the plan of care, the registered nurse (RN) engaged in Care Coordination and Transition Management (CCTM) recognizes the integral role patients, families, and caregivers have in ensuring the health and well-being of patients. Additionally, the RN in CCTM acknowledges that emotional, social, and developmental support are critical components in the delivery of health care (The Institute for Patient- and Family-Centered Care, 2014). Engaging patients and their designees in care plan development supports improved patient outcomes, increases patient and family satisfaction, restores dignity and control, and contributes to financial stewardship in the allocation of resources. Core concepts for patient-centered care planning include (a) respect and dignity: honor perspectives, choices, values, beliefs, and cultural backgrounds; (b) information sharing: timely, accurate, transparent, and complete communication; (c) participation: engagement and participation of patients and families in care and decision making; and (d) collaboration: inclusion of patients and families in program design, implementation, policy development, and professional education (The Institute for Patient- and Family-Centered Care, 2014). The degree of inclusion is determined by the patient and does not preclude the patient making care decisions independently if he or she is competent to do so (The Institute for Patient- and Family-Centered Care, 2014).

### I. Comprehensive Needs Assessment

A. Psychosocial Assessment Tool: this is a Patient Health Questionnaire with 2 or 9 questions (PHQ-2 or 9) that assesses patient for signs and symptoms of depression. According to Kroenke, Spitzer, and Williams (2003), "the purpose of the PHQ-2 is not to establish final diagnosis or to monitor depression severity, but rather to screen for depression in a first step approach" (p. 1). A score of 3 or more requires further inquiry using the PHQ-9 Questionnaire. Both questionnaires focus on the past 2 weeks. "The PHQ-9 is a multipurpose instrument for screening, diagnosing, monitoring and measuring the severity of depression" (Kroenke, Spitzer, & Williams, 2001, p. 1).

1. PHQ-2 or 9 is handed to the patient to complete.
2. It is scored by the primary care provider or another member of the team.
3. A positive screen PHQ-9 is further assessed for presence and duration of suicide ideation.
4. The questionnaire can be repeated at each visit to reflect improvement or worsening of depression and response to treatment.
5. Notify primary care provider for worsening signs and symptoms.
6. Emergent suicidal intervention for any planned interventions with adequate means to carry out intervention.

B. Functional assessment: the Katz Index of Independence in Activities of Daily Living (IADL) is the most appropriate instrument to use in assessing functional status when measuring a patient's ability to perform activities of daily living independently (Katz, Down, Cash, & Grotz, 1970). "One of the best ways to evaluate the health status of older adults is through functional assessment which provides objective data that may further indicate decline or improvement in health status, allowing the nurse to plan and intervene appropriately" (Shelkey & Wallace, 2012, p. 1).
   1. Tool is used to detect problems in performing ADLs.
   2. The index ranks adequacy of performing bathing, dressing, toileting, transferring, continence, and feeding.
   3. RN in CCTM should plan for increased services such as physical therapy, occupational therapy, and visiting nurse or aide services for patients who have difficulties with ADLs.

C. Cage and Cage-AID: the CAGE-AID is a questionnaire that focuses on both drug and alcohol abuse. The CAGE-AID is a conjoint questionnaire where the focus of each item of the CAGE questionnaire was expanded from alcohol alone to include other drugs (Brown & Rounds, 1995). Regard one or more yes responses to a positive screen. There are four questions to be completed by the patient.
   1. Positive screen would follow-up with primary care provider about drug and alcohol rehabilitation.
   2. Behavior medicine or behavioral health consult as needed.
   3. Monitor at each visit to promote dialogue about the problem.
   4. Recommend referral to Alcoholics Anonymous.
   5. Recommend referral to other drug or alcohol treatment programs in the area.

D. The Mini-Cog – Mental Status Assessment of Older Adults: "Five and a third million Americans of all ages have Alzheimer's disease or other dementias. The increased availability of successful treatments for dementia and dementia-related illnesses means there is a substantial need for increased early identification of cognitive impairment, particularly in the geriatric population" (Doerflinger, 2013, p. 1).
   1. The Mini-Cog is a simple screening tool that takes 3 minutes to administer.
   2. Effective triage tool to identify patients in need of further evaluation by a neurologist.
   3. Clock Drawing Test (CDT) is scored as normal or abnormal.
   4. CDT is considered normal if all numbers are present in correct sequence and position; hands are readably displayed at the correct time. (Length of hands is not a factor.)
   5. Instruct patient to remember three words such as table, pencil, and apple.
   6. Next, ask him or her to draw a clock showing the time of 11:15.
   7. Next, ask him of her to state the three recalled words.
   8. Award 1 point for each recalled word and 2 points for correct CDT.
   9. Score 0-2 is considered positive screen for dementia and requires prompt evaluation.
   10. Early identification and intervention should lead to better outcomes.

E. Modified Caregiver Strain Index: "Caregivers may be prone to depression, grief, fatigue, financial hardship, and changes in social relationships. Screening tools are useful to identify families who would benefit from a more comprehensive assessment of the care giving experience" (Onega, 2013, p. 1).
   1. Thirteen question tool that measures strain related to care provision.
   2. Covers five domains: financial, physical, psychological, social, and personal.
   3. Higher the score the higher the strain.
   4. Self-administered instrument by the client/caregiver.
   5. Appropriate interventions are needed to help the caregiver.
   6. Further assessment of the caregiver by his or her primary care provider.
   7. Early intervention could prevent further deterioration in the patient and caregiver.

F. Get Up and Go Test: "The timed Get Up and Go Test is a measurement of mobility. It includes a number of tasks such as standing from a seating position, walking, turning, stopping, and sitting down which are all important tasks needed for a person to be independently mobile" (Mathias, Nayak, & Issacs, 1986, p. 387).
   1. Test is performed when patient is wearing regular footwear, using usual walking aid, and sitting in chair with an armrest.

2. On the word "go" patient is asked to get up, walk 3 meters, turn, walk back to chair, and sit down.
3. Time the second effort only.
4. Observe patient for postural stability, step pace, stride length, and sway.
5. Normal scoring is ≤ 10 seconds.
6. Low score indicates good functional independence.
7. High score indicates need for physical therapy consult for fall risk.
8. Baseline should be done annually and repeated when any changes occur.

G. Patient Activation Measure: "The Patient Activation Measure® (PAM®) assessment gauges the knowledge, skills and confidence essential to managing one's own health and healthcare. The PAM assessment segments consumers into one of four progressively higher activation levels. Each level addresses a broad array of self-care behaviors and offers deep insight into the characteristics that drive health activation. A PAM score can also predict healthcare outcomes including medication adherence, ER utilization and hospitalization" (Insignia Health, 2014, p. 1).
1. Level 1: no confidence in their ability to change.
2. Level 2: lack confidence or understanding of their health.
3. Level 3: have knowledge and may begin to develop confidence.
4. Level 4: adopted new behaviors to effect change in their health status.
5. Engaged patients are more able to make positive changes in their health outcomes.

## II. Pre-Visit Chart Review and Visit Planning to Identify Gaps in Care and Individualize the Plan Focus

A. The patient's medical record or electronic health record is a useful tool in the early phase of patient assessment. Questions to be posed are:
1. When was the patient last seen by his or her primary care provider (PCP)?
2. Has he or she missed several appointments?
3. Has it been over 13 months since his or her last preventive care visit?
4. Are the patient's recommended preventive care guidelines up to date?
5. Has the patient had a hemoglobin A1c (HbA1c) that is less than 7% in the last 6 months?
6. What are the patient's most recent biometric data?
7. What is his or her body mass index (BMI)?
8. Are medications up to date (expired or need refill)?

B. The U. S. Preventive Services Task Force (USPTF) "works to improve the health of all Americans by making evidence-based recommendations about clinical preventive services such as screenings, counseling services, and preventive medications" (USPTF, 2013, p. 1).
1. Pre-visit chart review: examine patient's chart 24-48 hours before visit with PCP.
   a. Based on patient's age and sex, what are the recommended screenings and tests completed (e.g., colorectal screening ages 50-75)?
   b. Based on above, what screenings and/or tests are outstanding (missing screening such as Pap test)?
   c. Based on above, are there currently any pending orders for these tests (orders for screen pending)?
   d. Vaccine history and recommended vaccines needed at this appointment (flu vaccine during flu season)?
   e. Specialist appointments needed (e.g., yearly dilated eye exam for all diabetics related to diabetic retinopathy)?
   f. Abnormal lab work or test results to review with PCP?
   g. Is there a pattern of routinely missed appointments?
   h. Presence/absence of life-planning resources such as advanced directives, health care proxy/durable power of attorney for health care?
   i. Meaningful use core objectives as outlined by Centers for Medicare & Medicaid Services (2010) should be included in chart review as indicated (e.g., smoking status for all patients 13 years or older).
   j. Psychosocial information such as need for caregiver, housing assistance?
2. Visit planning: it is necessary to plan for the patient's visit in advance so outstanding test results, recommended preventive care, and PCP orders are obtained before visit.
   a. Identify missing lab results obtained from outside lab (need to record results from outside lab into medical record).
   b. Reports from outside ophthalmologist, endocrinologist, and discharge summary from hospital or ER; dentist and pharmacy information should be obtained and updated in patient's chart.
   c. Review missing labs, x-rays, and immunizations with PCP before visit, so orders can be obtained.
   d. Notify patient of any outstanding lab results, x-rays, etc.; schedule these tests before appointment with PCP.
   e. Print life-planning resource documents for patient to review during visit.
   f. Print screening tools to be used during visit (e.g., PHQ-2 or 9).

3. Gaps in care: if any gaps in care are noticed, be sure to review with PCP before appointment, so these issues can be addressed at time of appointment.
   a. Missed appointments.
      (1) Ascertain with patient why he or she missed appointment.
   b. No recent lab work (routine labs to check progression of their chronic disease).
   c. Discharge and pharmacy.
      (1) Meet with multidisciplinary team throughout discharge process.
      (2) Ensure inpatient case management and social work are included in plan.
      (3) Ensure PCP is aware of discharge plan through electronic or face-to-face communication.
      (4) Family and caregivers are aware and understand care plan.
      (5) Care plan is easily accessible to all involved.
      (6) Care plan is updated as needed.

## III. Risk Stratification

Proactively identify and outreach to at-risk patients to develop patient-centered care planning.

A. Different ways to identify patients at risk.
   1. Predictive modeling software, such as athenaClarity$^{sm}$, IBM Premier.
   2. Chronic disease based models, such as diabetes specific.
   3. Age-specific models, chronic disease registries, and risk scoring using different methodologies (e.g., LACE Index, Interact, BOOST Tools to predict re-admission risk).
   4. Once identified as a high-risk patient, one can be further risk stratified as high, moderate, and low risk. A common model is to focus on high-risk diabetics with HbA1c ranges greater than 8.0 with 2 or more associated co-morbidities.
   5. High-risk populations include recently discharged patients from any site including acute care and post-acute care.
   6. Patients in transition are at risk especially if they have multiple chronic diseases, polypharmacy, limited social support, age greater than 80, and decline in functional status after lengthy hospitalization.
   7. Example of chronic disease risk stratification model of care (see Table 2).

B. High-risk patients are identified through comprehensive chart review, consultation with PCP, and patient agreement. The RN in CCTM assesses the following to develop the foundation for care planning.
   1. Chart review.
      a. Does the patient meet high-risk criteria?
         (1) The patient is unstable.
         (2) The patient needs psychosocial support.
         (3) The patient does not have access to medications prescribed.
         (4) The patient has increased utilization of hospital and ED services.
         (5) Home situation has recently deteriorated.
      b. The patient meets high-risk criteria, but all needs are already met.
      c. Patient has additional care needs that require coordination.
         (1) Caregiver support.
         (2) Community resources or ancillary services.
         (3) Primary care and specialty medical management.
         (4) Psychosocial support.
         (5) Pharmacist support to optimize medication management.

C. Review patient list with PCP.
   1. Provider feels patient would not benefit from interventions.
   2. Provider knows patient is moving out of state in the next few months.
   3. Provider knows patient, physically and mentally well.
   4. Provider recommends additional patients not on registry.
   5. Patients are actively using ED and inpatient services.
   6. History of nonadherence to hospital follow-up appointments.
   7. Frequent calls to the practice with minor complaints.

D. Patient engagement: once the patient is identified as high-risk, next step is to contact the patient and/or caregiver for intake and assessment.
   1. Send an introductory letter explaining the program and identify patient PCP.
   2. Meet the patient at an upcoming appointment.
   3. Meet the patient when he or she is admitted to the hospital.
   4. Assign a team member to do outreach calls when available.
      a. State you work with PCP _____, and he or she requested you set up an appointment.
      b. Explain you are available to help with transportation, medications, disease-specific questions, and to coordinate care overall.
      c. Keep conversation simple.
      d. If patient is not responding to calls, engage team members to assist with outreach patient activation.
   5. Before calling patient, spend 5-10 minutes to do chart review.
      a. Focus on missed appointments, history, and behavioral health history.

    b. Medications.
    c. Symptoms/diagnoses.
    d. Assess areas you may be able to assist.

E. Barriers to patient engagement.
   1. Psychosocial or mental illness.
   2. Low motivation.
   3. Time constraints for providers.
   4. Not ready to change.
   5. Insufficient provider training of RN in CCTM new role.
   6. Illness or pain.
   7. Functional deficits.
   8. Substance abuse.
   9. Low health literacy (education).
   10. Religious beliefs.
   11. Culture differences.

## IV. Motivational Interviewing (MI)

A skillful clinical communication style for eliciting from patients their own motivations for making behavior changes in the interest of their health (Rollnick, Miller, & Butler, 2008).

A. MI is described as a form of collaborative conversation for strengthening a patient's own motivation and commitment to change. It is a patient-centered counseling style for addressing the common problem of ambivalence about change by paying particular attention to the language of change.

B. MI is designed to strengthen an individual's motivation for and movement toward a specific goal by eliciting and exploring the patient's own reasons for change within an atmosphere of acceptance and compassion (Motivational Interviewing Network of Trainers, 2013a, 2013b).

C. MI is characterized as collaborative, evocative, and supporting of a patient's autonomy.

D. Utilize the four guiding principles of MI: acronym RULE (Rollnick et al., 2008).
   1. Resist the righting reflex.
   2. Understand and explore the patient's own motivations.
   3. Listen with empathy.
   4. Empower the patient, encouraging hope and optimism.

E. Key listening skills.
   1. Listen in an empathetic, attentive, nonjudgmental, warm, and supportive way. Good listening begins with following. Following the patient's lead at the beginning of a conversation allows for understanding of the patient's symptoms and how these fit into the larger picture of his or her life and health (Rollnick et al., 2008).
   2. Summarize what the patient said. This is key to demonstrate to the patient you are listening while verifying you understood correctly. Offer periodic brief summaries to highlight the "pearls."

## V. Keys to Successful MI

A. Build rapport: 20% of conversation time is spent on building rapport.
   1. Engage the patient and invest in the beginning.
   2. The relationship is the most powerful tool in MI.
   3. The interaction between provider and patient powerfully influences patient resistance, compliance, and change.
   4. Ask mainly open-ended questions: *"Tell me more about…"*
   5. Use agenda setting to give the patient as much decision-making freedom as possible (Rollnick et al., 2008). A useful tool to achieve this is the bubble sheet, in which several relevant topics are outlined and the patient chooses which one to focus on. This brief conversation takes about 1 minute.

B. Resist the urge to "fix" things. This gets in the way of change.

C. Informing: knowledge about the risks and benefits is an important element in deciding to change. Provide personal feedback, advice, and/or education in a neutral manner (Rollnick et al., 2008). When informing, it is important to be aware of the "righting reflex."

D. Stages of change: recognize patients may relapse and progress through the stages several times before successfully maintaining the change; patients may not move through the stages in a linear fashion; stages may be skipped or they may revert to an earlier stage (Levensky, Forcehimes, O'Donohue, & Beitz, 2007).

E. "Change talk:" patients who express motivation to change (change talk) are more likely to change; those who argue against change (sustained talk) are less likely to change.
   1. Listen for "change talk." One of the first steps in helping patients make the arguments for change is being able to recognize change talk (Rollnick et al., 2008).

F. Resistance: an observable behavior, it is not a trait of the patient.

G. Explore, offer, and explore.
   1. Explore: ask what the patient knows or what he or she would like to know.
   2. Offer: offer information in a neutral and nonjudgmental manner.
   3. Explore: ask about the patient's thoughts, feelings, and reactions.

H. Next steps: patients who set goals for themselves are more likely to achieve behavior change than those who do not. In MI, this is called "next steps."

I. Becoming proficient in MI.
   1. Utilize a provider who is proficient in MI as a mentor.
   2. Practice in short blocks of time with an expert coach if possible.
   3. Attend a formal training (a list of trainers can be found at Motivational Interviewing Network of

Trainers, 2013b). When practicing with patients, pay attention to clues from them as to how you are doing.

4. Understand it takes time and practice to be proficient in MI (Rollnick et al., 2008).

## VI. Plan of Care

A. "Planning is the third part of the nursing process" (Nettina, 1996, p. 5). Planning is the development of goals and a plan of care designed to assist the patient in resolving the nursing diagnosis.

B. Care plans are developed based on mutually agreed upon goals, founded on evidence-based guidelines and begin and end with the patient.
   1. Care planning activities transcend barriers/transitions, keep the patient at the center, and provide patients and caregivers with information necessary to prevent redundant care, and ensure quality care across care settings.
   2. When the RN in CCTM meets with the patient and/or caregiver, perform a complete clinical and psychosocial assessment. Based on the assessment, chart reviews, and provider input, the RN in CCTM establishes small, incremental goals with the patient.

C. Assessment: start with a complete nursing assessment.
   1. Vital signs.
   2. Height, weight, BMI.
   3. Pain score.
   4. Risk assessments: patient safety, fall risk, functional status, Mini-Cog exam, Patient Health Questionnaire 2 or 9 questions, CAGE or CAGE-AID, Get Up and Go Test, tobacco history, sexual history, caregiver strain index, abuse, or neglect.
   5. Medication review and reconciliation including all over-the-counter and herbals.
   6. All the care devices used and current readings including glucometers, peak flow devices, scales, BP monitors.
   7. Special diet or restrictions.
   8. Current complaints or concerns.
   9. Psychosocial assessment, living situation, community services currently used, exercise or activity, sleep routine, trouble voiding or moving bowels, dental issues, swallowing issues.
   10. Advanced directives or life-planning documents.
   11. Immunization history, vaccines needed based on preventive care guidelines.
   12. Any support groups involved.
   13. Referrals to specialists needed.
       a. Goal setting: based on assessment, discuss goals that are agreeable to the patient and/or caregiver. The care plan is patient driven and all goals are patient, not provider, centered. Examples of goals:
          (1) I will become more active by________.
          (2) I will obtain my provider's approval before beginning an exercise program.
          (3) I will check my feet and skin after exercise.

D. Patient communication with providers, family, and friends.
   1. I will organize my questions in advance before I see my provider.
   2. I will be assertive and not afraid to ask questions about my care.
   3. I will communicate my needs to my provider.
   4. I will contact my provider with questions, concerns, and issues that arise between visits.

E. Patient coping and relaxation.
   1. I will identify a support person in my life.
   2. I will work on stress management and relaxation.
   3. I will seek help from a behavioral health specialist.
   4. I will add relaxation techniques into my daily routine.

F. Patient healthy eating and weight management.
   1. I will reduce my portion sizes.
   2. I will add more fruits and vegetables to my diet.
   3. I will add more fiber to my diet.
   4. I will read food labels to identify serving size and total carbohydrates.
   5. I will keep a food log.

G. Patient medication management.
   1. I will carry a complete medication list with me at all times.
   2. I will take all medications at the prescribed dosage with appropriate timing and frequency.
   3. I will wear a medical alert bracelet/necklace.
   4. I will refill my medications on time.

H. Patient pain, fatigue, and sleep goals.
   1. I will treat my acute pain aggressively to prevent chronic pain.
   2. I will identify and address the cause of my pain.
   3. I will participate in a pain management program.
   4. I will limit caffeine and reduce environmental stimuli 2-4 hours before sleep.

I. Patient personal safety.
   1. I will look for opportunities to prevent accidents, falls, and injuries in my home.
   2. I will use a cane, walker, or other device when walking short distances to prevent potential falls.
   3. I will transition slowly between sitting/standing in case of dizziness or loss of balance.
   4. I will report any bleeding or bruising to my provider while taking coumadin.

J. Patient problem solving.
   1. I will notify my provider for any changes in my blood sugar readings, weight changes, blood pressure (BP) changes, or peak flow readings.
   2. I will follow-up on life-planning resources.
   3. I will engage in activities to remedy or reduce financial concerns.
   4. I will manage my home equipment issues by ________.

K. Patient self-monitoring.
   1. I will check my blood sugar first thing in the morning.
   2. I will check my weight daily.
   3. I will check my feet regularly for signs of breakdown.
   4. I will check my BP ________ times per week.
L. Education: once the goals have been determined, the patient and RN in CCTM agree on a specified date and time for follow-up. The patient leaves with an action plan outlining goals, recommended referrals, educational materials illness, and educational needs.
   1. Patient will have action plan before leaving the office.
   2. Patient will have follow-up appointments booked.
   3. Patient will have culturally specific, literacy-based education material to review.
   4. Patient will understand who to call with questions.
   5. Patient will get follow-up community services discussed during the visit.
   6. Patient will call the case manager before going to the ED or hospital.
   7. Patient will have medication list updated.
   8. Patient will have all prescriptions filled on time.
   9. Patient will "teach back" all new learning.
   10. RN in CCTM will document patient's understanding through "teach back" and any areas of need for review.

## VII. Multidisciplinary Approach

An essential aspect of partnering with families is providing them with adequate information, tools, training, and resources to assist in the provision of care (Frampton & Wahl, 2012). Patients whose family caregivers thoroughly understand discharge instructions are less vulnerable to hospital re-admissions and gaps in care if caregivers are actively involved. "Marrying health care professionals clinical expertise with the knowledge of the family member (and patient) lays the foundation for patient-centered care planning that is focused on the patient's personal health goals and the necessary steps to attain them" (Frampton & Wahl, 2012, p. 11).

A. Interprofessional team members communicate regularly to discuss care focusing on the unique needs of the individual patient.
B. The development of an interdisciplinary care plan requires the following guiding principles (Jones, Jamerson, & Pike, 2012).
   1. Patient problems linked to mutual goals.
   2. Goals with outlined expectations.
   3. Outcomes (indicators) that document patient progress toward the goal.
   4. Evidence-based interventions that align with assessment and treatments.
   5. Education to prepare the patient and family for transitions in care.
C. Role functions: the diversity of titles and role functions related to cross continuum care management and patient-centered care planning has become complex. In an attempt to clarify, The Advisory Board (2012) has created a "Staff Audit Tool" to be used as a framework for deploying the most appropriate site-specific resources to meet the individual patient's needs.
   1. Inpatient care coordinator: serves as a primary contact for physicians and other care providers; responsible for managing patient care needs and progress, care plan development, and discharge planning while in acute care setting.
      a. Core tasks: develop patient care plan, navigate patient through inpatient setting and discharge planning.
      b. Potential tasks: quality measurement concurrent review, utilization review, payment review/pre-authorization, manage behavioral health and social needs.
      c. Common names: inpatient case manager, primary care coordinator, patient care coordinator, unit-based care manager, hospital-based care manager.
      d. Individual commonly deployed: RN, clinical nurse leader, licensed clinical social worker (LCSW), case manager.
   2. Transition partner: follows patients from the hospital to home or post-acute care facility after discharge, supports patient self-management during the transition.
      a. Core tasks: visit all sites of care with patient, coordinate patient care, promote care plan consistency.
      b. Common names: transition coach duties may fall under purview of high-risk outpatient care manager for high-risk patients.
      c. Individual commonly deployed: nurse practitioner (NP), RN, nursing student, community member.
   3. Nonurgent ED navigator: connects patients using the ED for nonacute needs with primary care, nonclinical assistance; promotes right-site utilization.
      a. Core tasks: engage nonacute patients in ED, assess primary care status, address nonclinical needs, schedule appointments and consults as needed, evaluate payment status.
      b. Potential tasks: assist with transfer to other care sites, follow-up call.
      c. Common names: life coach, transfer coordinator.
      d. Individual commonly deployed: RN, licensed practical nurse (LPN), LCSW.
   4. Clinical patient guide (catastrophic illness): provides guidance to patients, families, and physicians during acute inflection points (such as cancer diagnosis) or catastrophic illness; coordinates care and expedites scheduling in acute care setting.

a. Core tasks: evaluate various treatment options with patient, navigate patient across sites of care, coordinate with staff to ensure patient comfort, provide clarity around diagnosis.
b. Potential tasks: appointment scheduling.
c. Common names: nurse navigator, nurse life care planner.
d. Individual commonly deployed: RN, NP, LCSW, survivor.

5. Co-morbidity chronic care coordinator/high-risk outpatient care manager: this is the role of the RN in CCTM. Follows patients deemed heavy users of expensive inpatient care due to multiple chronic illnesses, high ED utilization, or recent discharge from a skilled nursing facility; promotes more active and informed role in patient self-care; navigates patients identified as high-risk across the continuum, longitudinally; activates complex patients.
   a. Core tasks: longitudinal support, disease management or referral to disease management, referrals to ancillary providers (pharmacy, social work, palliative, community organizations, nonclinical services), patient monitoring, education, supports patient care plan adherence; helps develop care plan in coordination with PCP; ensures care plan consistency across providers.
   b. Potential tasks: disease management, inpatient visit, home visit, appointment scheduling.
   c. Common names: chronic disease manager, health coach, RN chronic care coordination coordinator, team member, faith-based community liaison RN care manager, outpatient care manager, ambulatory case/care manager.
   d. Individual commonly deployed: RN, LCSW, case manager experienced RN, LCSW, staff with case management certification.
6. Disease-specific chronic care coach: counsels patients regularly regarding disease-related symptom management, advises patients on lifestyle choices to improve prognosis. Could be in assisted living, home health care nurse, or RN in CCTM.
   a. Core tasks: patient education, disease monitoring, promotion of self-management.
   b. Potential tasks: coordinate patient care appointments, telemonitoring.
   c. Common names: chronic disease manager; title may be disease specific (e.g., diabetes coach, cardiac disease manager, asthma coach).
   d. Individual commonly deployed: RN, NP, pharmacist, community member (peer coach).
7. Outpatient care coach: ambulatory care RNs promote disease management, preventative care, and wellness; may currently be managing patients of all risk levels, or managing lower-risk patients not attributed to the high-risk outpatient care manager.
   a. Core tasks: manage disease registry, disease management education, patient engagement and activation, fill gaps in preventative and chronic care.
   b. Potential tasks: coordinate patient care appointments, fulfill nonclinical needs, remote monitoring.
   c. Common names: health coach, health promoters (promotoras), chronic disease educator (diabetes, cardiac, asthma), low-risk care manager, outpatient care manager, ambulatory case/care manager.
8. Individual commonly deployed: RN (may divide tasks with MA), LPN, medical assistant.

## VIII. Evidence-Based Care Resources

"The term evidence-based practice is used to describe activities or treatments that are based on the results of clinical research, not on hunches or suspicions" (Tabloski, 2009, p. 53). The Agency for Healthcare Research and Quality (AHRQ, 2010) publishes guidelines on a variety of sources including nursing and medical topics. It is important for nurses to use research findings that affect patient care. Consumers and governing bodies expect professional nurses to provide care that is substantiated in research studies (Tabloski, 2012).

A. Keep up to date on latest research findings.
   1. Government agencies have free resources for evidence-based practice.
      a. Administration on Aging (www.aoa.gov).
      b. Centers for Disease Control and Prevention (www.CDC.gov).
      c. Agency for Healthcare Research and Quality (www.AHRQ.gov).
         (1) Hughes, R. (Ed.), *Patient safety and quality: An evidence-based handbook for nurses.* (This book is available online at the Agency for Healthcare Research and Quality website (http://www.ahrq.gov/qual/nurseshdbk/). In addition, this three-volume text is free to nurses as a CD).
   2. Nongovernmental sources on evidence-based practice.
      a. Institute for Healthcare Improvement (ww.ihi.org).
      b. Hartford Institute of Geriatric Nursing (www.hartfordign.org).
      c. NICHE (Nurses Improving Care for Health system Elders) (www.NICHE.org)

   d. American Geriatric Society (www.americangeriatrics.org).
   e. American Nurses Association (www.ANA.org).
3. Google best evidence-based practice for (list your problem and preferably your patient population, you will find latest evidence-based guidelines that may not be in library databases).
4. Develop evidence-based guidelines based on current research findings; an excellent resource for methods is Dearholt and Dang (2012).

## IX. Monitoring and Measuring Patients for Progress and Early Signs of Exacerbation/Increased Facility Utilization

A. Periodic reassessment of the patient's "needs for care and for coordination, including physical, emotional and psychological health; functional status; current health and health history; self-management knowledge and behaviors; current treatment recommendations, including prescribed medications; and need for support services" (AHRQ, 2010, p. 22).
B. Partnering with the patient, the RN in CCTM identifies incremental patient improvement measures, including medication adherence.
C. The RN in CCTM revises and refines care plan as needed to accommodate new information or circumstances and to address failures (AHRQ, 2010).
D. Common "red flags" when monitoring a patient's progress include:
   1. Hospital re-admissions including all-cause 30-day re-admissions.
   2. Increased complications associated with disease process (new kidney disease associated with uncontrolled diabetes).
   3. Missed appointments (hospital follow-up appointments with specialist after new diagnosis of heart failure).
   4. Underutilized prescriptions including missed refills.
   5. Frequent ED visits.
   6. Frequent falls.

## X. Quality Measures and Outcomes

Structured monitoring developed to measure both RN in CCTM and patient performance.

A. Close collaboration with patients is instrumental in achieving quality improvements in health care on all levels: individual, institutional, and system-level (Nickel, Trojan, & Kofahl, 2012).
B. The RN in CCTM establishes incremental goals and monitors patient progress via process and outcome indicators imbedded in nurse documentation.
C. Measures are tracked utilizing the Healthcare Effectiveness Data and Information Set (HEDIS), a tool used by more than 90% of America's health plans to measure performance on important dimensions of care and service (National Committee for Quality Insurance, 2014). Measures include breast cancer screening, colorectal cancer screening, and Chlamydia screening. These measures are tracked by the team; any outstanding measures are completed by patient outreach. The RN in CCTM will assist as needed to get patients in for testing based on age and diagnoses.

## XI. Communicating the Plan of Care

A. The care plan should be available for all care providers to observe in the patient's electronic medical record (EMR). The RN in CCTM should communicate changes to the care plan across the continuum to all interprofessional team members. The patient and family should have a copy of their most recent care plan with them at all times. An EMR with patient portal is ideal to encourage data exchanges across sites of care.

**Table 1.**
**Patient-Centered Care Planning: Knowledge, Skills, and Attitudes for Competency**

"Recognize the patient or designee as the source of control and full partner in providing compassionate and coordinated care based on respect for patient's preferences, values, and needs" (Cronenwett et al., 2007, p. 123).

| Knowledge | Skills | Attitudes | Sources |
|---|---|---|---|
| Integrate understanding of multiple dimensions of patient-centered care:<br>• patient/family/community preferences, values<br>• coordination and integration of care<br>• information, communication, and education<br>• physical comfort and emotional support<br>• involvement of family and friends<br>• transition and continuity.<br><br>Describe how diverse cultural, ethnic and social backgrounds function as sources of patient, family, and community values. | Elicit patient values, preferences, and expressed needs as part of clinical interview, implementation of care plan and evaluation of care.<br>Communicate patient values, preferences, and expressed needs to other members of health care team.<br>Provide patient-centered care with sensitivity and respect for the diversity of human experience. | Value seeing health care situations 'through patients' eyes.'<br>Respect and encourage individual expression of patient values, preferences, and expressed needs.<br>Value the patient's expertise with own health and symptoms.<br>Seek learning opportunities with patients who represent all aspects of human diversity.<br>Recognize personally held attitudes about working with patients from different ethnic, cultural, and social backgrounds.<br>Willingly support patient-centered care for individuals and groups whose values differ from own. | Cronenwett et al., 2007 |
| Demonstrate comprehensive understanding of the concepts of pain and suffering, including physiologic models of pain and comfort. | Assess presence and extent of pain and suffering.<br>Assess levels of physical and emotional comfort.<br>Elicit expectations of patient and family for relief of pain, discomfort, or suffering.<br>Initiate effective treatments to relieve pain and suffering in light of patient values, preferences, and expressed needs. | Recognize personally held values and beliefs about the management of pain or suffering.<br>Appreciate the role of the nurse in relief of all types and sources of pain or suffering.<br>Recognize that patient expectations influence outcomes in management of pain or suffering. | Cronenwett et al., 2007 |
| Examine how the safety, quality, and cost effectiveness of health care can be improved through the active involvement of patients and families.<br>Examine common barriers to active involvement of patients in their own health care processes.<br>Describe strategies to empower patients or families in all aspects of the health care process. | Remove barriers to presence of families and other designated surrogates based on patient preferences.<br>Assess level of patient's decisional conflict and provide access to resources.<br>Engage patients or designated surrogates in active partnerships that promote health, safety and well-being, and self-care management. | Value active partnership with patients or designated surrogates in planning, implementation, and evaluation of care.<br>Respect patient preferences for degree of active engagement in care process.<br>Respect patient's right to access to personal health records. | Cronenwett et al., 2007 |

*continued on next page*

**Source Note:** Cronenwett et al. (2007) reprinted from *Nursing Outlook, 55*(3), 122-131, with permission from Elsevier.

**Table 1. (continued)**
**Patient-Centered Care Planning: Knowledge, Skills, and Attitudes for Competency**

| Knowledge | Skills | Attitudes | Sources |
|---|---|---|---|
| Explore ethical and legal implications of patient-centered care.<br>Describe the limits and boundaries of therapeutic patient-centered care. | Recognize the boundaries of therapeutic relationships.<br>Facilitate informed patient consent for care. | Acknowledge the tension that may exist between patient rights and the organizational responsibility for professional, ethical care.<br>Appreciate shared decision making with empowered patients and families, even when conflicts occur. | Cronenwett et al., 2007 |
| Discuss principles of effective communication.<br>Describe basic principles of consensus building and conflict resolution.<br>Examine nursing roles in assuring coordination, integration, and continuity of care. | Assess own level of communication skill in encounters with patients and families.<br>Participate in building consensus or resolving conflict in the context of patient care.<br>Communicate care provided and needed at each transition in care. | Value continuous improvement of own communication and conflict resolution skills. | Cronenwett et al., 2007 |
| Describe strategies for learning about the outcomes of care in the setting in which one is engaged in clinical practice. | Seek information about outcomes of care for populations served in care setting. Seek information about quality improvement projects in the care setting. | Appreciate that continuous quality improvement is an essential part of the daily work of all health professionals. | Cronenwett et al., 2007 |
| Recognize that nursing and other health professions students are parts of systems of care and care processes that affect outcomes for patients and families. Give examples of the tension between professional autonomy and system functioning. | Use tools (such as flow charts, cause-effect diagrams) to make processes of care explicit. Participate in a root cause analysis of a sentinel event. | Value own and others' contributions to outcomes of care in local care settings. | Cronenwett et al., 2007 |
| Explain the importance of variation and measurement in assessing quality of care. | Use quality measures to understand performance.<br>Use tools (such as control charts and run charts) that are helpful for understanding variation.<br>Identify gaps between local and best practice. | Appreciate how unwanted variation affects care. Value measurement and its role in good patient care. | Cronenwett et al., 2007 |
| Describe approaches for changing processes of care. | Design a small test of change in daily work. | | Cronenwett et al., 2007 |

*continued on next page*

**Table 1. (continued)**
**Patient-Centered Care Planning: Knowledge, Skills, and Attitudes for Competency**

| Knowledge | Skills | Attitudes | Sources |
|---|---|---|---|
| Community Dimensions of Practice Skills | "Identifies the health status of populations and their related determinants of health and illness (e.g., factors contributing to health promotion and disease prevention, the quality, availability, and use of health services).<br>Describes the characteristics of a population-based health problem (e.g., equity, social determinants, environment).<br>Uses variables that measure public health conditions." | | The Council on Linkages Between Academia and Public Health Practice, 2010, p. 7 |
| Analytic/Assessment Skills | "Uses methods and instruments for collecting valid and reliable quantitative and qualitative data.<br>Identifies sources of public health data and information.<br>Recognizes the integrity and comparability of data.<br>Identifies gaps in data sources.<br>Adheres to ethical principles in the collection, maintenance, use, and dissemination of data and information." | | The Council on Linkages Between Academia and Public Health Practice, 2010, p. 7 |
| Analytic/Assessment Skills | "Describes the public health applications of quantitative and qualitative data.<br>Collects quantitative and qualitative community data (e.g., risks and benefits to the community, health and resource needs).<br>Uses information technology to collect, store, and retrieve data.<br>Describes how data are used to address scientific, political, ethical, and social public health issues." | | The Council on Linkages Between Academia and Public Health Practice, 2010, p. 8 |

*continued on next page*

**Table 1. (continued)**
**Patient-Centered Care Planning: Knowledge, Skills, and Attitudes for Competency**

| Knowledge | Skills | Attitudes | Sources |
|---|---|---|---|
| Communication Skills | "Identifies the health literacy of populations served.<br>Communicates in writing and orally, in person, and through electronic means, with linguistic and cultural proficiency.<br>Solicits community-based input from individuals and organizations.<br>Conveys public health information using a variety of approaches (e.g., social networks, media, blogs).<br>Participates in the development of demographic, statistical, programmatic, and scientific presentations.<br>Applies communication and group dynamic strategies (e.g., principled negotiation, conflict resolution, active listening, risk communication) in interactions with individuals and groups." | | The Council on Linkages Between Academia and Public Health Practice, 2010, p. 11 |
| Cultural Competency Skills | "Incorporates strategies for interacting with persons from diverse backgrounds (e.g., cultural, socioeconomic, educational, racial, gender, age, ethnic, sexual orientation, professional, religious affiliation, mental and physical capabilities).<br>Recognizes the role of cultural, social, and behavioral factors in the accessibility, availability, acceptability, and delivery of public health services.<br>Responds to diverse needs that are the result of cultural differences.<br>Describes the dynamic forces that contribute to cultural diversity." | | The Council on Linkages Between Academia and Public Health Practice, 2010, p. 12 |

*continued on next page*

 

**Table 1. (continued)**
**Patient-Centered Care Planning: Knowledge, Skills, and Attitudes for Competency**

| Knowledge | Skills | Attitudes | Sources |
|---|---|---|---|
| Cultural Competency Skills *(continued)* | "Describes the need for a diverse public health workforce.<br>Participates in the assessment of the cultural competence of the public health organization." | | |
| Values/Ethics for Interprofessional Practice<br>"Work with individuals of other professions to maintain a climate of mutual respect and shared values." | "VE 5. Work in cooperation with those who receive care, those who provide care, and others who contribute to or support the delivery of prevention and health services.<br>VE 6. Develop a trusting relationship with patients, families, and other team members.<br>VE 7. Demonstrate high standards of ethical conduct and quality of care in one's contributions to team-based care.<br>VE 8. Manage ethical dilemmas specific to interprofessional patient/population-centered care situations.<br>VE 9. Act with honesty and integrity in relationships with patients, families, and other team members.<br>VE 10. Maintain competence in one's own profession appropriate to scope of practice." | "VE1. Place the interests of patients and populations at the center of interprofessional health care delivery.<br>VE 2. Respect the dignity and privacy of patients while maintaining confidentiality in the delivery of team-based care.<br>VE 3. Embrace the cultural diversity and individual differences that characterize patient populations and the health care team.<br>VE 4. Respect the unique cultures, values, roles/responsibilities, and expertise of other health professions." | Interpersonal Education Collaborative (IPEC), 2011, p. 19 |

*continued on next page*

**Table 1. (continued)**
**Patient-Centered Care Planning: Knowledge, Skills, and Attitudes for Competency**

| Knowledge | Skills | Attitudes | Sources |
|---|---|---|---|
| Roles and Responsibilities for Interprofessional Practice<br>"Use the knowledge of one's own role and those of other professions to appropriately assess and address the healthcare needs of the patients and populations served." | "RR1. Communicate one's roles and responsibilities clearly to patients, families, and other professionals.<br>RR3. Engage diverse health care professionals who complement one's own professional expertise, as well as associated resources, to develop strategies to meet specific patient care needs.<br>RR4. Explain the roles and responsibilities of other care providers and how the team works together to provide care.<br>RR5. Use the full scope of knowledge, skills, and abilities of available health professionals and health care workers to provide care that is safe, timely, efficient, effective, and equitable.<br>RR6. Communicate with team members to clarify each member's responsibility in executing components of a treatment plan or public health intervention.<br>RR7. Forge interdependent relationships with other professionals to improve care and advance learning.<br>RR8. Engage in continuous professional and interprofessional development to enhance team performance.<br>RR9. Use unique and complementary abilities of all the team to optimize patient care." | "RR2. Recognize one's limitations in skills, knowledge, and abilities." | IPEC, 2011, p. 21 |

*continued on next page*

**Table 1. (continued)**
**Patient-Centered Care Planning: Knowledge, Skills, and Attitudes for Competency**

| Knowledge | Skills | Attitudes | Sources |
|---|---|---|---|
| "Describe IP team dynamics as they related to individual team member's values and the impact on team functioning in ethical dilemmas.<br>Describe the nature of IP ethical reasoning and justification." | "Identify IP ethical issues within a team context.<br>Utilize the basic skills of reasoning and justification as it relates to identified ethical issue within an IP team.<br>Guided by an ethics framework, contribute to IP ethical reasoning and decision making.<br>Perform effectively to develop shared team values.<br>Practice ethically in an IP environment.<br>Able to use a framework for ethical decision-making to guide ethical reasoning within an IP team." | "Reflect on own values, personal and professional, and respect those of other IP team members/clients/families.<br>Clarify values including accountability, respect, confidentiality, trust, integrity, honesty, and ethical behavior, equity as it relates to IP team functioning to maximize quality, safe patient care.<br>Advance values including accountability, respect, confidentiality, trust, integrity, honesty, and ethical behavior, equity as it relates to IP team functioning to maximize quality, safe patient care.<br>Accept, through respect and value, others and their contributions in relational-centered care." | IPEC, 2011, p. 31 |
| "Describe frameworks for ethical decision-making within an IP team." | | | IPEC, 2011, p. 31 |

**Table 2.**
**Chronic Disease Risk Stratification Tool**

| Low (8-12 visits) | High (18-24 visits) |
|---|---|
| • Chronic renal failure (CRF) stage 1-2 with glomerular filtration rate (GFR) 60 or greater<br>• A1C > or = 7.0<br>• Positive tobacco use<br>• Controlled HTN <BP 140/90<br>• No appointment with PCP within 1 year<br>• One ER visit and/or hospitalization in preceding 12 months | • CRF stages 4 or 5 GFR less than 29<br>• A1C > 8.0<br>• HTN stage 2:2 or more > or = 160; or ≥ 100<br>• History of CAD<br>• Prescribed eight or more medications<br>• Re-admission within 30 days<br>• Mental health diagnosis<br>• Age greater than 80<br>• Greater than one ER visit and/or hospitalization in preceding 3 months |
| **Moderate (12-18 visits)** | **Variances** |
| • CRF stage 3 GFR 30-59<br>• AIC > 7-8<br>• Uncontrolled HTN 2 or more readings > 140-159; or 90-99<br>• History of CAD<br>• Prescribed eight or more medications<br>• One ER visit and/or hospitalization in preceding 6 months | • Co-morbid disease exacerbation requiring medication initiation/titration<br>• Cognitively impaired with caregiver support<br>• Cognitively impaired without caregiver support<br>• ER or inpatient re-admission after program initiation<br>• Established adherence with program goals met<br>• Established history of nonadherence<br>• Identified barrier to learning<br>• Mental health diagnosis, undertreated or unstable<br>• New diagnosis<br>• Reinforcement of treatment plan objectives needed<br>• Risk stratification classification change to more complicated level |

**Source:** Lahey Hospital & Medical Center, Burlington, MA. Reprinted with permission.

## References


Advisory Board Company, The. (2012). *High-risk patient care management.* Washington, DC: Author.

Agency for Healthcare Research and Quality (AHRQ). (2010). *Care coordination measures atlas.* Rockville, MD: U.S. Department of Health and Human Services.

Brown, R.., & Rounds, L. (1995). Conjoint screening questionnaires for alcohol and other drug abuse: Criterion validity in a primary care practice. *Wisconsin Medical Journal, 94*(3), 135-140.

Centers for Medicaid & Medicare Services. (2010). *EHR incentive program meaningful programs.* Retrieved from www.cms.gov/EHRincentive-Programs

Council on Linkages Between Academia and Public Health Practice, The. (2010). *Core competencies for public health professionals.* Retrieved from http://www.phf.org/resourcetools/Documents/Core_Competencies_for_Public_Health_Professionals_2010May.pdf

Cronenwett, L., Sherwood, G., Barnsteiner, J., Disch, J., Johnson, J., Mitchell, P., ... Warren, J. (2007). Quality and safety education for nurses. *Nursing Outlook, 55*(3), 122-131.

Dearholt, S., & Dang, D. (2012). *Johns Hopkins nursing evidence-based practice model and guidelines* (2nd ed.). Indianapolis, IN: Sigma Theta Tau International.

Doerflinger, D. (2013). *Mental status assessment of older adults: The Mini-Cog.* New York, NY: The Hartford Institute for Geriatric Nursing.

Frampton, S., & Wahl, C. (2012). Partnering with families: Those that know the patient best can help bridge the gap between hospital to home. *American Journal of Nursing, 112*(10), 11.

Insignia Health. (2014). *Four levels of health activaton. Patient Activation Model (PAM).* Retrieved from http://www.insigniahealth.com/solutions/patient-activation-measure

Institute for Patient- and Family-Centered Care. (2014). *What is patient and family centered care?* Retrieved from http://www.ipfcc.org/faq.html

Interprofessional Education Collaborative (IPEC). (2011). *Core competencies for interprofessional collaborative practice.* Retrieved from http://www.aacn.nche.edu/education-resources/ipecreport.pdf

Jones, K., Jamerson, C., & Pike, S. (2012). The journey to electronic interdisciplinary care plans. *Nursing Management, 43*(12), 9-12.

Katz, S., Down, T.D., Cash, H.R., & Grotz, R.C. (1970). Progress in the development of the index of ADL. *The Gerontologist, 10*(1), 20-30.

Kroenke, K., Spitzer, R., & Williams, W. (2001). The PHQ-9: Validity of a brief depression severity measure. *Journal of General Internal Medicine, 16*(9), 606-616.

Kroenke, K., Spitzer, R., & Williams, W. (2003). The patient health questionnaire-2: Validity of a two-tier depression screener. *Medical Care, 4*(11), 1284-1292.

Levensky, E.R., Forcehimes, A., O'Donohue, W.T., & Beitz, K. (2007). Motivational interviewing: An evidence-based approach to counseling helps patients follow treatment recommendations. *American Journal of Nursing, 107*(10), 50-58.

Mathias, S., Nayak, U.S., & Isaacs, B. (1986). Balance in elderly patient: The "get up and go" test. *Archives Physical Medicine and Rehabilitation, 67*(6), 387-389.

Motivational Interviewing Network of Trainers. (2013a). *Motivational interviewing training for new trainers (TNT).* Retrieved from http://www.motivationalinterview.org/Documents/TNT_Manual_Nov_08.pdf

Motivational Interviewing Network of Trainers. (2013b). *What is motivational interviewing?* Retrieved from http://www.motivationalinterviewing.org/

National Committee for Quality Assurance. (2014). *HEDIS & performance measurement.* Washington, DC: Author. Retrieved from www.ncqa.org/tabid/59/Default.aspx

Nettina, S. (1996). *The Lippincott manual of nursing practice* (6th ed). Philadelphia, PA: Lippincott, Williams & Wilkins.

Nickel, S., Trojan, A., & Kofahl, C. (2012). Increasing patient centeredness in outpatient care through closer collaboration with patient groups? An exploratory study on the views of health care professionals working in quality management for office-based physicians in Germany. *Health Policy, 107*(2-3), 249-257.

Onega, L. (2013). *The modified caregiver strain index (MCSI).* New York, NY: The Hartford Institute for Geriatric Nursing.

Rollnick, S., Miller, W., & Butler, C. (2008). *Motivational interviewing in health care.* New York, NY: The Guilford Press.

Shelkey, M., & Wallace, M. (2012). *Katz index of independence in activities of daily living (ADL).* New York, NY: The Hartford Institute for Geriatric Nursing.

Tabloski, P.A. (2012). *Gerontological nursing review and resource manual* (3rd ed.). Silver Spring, MD: Pearson Higher Ed.

U.S. Preventive Services Task Force (USPSTF). (2013). *Recommendations.* Retrieved from http://www.uspreventiveservicestaskforce.org/recommendations.htm


## Additional Readings


Laughlin, C. (Ed.). (2013). *Core curriculum for ambulatory care nursing* (3rd ed). Pitman, NJ: American Academy of Ambulatory Care Nursing.

Quality and Safety Education for Nurses Institute. (2012). *Graduate KSA.* Retrieved from http://qsen.org/competencies/graduate-ksas/

Quality and Safety Education for Nurses Institute. (2012). *Pre-licensure KSA.* Retrieved from http://qsen.org/competencies/pre-licensure-ksas/

Wasson, J.H., Godfrey, M.M., Nelson, E.C., Mohr, J.J., & Batalden, P.B. (2003). Microsystems in health care: Part 4. Planning patient centered care. *Joint Commission Journal on Quality & Safety, 29*(5), 227-237.

# CHAPTER 6

# Support for Self-Management

*Stephanie G. Witwer, PhD, RN, NEA-BC*
*Candia Baker Laughlin, MS, RN-BC*
*Kari J. Hite, MN, RN, CDE*

## Learning Outcome Statement

The purpose of this chapter is to enable the reader to articulate the primary components of self-management support, including the importance of a comprehensive needs assessment, common strategies for collaborative goal setting, and concepts important to self-management.

## Learning Objectives

After reading this chapter, the registered nurse (RN) working in the Care Coordination and Transition Management (CCTM) role will be able to:

- Describe the concepts associated with support of self-management by ambulatory care RNs who are providing care coordination and transition management within the CCTM Model including:
  - Knowledge and understanding of chronic condition(s).
  - Ability to positively impact health promotion and disease-prevention activities.
  - Recognition of the importance of social and lifestyle adaptation.
  - Support for development of self-regulation skills.
- Discuss the need for patient-centered assessment, and incorporation of patient values, goals, and preferences into planned care activities and approaches.
- Identify patient self-management skills, and gaps or barriers often encountered by members of the health care team.
- Outline the importance of recognizing the patient and health care team as equal partners in managing chronic conditions, with the RN in CCTM focused on building the patient's and family's knowledge, skills, and attitudes for self-management.
- Demonstrate understanding of knowledge, skills, and attitudes required for the support for the self-management dimension (see Table 1).

## Competency Definition

*Self-management support* is defined as the "systematic provision of education and supportive interventions by health care staff to increase patients' skills and confidence in managing their health problems, including regular assessment of progress and problems, goal setting, and problem-solving support" (Pearson, Mattke, Shaw, Ridgely, & Wiseman., 2007, p. 1). Patients self-manage by performing behaviors (or behaviors performed by their families) to manage their condition and maximize their health (Grey, Knafl, & McCorkle, 2006). Self-management requires "having the confidence to deal with medical management, role management, and emotional management of their conditions" (Pearson et al., 2007, p. 7). For children and adolescents with chronic conditions, self-management activities and decision making are shared by the youth and parents with a goal that as the child develops and matures, responsibility is progressively transferred (Schilling, Grey, & Knafl, 2002). For some adults, decision-making activities may also be shared with significant others or become the responsibility of a designated decision-making surrogate.

Self-management support is an essential dimension of the role of the registered nurse in Care Coordination and Transition Management (CCTM). In a comparative effectiveness review of studies related to outpatient case management for adults with complex care needs, Hickman and colleagues (2013) found evidence that successful interventions for a variety of chronic conditions included providing support of self-management. Enhanced self-, and family-management can improve physical outcomes for some conditions and improve personal outcomes such as self-efficacy, empowerment, adherence to treatment regimens, and quality of life (Grey et al., 2006). Ryan and Sawin (2009) noted the critical relationship among patient self-management behaviors, improvement of health outcomes, increased quality of life, and reduction in demand for health services. Interactions between patients and the health care system occur in only a small fraction of each patient's life. Consequently, patients are making critical health care decisions every day. As noted by Bodenheimer, Lorig, Holman, and Grumbach (2002), "The question is not whether patients with chronic conditions manage their illness, but how they manage" (p. 2470). Given all patients are chronic disease self-managers, the role of the RN in CCTM in self-management support is to positively impact *how* self-management occurs. This process begins with an assessment of patient knowledge, skills, behaviors, and confidence in managing chronic conditions and maintaining health. Next, the RN in CCTM works directly with the patient and/or family and the health care team to develop a collaborative plan of care, building the plan around the values and preferences of the patient. Another critical component of the assessment and plan are the key supports and resources required to address social and lifestyle needs. Finally, the RN in CCTM helps the patient develop important self-regulatory skills to support critical self-management decisions. Self-management support occurs in a variety of settings and venues, individual or group, face to face or utilizing an ever-expanding arsenal of telehealth tools.

## I. Support Knowledge and Understanding of Chronic Condition(s)

A. Perform comprehensive assessment of understanding of chronic condition(s) and initiate discussion of self-management techniques.

B. Develop tailored education for the patient/family considering (Grey et al., 2006):
   1. Health literacy.
   2. Educational level.
   3. Cognitive/Developmental level.
   4. Language.
   5. Preferences.
   6. Family/Significant other.
   7. Learning style.
   8. Adult learning principles.
   9. Readiness to learn.
      a. Information may need to be repeated.
      b. When the patient is ready to learn.

C. Emphasize self-management concepts (Lorig et al., 2012).
   1. Cause of chronic condition: often multiple causes and contributing factors.
      a. Heredity.
      b. Lifestyle.
      c. Exposure to environmental factors (e.g., secondhand smoke).
      d. Physiological changes (e.g., electrolyte imbalance, low levels of thyroid hormone, changes in brain chemistry).
   2. Patient expertise in living with chronic condition(s) and social situation.
   3. Symptoms and symptom management: even though diseases may differ, symptoms may be similar. Understanding symptoms and self-management strategies is essential to improve quality of life. Assess and support patient's and family's problem solving around these common symptoms.
      a. Fatigue: may be caused by the disease process, inactivity, poor nutrition, ineffective sleep, stress, or medications.
         (1) Increase physical activity.
         (2) Stress management.
         (3) Screen for depression.
         (4) Improve nutrition.
         (5) Improve sleep quality.
      b. Pain/physical discomfort: may be caused by the disease process, muscle tension, deconditioning, stress and emotional responses, and medications.
         (1) Chronic pain has a strong emotional component that can increase perceived pain levels.
         (2) Encourage stretching, increased activity.
         (3) Ice, heat, massage.
         (4) Integrative techniques: distraction, music, relaxation, etc.
         (5) Medication use.
      c. Shortness of breath: may be caused by multiple disease processes that interfere with pulmonary or cardiac function, being overweight or obese, a deconditioned state, smoking.
         (1) Teach breathing management techniques such as diaphragmatic or pursed-lip breathing, huffing, and positions that ease breathing.
         (2) Follow low-sodium diet.
         (3) Prop up with pillows to aid sleeping.
         (4) Monitor fluid retention and weight gain.
         (5) Encourage fluid intake unless restricted.
         (6) Eliminate smoke exposure.
         (7) Increase activity if possible.
         (8) Reduce weight if contributing factor.
      d. Sleep disturbances: high-quality sleep very important.
         (1) Comfortable bed and room temperature.
         (2) Comfort positions in bed (pillows, head of bed).
         (3) Regular routine.
         (4) Safe environment: lighting, assistive devices handy.
         (5) Avoid alcohol and eating at bedtime.
         (6) Avoid caffeine late in the day or other stimulating activities near bedtime.
         (7) Avoid sleeping pills or diuretics at bedtime.
         (8) Professional help for sleep apnea.
      e. Memory loss.
         (1) Professional help if memory loss interferes with life activities.
      f. Itching (pruritus) – may be difficult to pinpoint cause.
         (1) Keep skin dry.
         (2) Comfortable clothes.
         (3) Soothing medications.
         (4) Stress management.
         (5) Minimize scratching.

g. Urinary incontinence: more common in women (Lorig et al., 2012).
   (1) Use of Kegel exercises, bladder emptying techniques, scheduled urination.
   (2) Consume fewer beverages at bedtimes, especially those that stimulate urine production.
   (3) Use of absorbent pads.
   (4) Medications.

4. Impact of disease and treatment (Newman, Steed, & Mulligan, 2004).
   a. Physiological.
   b. Psychological.
   c. Social.
5. Disease trajectory (Grey et al., 2006).
   a. Full recovery often not possible.
   b. Disease pattern may be unpredictable.
   c. Symptoms can contribute to development of additional symptoms.

D. Set goals collaboratively (Battersby et al., 2010).
   1. Patient as full partner.
   2. Health care team.
   3. Community providers.
   4. Incorporate end-of-life wishes.

E. Train and develop skills (Hill-Briggs & Gemmell, 2007).
   1. Medication use.
   2. Monitoring and medication adjustment.
   3. Use of medical equipment.
   4. Dietary changes.
   5. Adaptive devices and supports.

F. Recognize acute symptoms and emergencies (Lorig & Holman, 2003).
   1. Sick day plans.
   2. Collaborative plan for patient-initiated activities to address symptom exacerbation.
   3. When and how to seek care.

G. Use medications safely (Marek et al., 2013).
   1. Use of reminder devices (e.g., blister packs, med-planners, reminder devices, and machines that dispense medication).

H. Communicate effectively with health care team (Ilioudi, Lazakidou, & Tsironi, 2010).
   1. Effective communication strategies for planned visits.
   2. Understanding who and how to contact regarding health care needs and questions.
   3. Use of the plan of care and end-of-life care (health care power of attorney, living will, Physician Orders for Life-Sustaining Treatment [POLST], wishes with health care providers).

I. Incorporate care regimen into daily practices (May, Montori, & Mair, 2009).
   1. Minimal disruption principles.
   2. More complex regimens less likely to be followed.

J. Support transitions of care (Naylor et al., 1999).
   1. Update plan of care at transitions.
   2. Patient wishes follow patient across transitions.

## II. Support Knowledge and Understanding of Health Promotion and Disease Prevention

A. Assess current health promotion and disease prevention knowledge and unmet preventive service needs.

B. Assess health behavior/lifestyle risks (Pearson et al., 2007).

C. Advising/coaching regarding healthy behaviors/lifestyle (Olsen & Nesbitt, 2010).
   1. Regular physical activity.
   2. Nutritious diet.
   3. Weight management.
   4. Adequate sleep and rest.
   5. Tobacco cessation.
   6. Avoidance of excess alcohol consumption or mood altering substances.
   7. Stress management.
   8. Medication adherence.

D. Incorporate planned lifestyle changes into collaborative plan of care.

E. Encourage self-monitoring of behavior changes (see Section IV Support Development of Self-Regulation Skills).

## III. Support Social and Lifestyle Adaptations

A. Perform comprehensive assessment of barriers to self-care in the home setting (Baumann & Dang, 2012) including physical, psychological, cognitive, economic, social, and cultural barriers.
   1. Physical barriers.
      a. Assess for physical disability/perform functional assessment including Get Up and Go test (Mathias, Nayak, & Isaacs, 1986).
      b. Assess for safety and accessibility of the home setting.
         (1) Stairs.
         (2) Narrow doorways.
         (3) Bathroom accessibility.
         (4) Kitchen/food preparation access.
      c. Assess need for adaptive devices.
         (1) Wheelchair, walker, hospital bed, grab bars, raised toilet seat, commode, etc.
         (2) Assess need for durable medical equipment.
            (a) Oxygen, continuous positive airway pressure, etc.
      d. Assess family/significant other involvement/support in care.
      e. Assess need for support services.
         (1) Home health nursing, home health aides, palliative care, etc.
      f. Assess transportation concerns.
         (1) Ability to obtain health care services.
         (2) Ability to receive other necessary goods and services.

2. Psychological barriers.
   a. Assess for depression or emotional distress that may impact the patient's ability to work and/or perform self-care.
   b. Assess for barriers related to the disease or illness that will interfere with the patient's ability to maintain long-term employment (post-traumatic stress disorder, schizophrenia, major depression, mania, substance abuse, etc.).
      (1) Consider use of standardized assessment tools (e.g., Patient Health Questionnaire [PHQ-9], Drug Abuse Screening Test [DAST], Generalized Anxiety Scale [GAD-7]).
   c. Assess for family member/caregiver burden related to supporting the patient in the home setting.
      (1) Use standardized screening tools such as the Zarit Burden Interview or other tool deemed by your institution.
   d. Determine if social networks or peer support groups, including reflecting on shared experiences, would be beneficial to the patient, family, and/or caregivers.
3. Cognitive barriers.
   a. Perform cognitive assessment.
      (1) Determine patient's cognitive ability.
      (2) Recognize early impairment in cognitive functioning.
      (3) Monitor cognitive response to various treatments or longitudinally.
      (4) Cognitive impairment associated with greater morbidity and mortality (Inouye, Foreman, Mion, Katz, & Cooney, 2001).
         (a) Examples of conditions associated with cognitive deterioration: dementia, Alzheimer's disease, delirium.
         (b) Tools used to assess cognitive functioning.
            i. Mini-Mental State Examination (MMSE).
            ii. Mini-Cog.
            iii. Montreal Cognitive Assessment (MoCA).
   b. Assess for history of traumatic brain injuries, stroke, and anoxic brain injuries along with serious mental illnesses that can affect the patient's ability to understand and/or apply health care information to self-care measures and lifestyle adaptation.
   c. Review medications prescribed that potentially can change work roles due to sedation or other side effects and legal constraints.
4. Economic barriers.
   a. Assess for any physical and/or cognitive changes that will impact the patient's ability to seek/maintain employment.
      (1) In diseases like epilepsy and insulin-dependent diabetes, people who drive commercial vehicles may lose their ability to maintain commercial and/or regular driving licenses.
      (2) Is there public transportation available or family or friends who can assist with transportation?
         (a) Is there a need for application to special transportation services?
      (3) If the patient is homebound, determine if home health services such as home-based primary care, skilled home health services, or technologically based supports such as home telemonitoring are available to assist with care management.
      (4) Are there concerns or fear regarding premature death, disability, and consequences for the family?
         (a) Refer to social service staff to assist with applications processes for social security disability, and other assistance that may be available.
         (b) Suggest that family review insurance policies and work-related benefits that may be available to provide support.
5. Social and cultural barriers.
   a. Assess patient/family's cultural norms.
      (1) Identify cultural barriers related to the disease process or illness within the patient's specific culture and incorporate into plan of care.
      (2) Does the patient or family have religious beliefs? Can the religious community assist with providing family support?
      (3) Are culturally specific services such as community-based health educators (e.g., promotoras) available in the community? Would the patient and family be willing to have culturally specific staff visit the home? (McEwen, Pasvogel, Gallegos, & Barrera, 2010).

B. Care coordinators collaborate with many other disciplines to assist with meeting the patient's needs.
   1. Referral to other members of the multidisciplinary health care team should be completed when appropriate.
   2. Technology-based support such as telehealth (Baldonado et al., 2013), use of social media, and computer-based support should be considered.
   3. Service animals and/or other pets may be a helpful source of support for patients.

## IV. Support Development of Self-Regulation Skills

A. Self-regulation.
   1. Emphasizes the patient's central role in managing his or her health.
   2. Is based in Social Learning or Social Cognitive Theory (Bandura, 1986).
   3. Results from combined impacts of a person's cognitive processes, social and physical environment, and behavior.
   4. Is developed by the patient and family with the support of health care team members.
   5. Involves development of the following skills (Lorig & Holman, 2003; Ryan & Sawin, 2009).
      a. Goal setting and self-monitoring.
      b. Reflective thinking.
      c. Decision making.
      d. Development of an action plan and implementation.
      e. Self-evaluation and tailoring.
      f. Management of physical, emotional, and cognitive responses related to the behavior change.

B. Goal setting and self-monitoring by the patient and family.
   1. Self-care goals must be the goals of the patient or family, not those of the health care team.
   2. Goals are developed in collaboration with members of the health care team, directed toward positively influencing health outcomes (Funnell et al., 2011).
   3. Types of patient and family goals may include:
      a. Learning goals.
      b. Goals to change behaviors, such as physical activity, diet, medication compliance, health promotion, or risk reduction.
      c. Clinical status goals, such as better control of glycemia or blood pressure.
   4. I-SMART goals (Tang, Funnell, Gillard, Nwankwo, & Heisler, 2010).
      a. Inspiring.
         1. "What is most important for you (patient/family) to work on?"
         2. "On a scale of 1-10, how important is this to you?"
      b. Specific: "What will you do? Where? When?"
      c. Measurable: "How much will you do? How often?"
      d. Achievable.
         1. "What barriers might you face? How will you deal with them?"
         2. "On a scale of 1-10, how confident are you that you can complete this specific plan?"
      e. Relevant: "How will this step help you achieve your overall goal?"
      f. Time-specific: "How long will you try this experiment?"
   5. Self-monitoring.
      a. Success with solving problems and reaching goals leads to increased confidence in self-efficacy.
      b. Regular contact with the health care team assists the patient and family with removing barriers, modifying goals and strategies, and acknowledging accomplishments.

C. Reflective thinking by the patient and family.
   1. In considering self-management tasks and changes, patients and families engage in self-reflection about readiness and ability to change, beliefs, and barriers.
   2. Self-efficacy: a person's confidence in his/her ability to carry out behaviors necessary to achieve the desired goal (Ilioudi et al., 2010).
      a. Is a continuum, not simply present or absent.
      b. Enhanced by success in solving own problems.
      c. Self-assess on a scale of 1-10. Explore why they scored themselves that score and what it would take to improve the score.
   3. Five stages of readiness for change (Fava, Velicer, & Prochaska, 1995).
      a. Pre-contemplation ("I'm not seriously thinking about quitting smoking").
      b. Contemplation ("I will quit smoking sometime in the next 6 months").
      c. Preparation ("I will quit in the next month").
      d. Action ("I have quit and am using nicotine replacement").
      e. Maintenance ("I have not smoked for more than 6 months").
   4. Health beliefs and attitudes (Janz & Becker, 1984).
      a. The extent to which a person believes he or she is susceptible to the ill health condition ("Will smoking cause me to have heart or lung disease or cancer?").
      b. If he or she would develop it, how serious does the person believe the consequences will be in his or her life ("If I have cancer due to smoking, how sick will I be? Could I possibly die?").
      c. The extent to which benefits to the person outweigh the barriers ("It is really hard to quit and I like smoking. Is it worth the effort?").
      d. The sense of confidence that the person can perform the action ("I have quit before, but started again. Can I do it this time?").

D. Decision making by the patient and family.
   1. In collaboration with the health care team, the patient and family weigh priorities.
      a. Build on individualized assessment of strengths and weaknesses.
      b. Identify what is valued by the patient and family.
      c. Build on small incremental steps of change.

2. Problem-solving skills.
   a. Clearly define the problem.
   b. Generate options of possible solutions.
      (1) Can base options on own prior experiences.
      (2) May seek input from health care team members.
      (3) May seek input from family members or friends.
      (4) Avail self of other resources online or in the community.
   c. Implementation of solution.
   d. Evaluation of solution (Lorig & Holman, 2003).

E. Development of an action plan and implementation.
1. Collaborative plan identifies actions to be taken, person responsible, and time frame for review.
2. Health care team takes responsibility for ordering of tests and treatments, support, and follow-up.
3. Patient or family activities for self-management may include development of the following knowledge, skills, or abilities (Petkov, Harvey, & Battersby, 2010).
   a. Knowledge of condition(s).
   b. Knowledge of treatment(s).
   c. Ability to take medication.
   d. Ability to share in decisions.
   e. Ability to arrange appointments.
   f. Ability to attend appointments.
   g. Understanding of monitoring and recording.
   h. Ability to monitor and record.
   i. Understanding of symptom management.
   j. Ability to manage symptoms.
   k. Ability to manage the physical impact.
   l. Ability to manage the social impact.
   m. Ability to manage the emotional impact.
   n. Progress toward a healthy lifestyle.

F. Self-evaluation and tailoring by the patient and family.
1. Requires the patient and family to measure success against individualized goals.
   a. Success should not be measured strictly according to compliance or adherence to medical treatment plan.
   b. Frustration or perceptions of failure may indicate need to modify the goals and/or the action plan.
   c. Progress toward goals may not be appreciated by the patient and family, and the health care team may provide valuable feedback and encouragement.
2. Exacerbation or progression of the condition may require a shift in the goals and different interventions and self-care behaviors, as well as support of coping (Grey et al., 2006).

G. Management of physical, emotional, and cognitive responses related to the behavioral change by the patient and family.
1. Individuals and families vary in their ability to incorporate management of chronic conditions into their routines.
2. Little research has been done on the impact of health care team members on management of illness by families (Grey et al., 2006).
3. Studies have shown that, over time, families view themselves as capable of managing the treatment regimen well, and disruption on their family life is minimized.

H. Methods for supporting self-regulation.
1. Motivational interviewing (Miller & Rollnick, 2002).
   a. Requires development of partnership with patient and exchange of information for informed decision making by the patient.
   b. Explores and resolves ambivalence about changing health behaviors, and elicits commitment.
   c. Uses communication techniques, such as open-ended questions, affirmation, reflection, and encouraging "change talk."
   d. Requires the clinician to be trained, to practice, and receive feedback in order to master the technique.
   e. Is shown effective with some patient populations, but not others.
2. Empowerment approach (Anderson & Funnell, 2010; Feste & Anderson, 1995).
   a. Primarily used for patients with type 2 diabetes because the behavioral changes are integral aspects of patients' daily lives.
   b. Designed to help patients choose personally meaningful goals that result in behavioral changes that are internally motivated.
   c. Emphasizes patient autonomy, while helping patients examine the social, cognitive, and emotional aspects of their lives and the influences on their decision making.
3. Five A's approach (McGowan, 2013).
   a. Assess, advise, agree, assist, and arrange.
   b. Used to develop an individualized, collaborative plan to attain goals.
   c. Not a linear process, in which steps overlap.
   d. Has been applied successfully and in combination with other approaches with a variety of patient populations.
4. Peer coaching (Tang et al., 2011).
   a. Peers can function as educators, advocates, cultural translators, mentors, case managers, or group facilitators.
   b. Peers can teach patients and families to do many things.
      (1) Communicate with providers.
      (2) Obtain resources.
      (3) How to seek emotional support.
      (4) Set goals, make decisions, develop action plans, and solve problems.

c. Training of peer counselors may vary greatly.
d. Stanford model (Lawn & Schoo, 2009; Lorig & Holman, 2003).
(1) Structured 6-week group course with both a health professional and a trained peer leader.
(2) Teach participants self-regulation skills.
(3) Objectively measures participants' knowledge, skills, and abilities pre- and post-course and provides feedback tools.
(4) Scientifically evaluated with a variety of chronic conditions for over 25 years.

5. Information technologies (Ilioudi et al., 2010).
a. Online diary with feedback on self-management.
b. Self-monitoring tools to inform decision making.
c. In-home monitoring.
d. Patient education to enhance knowledge.
e. Webinars (Yank, Laurent, Plant, & Lorig, 2013).

6. Traditional health coaching and counseling programs.
a. Individually with health professional or group.
b. Disease specific or generic about living with chronic conditions.
c. Variability exists in referral sources to programs, characteristics of the participants, and in the counseling process itself, which confounds the ability to measure effectiveness of the approaches (Packer et al., 2011).
d. The Flinders Program™ (2014).
(1) Individual, patient-centered assessment and care planning, using various tools incorporating motivational interactions.
(2) Standardized tools and forms for patient self-assessment of capacity to change, guide for the motivational interview, development and prioritization of goals, and construction of the self-management plan.
(3) Has undergone multiple trials in Australia, New Zealand, Canada, and the United States (Harvey et al., 2008; Lawn & Schoo, 2010; Petkov et al., 2010).

I. Follow-up.
1. Evidence supports systematic follow-up increases rates of patients' behavioral changes, both in chronic condition self-management and risk factor reduction (Battersby et al., 2010).
2. Successful methods include:
a. Follow-up appointments.
b. Case management via telephone; teleconferencing.
c. Telemonitoring.
d. Personalized reminders.
3. Value of follow-up enhanced if it specifically addresses review of the patients' data, monitoring of progress toward goals, and problem solving to address barriers to goals (Battersby et al., 2010).
4. The National Standards for Diabetes Self-Management Education: collaboratively developed plan of care, must include follow-up plan for ongoing self-management to support the following (Funnell et al., 2011):
a. Lack of knowledge or understanding.
b. Low health literacy.
c. Impairment of cognitive functioning.
d. Economic barriers.
e. Social and cultural barriers.

**Table 1.**
**Support Self-Management: Knowledge, Skills, and Attitudes for Competency**

| Patient-Centered Care | | | |
|---|---|---|---|
| The RN in CCTM will provide comprehensive care that recognizes the patient or designee as the source of control and full partner in providing compassionate and coordinated care based on respect for patient's preferences, values, and needs (Cronenwett et al., 2009). | | | |
| **Knowledge** | **Skills** | **Attitudes** | **Sources** |
| Demonstrate comprehensive knowledge about chronic conditions, including skills and techniques for monitoring and managing common symptoms. | Apply knowledge of chronic conditions in all patient interactions.<br><br>Teach/demonstrate self-management techniques to patients.<br><br>Develop educational resources if needed. | Understand knowledge limitations and utilizes resources effectively.<br><br>Value resources of the interdisciplinary team to augment self-management support (e.g., MD, nurse practitioner, physician assistant, pharmacist, diabetes educator, dietitian, social worker).<br><br>Value peer-provided support. | Lorig et al., 2012 |
| | Understand references/resources for enhancing knowledge of chronic conditions. | Value team-based approach to patient care.<br><br>Value individualized approach to address patient-identified needs. | Pearson et al., 2007 |
| | Assess patient and family understanding of chronic condition, causes, treatment options, and self-management requirements.<br><br>Address identified needs and gaps in understanding through planned learning activities. | Respect patient values, preferences, and choices. | Glasgow et al., 2003 |
| Demonstrate knowledge regarding evidence-based standards or guidelines in the care of patients with chronic conditions. | Critically seek and review evidence-based guidelines or standards of care and incorporates into care. | Value the use of evidence-based approach to care. | Battersby et al., 2010 |
| | Understand and apply theoretical models related to self-management support (e.g., social cognitive theory, transtheoretical model, adult learning theory, etc.). | | Pearson et al., 2007 |
| | | Commit to ongoing personal development. | Funnell et al., 2011 |

*continued on next page*

**Source Note:** Cronenwett et al. (2007) reprinted from *Nursing Outlook, 55*(3), 122-131, with permission from Elsevier.

**Table 1. (continued)**
**Support Self-Management: Knowledge, Skills, and Attitudes for Competency**

| Knowledge | Skills | Attitudes | Sources |
|---|---|---|---|
| Describe how the strength and relevance of available evidence influences the choice of interventions in provision of patient-centered care. | Participate in structuring the work environment to facilitate integration of new evidence into standards of practice.<br><br>Question rationale for routine approaches to care that result in less-than-desired outcomes or adverse events. | Value the need for continuous improvement in clinical practice based on new knowledge. | Cronenwett et al., 2007 |
| Understand the importance of health promotion and prevention activities applicable to the patient. | Promote completion of appropriate health promotion and preventive services.<br><br>Support the patient/ family in understanding need for preventive care. | Value the importance of health-promoting activities. Confronts any personal negative beliefs regarding lifestyle changes (smoking cessation, weight loss, etc.). | Lorig et al., 2012 |
| | Consider integrative approaches such as stress management, meditation, yoga, etc. | Appreciate the value of integrative therapies as self-management approaches. | Ryan & Sawin, 2009 |
| Identify potential barriers to self-care, including physical, psychological, cognitive, economic, and social. | Perform comprehensive assessment of barriers to self-care.<br><br>Provide coaching and identifies resources to diminish barriers to self-care. | Respect patient preferences for degree of active engagement in care process. | Marrero & Ackerman, 2007 |
| | | Acknowledge personal and situational limitations and seeks to maximize skills, abilities, and resources. | Cole et al., 2013 |
| | | Recognize patient expectations influence outcomes in management of pain or suffering. | Cronenwett et al., 2007 |
| Integrate understanding of multiple dimensions of patient-centered care:<br>• Patient/family/community preferences, values.<br>• Coordination and integration of care.<br>• Information, communication, and education.<br>• Physical comfort and emotional support.<br>• Involvement of family and friends.<br>• Transition and continuity. | Elicit patient values, preferences, and expressed needs as part of clinical interview.<br><br>Communicate patient values, preferences, and expressed needs to other members of the health care team.<br><br>Provide patient-centered care with sensitivity and respect for the diversity of the human experience. | Value seeing health care situations "through patients' eyes."<br><br>Respect and encourages individual expression of patient values, preferences, and needs.<br><br>Value the patient's expertise with own health and symptoms.<br><br>Willingly support patient-centered care for individuals and groups whose values differ from own. | Cronenwett et al., 2007 |

*continued on next page*

**Table 1. (continued)**
**Support Self-Management: Knowledge, Skills, and Attitudes for Competency**

| Knowledge | Skills | Attitudes | Sources |
|---|---|---|---|
| Understand concepts of self-regulation, and the patient's and family's central role in managing health conditions. | Support patient and family development of the following self-management skills:<br>1. Goal-setting and self-monitoring.<br>2. Reflective thinking.<br>3. Decision making.<br>4. Development of an action plan and implementation.<br>5. Self-evaluation and tailoring.<br>6. Management of physical, emotional, and cognitive responses related to the behavior change. | Support patients with skill development in these areas, but does not "perform for" them.<br><br>View patient as full partner in care.<br><br>Seek ways to promote independence.<br><br>Value patient decisions and accepts decisions not consistent with recommendations.<br><br>Recognize and encourages successes. | Ryan & Sawin, 2009 |
| | Utilize appropriate patient engagement/ activation skills such as motivational interviewing, 5 A's, positive psychology. | Value the use of patient engagement and activation skills. | Battersby et al., 2010 |
| | | Recognize the importance of practice in becoming expert in the application of these skills. | Olsen & Nesbitt, 2010 |
| Demonstrate the ability to perform a comprehensive self-management support assessment. | Employ effective Interviewing techniques.<br><br>Perform appropriate assessment activities, including use of standardized tools.<br><br>Utilize active listening principles. | Appreciate that a comprehensive assessment becomes the foundation of the collaborative plan of care.<br><br>View patients as experts in their own lives. | Battersby et al., 2010 |
| Synthesize critical information to develop a patient-centered collaborative plan of care. | Utilize adult learning principles when working with adult patients. | Value patient wishes and priorities for goal setting.<br><br>Value contributions of interdisciplinary team, including community team members.<br><br>Exercise creativity in plan development. | Battersby et al., 2010 |
| | | Identify own biases and values related to health behaviors and goals.<br><br>Respect and encourages patient expression of values, preferences, and needs.<br><br>Value the patient's expertise with own health and symptoms. | Ryan & Sawin, 2009 |
| | Develop goals that are SMART (specific, measureable, achievable, realistic, timely). | | Tang et al., 2011 |

**Table 1. (continued)**
**Support Self-Management: Knowledge, Skills, and Attitudes for Competency**

| Knowledge | Skills | Attitudes | Sources |
|---|---|---|---|
| Demonstrate the ability to identify, obtain, and coordinate resources needed (e.g., multiple health care providers, community, other caregivers) to provide integrated, comprehensive care. | Identify resources available to assist patient/family in meeting needs.<br><br>Identify safety issues and follows up as appropriate. | Accept that patient needs can be met in a variety of ways and through multiple agencies/groups.<br><br>Honor patient's wishes regarding use of community support. | Battersby et al., 2010<br><br>Lorig & Holman, 2003 |
| Evaluate collaborative plan of care, progress toward goal achievement, and effectiveness of planned interventions; modifies as needed. | Elicit cooperation of patient/family and health care team in review and revision of plan of care as needed. | Value importance of patient-centered interdisciplinary plan.<br><br>Exercise creativity in meeting patient needs.<br><br>Value keeping team informed of changes. | Battersby et al., 2010 |

| Self-Management Support Outcome Measure | | |
|---|---|---|
| **Chronic Disease Self-Care Behavior** | **Measures** | **Validated Scale** |
| Self-efficacy in the management of chronic conditions. | Self-efficacy measure at enrollment, 6 months and 1 year. | Self-Efficacy for Managing Chronic Disease 6-Item Scale.<br><br>Stanford/Garfield Kaiser Chronic Disease Dissemination Study (Lorig et al., 2001). |

## References


Anderson, R.M., & Funnell, M.M. (2010). Patient empowerment: Myths and misconceptions. *Patient Education and Counseling, 79,* 277-282.

Baldonado, A., Rodriguez, L., Renfro, D., Sheridan, S., McElrath, M., & Chardos, J. (2013). A home telehealth heart failure management program for veterans through care transitions. *Dimensions of Critical Care Nursing, 34*(4), 162-165.

Bandura, A. (1986). *A social foundation of thoughts and action. A social cognitive learning theory.* Englewood Cliffs, NJ: Prentice-Hall.

Battersby, M., Von Korff, M., Schaefer, J., Davis, C., Ludman, E., Greene, S.M., ... Wagner, E.H. (2010). Twelve evidence-based principles for implementing self-management support in primary care. *The Joint Commission Journal on Quality and Patient Safety, 36*(12), 561-570.

Baumann, L.C., & Dang, T.T.N. (2012). Helping patients with chronic conditions overcome barriers to self-care. *The Nurse Practitioner, 37*(3), 32-38.

Bodenheimer, T., Lorig, K., Holman, H., & Grumbach, K. (2002). Patient self-management of chronic disease in primary care. *JAMA, 288*(19), 2469-2475.

Cole, J., Smith, N., & Cupples, M. (2013). Do practitioners and friends support patients with coronary heart disease in lifestyle change? A qualitative study. *BMC Family Practice, 14,* 126.

Cronenwett, L., Sherwood, G., Barnsteiner, J., Disch, J., Johnson, J., Mitchell, P., Sullivan, D.T., & Warren, J. (2007). Quality and safety education for nurses. *Nursing Outlook, 55*(3), 122-131.

Cronenwett, L., Sherwood G., Pohl, J., Barnsteiner, J., Moore, S., Sullivan, D., Ward, D., & Warren, J., (2009). Quality and safety education for advanced nursing practice. *Nursing Outlook, 57,* 338-348.

Fava, J.L., Velicer, W.F., & Prochaska, J.O. (1995). Applying the transtheoretical model to a representative sample of smokers. *Addictive Behaviors, 20*(2), 189-203.

Feste, C., & Anderson, R.M. (1995). Empowerment: From philosophy to practice. *Patient Education and Counseling, 26,* 139-144.

Flinders University. (2014). *The Flinders program™.* Retrieved from http://www.flinders.edu.au/medicine/sites/fhbhru/self-management.cfm

Funnell, M.M., Brown, T.L., Childs, B.P., Haas, L.B., Hosey, G.M., Jensen, B., ... Weiss, M.A. (2011). National standard for diabetes self-management education. *Diabetes Care, 34*(Suppl. 1), S89-S96.

Glasgow, R.E., Davis, C. L., Funnell, M.M., & Beck, A. (2003). Implementing practical interventions to support chronic illness self-management. *Joint Commission Journal on Quality and Safety, 29*(11), 563-574.

Grey, M., Knafl, K., & McCorkle, R. (2006). A framework for the study of self- and family management of chronic conditions. *Nursing Outlook, 54*(5), 278-286.

Harvey, P.W., Petkov, J.N., Missan, G., Fuller, J., Battersby, M., Cayetano, T.N. ... Holmes, P. (2008). Self-management support and training for patients with chronic and complex conditions improved health-related behavior and health outcomes. *Australian Health Review, 32*(2), 330-338.

Hickman, D.H., Weiss, J.W., Guise, J-M., Buckley, D., Motu'apuaka, M., Graham, E., ... Saha, S. (2013). *Outpatient care management for adults with medical illness and complex care needs.* ARHQ publication no. 13-EHC031-EF. Rockville, MD: Agency for Healthcare Research and Quality.

Hill-Briggs, F., & Gemmell, L. (2007). Problem solving in diabetes self-management and control. A systematic review of the literature. *The Diabetes Educator, 33*(6), 1032-1050.

Ilioudi, S., Lazakidou, A., & Tsironi, M. (2010). Information and communication technologies for better patient self-management and self-efficacy. *International Journal Electronic Healthcare, 5*(4), 337-339.

Inouye, S.K., Foreman, M.D., Mion, L.C., Katz, K.H., & Cooney, L.M. Jr. (2001). Nurses' recognition of delirium and its symptoms: Comparison of nurse and researcher ratings. *Archives of Internal Medicine, 161*(20), 2467-2473.

Janz, N.K., & Becker, M.H. (1984). The health belief model: A decade later. *Health Education Quarterly, 11*(1), 1-47.

Lawn, S., & Schoo, A. (2010). Supporting self-management of chronic health conditions: Common approaches. *Patient Education and Counseling, 80*(2), 205-211.

Lorig, K.R., & Holman, H.R. (2003). Self-management education: History, definition, outcomes, and mechanisms. *Annals of Behavioral Medicine, 26*(1), 1-7.

Lorig, K., Holman, H., Sobel, D., Laurent, D., Gonzalez, V., & Minor, M. (2012). *Living a healthy life with chronic conditions* (4th ed.). Boulder, CO: Bull Publishing Co.

Lorig, K.R., Sobel, D.S., Ritter, P.L., Laurent, D., & Hobbs, M. (2001). Effect of a self-management program for patients with chronic disease. *Effective Clinical Practice, 4,* 256-262.

Marek, K., Stetzer, F., Ryan, P.A., Bub, L. D., Adams, S.J., Schlidt, A., ... & O'Brien, A. (2013). Nurse care coordination and technology effects on health status of frail older adults via enhanced self-management of medication. *Nursing Research, 62*(4), 269-278.

Marrero, D., & Ackerman, R. (2007). Providing long-term support for lifestyle changes: A key to success in diabetes prevention. *Diabetes Spectrum, 20,* 205-209.

Mathias, S., Nayak, U.S., & Isaacs, B. (1986). Balance in elderly patients: The "get-up and go" test. *Archives of Physical Medicine and Rehabilitation, 67*(6), 387-389.

May, C., Montori, V., & Mair, F. (2009). We need minimally disruptive medicine. *British Medical Journal, 339,* 485-487.

McEwen, M., Pasvogel, A., Gallegos, G., & Barrera, L. (2010). Type 2 diabetes self-management social support intervention at the U.S.-Mexico border. *Public Health Nursing, 27*(4), 310-319.

McGowan, P. (2013). The challenge of integrating self-management support into clinical settings. *Canadian Journal of Diabetes, 37,* 45-50.

Miller, W.R., & Rollnick, S. (2002). *Motivational interviewing* (2nd ed.). New York, NY: Guilford.

Naylor, M.D., Brooten, D., Campbell, R., Jacobsen, B.S., Mezey, M.D., Pauly, M.V., & Shwartz, J.S. (1999). Comprehensive discharge planning and home follow-up of hospitalized elders. *Journal of the American Medical Association, 281*(7), 613-620.

Newman, S., Steed, L., & Mulligan, K. (2004). Self-management interventions for chronic illness. *The Lancet, 364,* 1523-1537.

Olsen, J.M., & Nesbitt, B.J. (2010). Health coaching to improve healthy lifestyle behaviors: An integrative review. *American Journal of Health Promotion, 25*(1), e1-e11.

Packer, T.L., Boldy, D., Ghahari, S., Melling, L., Parsons, R., & Osborne, R.H. (2011). Self-management programs conducted within a practice setting: Who participates, who benefits and what can be learned. *Patient Education and Counseling, 87*(1), 93-100.

Pearson, M.L., Mattke, S., Shaw, R., Ridgely, M.S., & Wiseman, S.H. (2007). Patient self-management support programs: An evaluation. *Agency for Healthcare Research and Quality,* Publication #08-0011. Retrieved from http://www.ahrq.gov/research/findings/final-reports/ptmgmt/index.html

Petkov, J., Harvey, P., & Battersby, M. (2010). The internal consistency and construct validity of the partners in health scale: Validation of a patient rated chronic condition self-management measure. *Quality of Life Research, 19,* 1079-1085.

Ryan, P., & Sawin, K.J. (2009). The individual and family self-management theory: Background and perspectives on context, process and outcomes. *Nursing Outlook, 57,* 217-225.

Schilling, L.S., Grey, M., & Knafl, K.A. (2002). The concept of self-management of type 1 diabetes in children and adolescents: An evolutionary concept analysis. *Journal of Advanced Nursing, 37*(1), 87-99.

Tang, T.S., Funnell, M.M., Gillard, M., Nwankwo, R., & Heisler, M. (2011). Training peers to provide ongoing diabetes self-management support (DSMS): Results from a pilot study. *Patient Education and Counseling, 85,*160-168.

Yank, V., Laurent, D., Plant, K., & Lorig, K. (2013). Web-based self-management support training for health professionals: A pilot study. *Patient Education and Counseling, 90*(1), 29-37.

# CHAPTER 7

# Nursing Process (Proxy for Monitoring and Evaluation)

*Traci S. Haynes, MSN, RN, CEN*
*Sheila A. Haas, PhD, RN, FAAN*
*Beth Ann Swan, PhD, CRNP, FAAN*

## Learning Outcome Statement

The purpose of this chapter is to enable the reader to use the required steps in the nursing process when performing in the role of the registered nurse (RN) in Care Coordination and Transition Management (CCTM).

## Learning Objectives

After reading this chapter, the RN working in the CCTM role will be able to:

- Outline the steps of the nursing process and how the steps promote critical thinking.
- Identify the skills necessary for application of the nursing process in ambulatory care.
- Apply the nursing process in ambulatory care.
- Explain how to determine if outcomes are achieved.
- Explain adaptations and additions to the steps in the nursing process required when performing as an RN in CCTM.
- Demonstrate the knowledge, skills, and attitudes required for the nursing process dimension (see Table 1).

## Competency Definitions

"Nursing is the protection, promotion, and optimization of health and abilities, prevention of illness and injury, alleviation of suffering through the diagnosis and treatment of human response, and advocacy in the care of individuals, families, communities, and populations" (American Nurses Association [ANA], 2014a, para. 1).

"The common thread uniting different types of nurses who work in varied areas is the nursing process – the essential core of practice for the registered nurse to deliver holistic, patient-focused care" (ANA, 2014b, para. 1).

The nursing process is an adaptation of the scientific method and involves five steps (ANA, 2014b):

*Assessment.* A registered nurse (RN) uses a systematic, dynamic way to collect and analyze data about a client, the first step in delivering nursing care. Assessment includes not only physiological data, but also psychological, sociocultural, spiritual, economic, and lifestyle factors as well.

*Diagnosis.* The nursing diagnosis is the nurse's clinical judgment about the client's response to actual or potential health conditions or needs. The diagnosis reflects not only what the patient is experiencing, but also specification of possible causes of the experience.

*Plan.* Based on the assessment and diagnosis, the nurse, in collaboration with the patient and/or family, sets measurable and achievable short and long-range goals for a patient. Assessment data, diagnosis, and goals are written in the patient-centered plan of care that also reflects the patient's values and preferences, so that nurses as well as other health professionals caring for the patient have access to it for continuity of care.

*Implementation.* Evidence-based nursing care is implemented according to the individualized patient plan of care. This ensures continuity of care for the patient. Care is documented in the patient's medical record.

*Evaluation.* Both the patient's status and the effectiveness of the nursing care must be evaluated continuously against expected outcomes of care and the plan of care and modified as needed.

The nursing process as defined above is the basic critical thinking method used by all nurses working in the ambulatory care setting. Therefore, the Application of the Nursing Process in Ambulatory Care authored by Kathy Kesner, MS, RN, CNS, and Wanda Mayo, MSN, RN, CPN, for the *Core Curriculum for Ambulatory Care Nursing* (Kesner & Mayo, 2013) has been reproduced and adaptations added to reflect expectations of the RN performing within the Care Coordination and Transition Management (CCTM) role. Please note the Institute of Medicine's (2010) recommendations and provisions of the Patient Protection and Affordable Care Act (2010) have expanded expectations of care planning such that there is now a separate dimension of the RN in CCTM role named Patient-Centered Care Planning (Chapter Five) that delineates assessments, interventions, and outcomes of the planning phase of the nursing process; so readers are referred to this chapter to understand expectations of RNs in CCTM in the care planning dimension.

Collaborative and interprofessional approaches significantly impact the role of the nurse in the provision of nursing care. Critical thinking is an essential nursing competency, and is applied to every step of the nursing process. Planning and implementation are based on scientific principles and evidence-based practice that are congruent with the overall plan of care. A goal for patient/family education is to empower the patient and family to be involved in assessments, planning, interventions, and evaluation of effectiveness pertaining to the management of his or her care. Outcomes are based on the evidence and established goals of care and are measured in the evaluation portion of the nursing process.

## I. The Nursing Process

A. Definition of the nursing process.
   1. Is guided by critical thinking.
   2. Leads to accurate and thorough data collection.
   3. Involves the integration of data and information at every step.
   4. Provides an organized framework for the delivery of nursing care.
   5. Is theory and research-based.
   6. Is not static, fixed, or linear.
   7. Provides a feedback loop until the patient's diagnosis(es) is/are resolved.
   8. Includes documentation, a crucial step in the process that has at times been identified as an additional step in the process (Healthcare Information and Management Systems, 2012).

B. The nursing process steps.
   1. Assessment.
   2. Diagnosis.
   3. Plan.
   4. Implementation.
   5. Evaluation.

C. Critical thinking: problem-solving and decision making are crucial skills for a nurse. Critical thinking is an essential nursing competency. Critical thinking in nursing is an essential component of professional accountability and quality nursing care. Critical thinkers in nursing exhibit these habits of the mind: confidence, contextual perspective, creativity, flexibility, inquisitiveness, intellectual integrity, intuition, open-mindedness, perseverance, and reflection. Critical thinkers in nursing practice the cognitive skills of analyzing, applying standards, discriminating, information seeking, logical reasoning, predicting, and transforming knowledge (Scheffer & Rubenfeld, 2000).
   1. There is no single, agreed upon definition of critical thinking. Benner, Hughes, and Sutphen (2008) discussed three main definitions.
      a. Bittner and Tobin's (1998) definition discussed critical thinking as being "influenced by knowledge and experience, using strategies such as reflective thinking as a part of learning to identify the issues and opportunities, and holistically synthesize the information in nursing practice" (p. 268).
      b. Scheffer and Rubenfeld (2000) discussed critical thinking in nursing as an essential component of professional accountability and quality nursing care. Critical thinkers in nursing exhibit these habits of the mind: confidence, contextual perspective, creativity, flexibility, inquisitiveness, intellectual integrity, intuition, open-mindedness, perseverance, and reflection. Critical thinkers in nursing practice the cognitive skills of analyzing, applying standards, discriminating, information seeking, logical reasoning, predicting, and transforming knowledge.
      c. The National League for Nursing Accreditation Commission (2002) defined critical thinking as: "the deliberate nonlinear process of collecting, interpreting, analyzing, drawing conclusions about, presenting, and evaluating information that is both factually and belief based. This is demonstrated in nursing by clinical judgment, which includes ethical, diagnostic, and therapeutic dimensions and research" (p. 8).
   2. Activities of the nurse require other types of thinking skills, such as clinical reflection (one asks questions of practices that need reform) and clinical reasoning (one reasons through a situation as it changes, taking into account context and concerns of the patient and family). Critical thinking is sometimes used to represent the myriad ways nurses interact with information and ideas (Benner, Sutphen, Leonard, & Day, 2010).
   3. Critical thinking is applied to every step in the nursing process (Maiocco, 2010).
      a. Assessment: Are the data complete?
      b. Diagnosis: What else could be happening? Is there more than a single problem affecting the patient and family?
      c. Plan: What are the goals for this patient? Has the patient shared in the establishment of these goals? What are the best interventions to meet these goals?
      d. Implementation: Can the patient tolerate the intervention? Should the intervention be altered to meet the needs of the patient? If so, will it still be effective?
      e. Evaluation: Did the interventions achieve the desired outcomes? Do more data need to be collected?

D. Assessment: systematic collection of data to determine the patient's health status and to identify any actual or potential health problems (Nettina, 2006). Through the assessment process, the deliberate collection of data is obtained by interviewing, observing, and examining the patient for evidence of health problems and risk factors. Incomplete or inaccurate data can lead to errors in decision making. In the assessment phase of the nursing process, obtaining, classifying, and organizing data is the main function of critical thinking (Nettina, 2006).
   1. Assessment occurs each time a patient enters the care system, whether in person, on the telephone, through electronic communications, or via remote technological monitoring.
   2. Situations in which assessment occurs:
      a. Comprehensive (such as pre-admission or pre-operative).
         (1) The RN in CCTM will complete a patient record review prior to the patient visit to identify needs and review/develop/update a plan of care.
      b. Problem-focused (symptomatic visit or call).
      c. Emergency assessment (triage).
      d. Time-lapsed reassessment: chronic care management. Continuously monitoring responses to treatment.
         (1) The RN in CCTM will assess patient and family's understanding of the condition and treatment plan; as well as the ability to manage care over time.
         (2) The RN in CCTM will continuously assess and stratify at-risk patients as high, moderate, or low risk.
   3. Assessment includes:
      a. Collection of data: continues with each nurse-patient interaction. Evidence-based assessment tools are available to collect both objective and subjective data. For more information on assessment tools, see Chapter Five: Patient-Centered Care Planning.
         (1) Objective: data are observed directly or indirectly through measurement or physical examination using sight, touch, sound, and smell. Includes collection of data about the body, the mind, and the environment.
         (2) Subjective: data that are stated, described, and verified by the patient and family through verbal and nonverbal communication. Can be collected during interviews, and portray the patient's and family's point of view. Subjective data include the patient's feelings, perceptions, and concerns.
      b. Verification of data to validate the understanding of the problem and determine all information is factual and complete.
         (1) Confirm observations through interview and examination.
         (2) Review data collected to identify if more in-depth or additional information is necessary using critical thinking skills.
         (3) Document data in a systematic manner.
      c. Organization and analysis of data to prioritize potential or actual problems by clustering data to identify patterns and assist with making inferences.
      d. Prediction, detection, prevention, and control of outcomes.
         (1) Consider cultural, spiritual, and environmental factors.
         (2) Assess patient and family wishes, strengths, and limitations.
      e. Documentation of data to form a database to communicate with other members of the health care team.

E. Diagnosis: organize, synthesize, and summarize assessment data (Nettina, 2006). The analysis results in the identification of the patient's problems, which may be expressed as nursing diagnoses. A nursing diagnosis includes the etiology and forms the basis for the plan of care. According to the North American Nursing Diagnosis Association (NANDA, 2009), a nursing diagnosis is a clinical judgment about individual, family, or community responses to actual or potential health problems/life processes. Nursing diagnoses provide the basis for selection of nursing interventions to achieve outcomes for which the nurse is accountable.
   1. Analyzes and synthesizes data collected for problem identification.
      a. Classifies data, grouping significant and related data.
      b. Creates a list of suspected problems.
      c. Identifies problems that must be managed by physicians or advanced practice nurses, or another member of the health care team (Alfaro-LeFevre, 2005).
      d. Rules out similar problems using critical thinking skills.
      e. Determines risk factors that must be managed.
      f. Identifies resources, strengths, and areas for health promotion.
   2. Defines the patient's problems, and problem characteristics and etiology.
      a. Development of nursing diagnosis may employ one of the 12 ANA-recognized terminologies that support nursing practice such as the

NANDA diagnoses, definitions, and classification.
    (1) Excludes all nonnursing diagnoses.
    (2) Includes environmental stressors.
    (3) Includes data identified during assessment.
3. The nurse is accountable for actions that occur within the scope of the nursing diagnosis framework.
4. The nursing diagnosis provides criteria for quality improvement through review and evaluation.
5. Nursing diagnoses are intended to improve communication between health care professionals.
   a. The RN in CCTM will integrate nursing diagnoses in the comprehensive plan of care used by the interdisciplinary care team.

F. Plan: prioritizes identified nursing diagnoses, and identifies the action the nurse should take to achieve the desired goals and outcomes. It is aimed at solving or alleviating the problems identified in the assessment process by setting realistic goals that are clear, concise, and established with the patient and family and in conjunction with the primary care provider and other members of the health care team. The plan is based on the patient and family's values, preferences, and needs and includes short and long-term patient-centered goals, strategies for outcome achievement, and nursing measures for the delivery of care (Lewis, Sheehan, & Jessie, 2014; Smith, Duell, & Martin, 2008).
1. A plan of care (Alfaro-LeFevre, 2005).
   a. Promotes communication among caregivers.
   b. Provides continuity of care.
   c. Directs care and documentation.
   d. Includes advocacy by promoting the patient's right to autonomy.
   e. Incorporates evidence.
   f. Is patient- and family-centered.
2. Clarification of goals and outcomes are guided by the use of:
   a. Protocols.
      (1) Provide basis for consistency.
      (2) Describe steps and actions in exact order.
      (3) Delineate responsibilities.
      (4) Do not supersede clinical judgment.
   b. Guidelines.
      (1) Based on standards of care that guide nursing actions.
      (2) Based on current best evidence.
      (3) Aimed at achieving outcomes.
      (4) Do not supersede clinical judgment.
   c. Patient and family preference.
      (1) Based on own values and concerns.
      (2) Readiness to change/motivation.
      (3) Do not supersede clinical judgment.
   d. Patient outcomes: reflected in expected changes in the patient.
      (1) Should be specific, measurable, attainable, realistic, time sensitive, and reportable.
      (2) Allow the nurse as well as the patient/family to evaluate outcome achievement and re-evaluate the plan of care as needed.

G. Implementation: refers to priority nursing actions performed to accomplish a specified goal. Coordinates activities of the patient, family, nursing team, and other health care professionals (Nettina, 2006), and is the action component of the nursing process.
1. Nursing interventions.
   a. May involve delegation.
      (1) The RN in CCTM will communicate with other members of the health care team.
   b. Assess patient response pre and post-action.
   c. Weigh risks and consequences of each action.
   d. Resolve, prevent, or manage problems.
   e. Promote optimum sense of physical, psychological, and spiritual well-being.
      (1) The RN in CCTM will use motivation interviewing technique honoring patient autonomy.
   f. Include safety measures: The Joint Commission National Patient Safety Goals and other safety needs.
2. Nursing Interventions may employ one of the 12 ANA-recognized terminologies that support nursing practice such as the Nursing Intervention Classification, which describes the interventions and treatments nurses perform (Bulechek, Butcher, & Dochterman, 2008).
   a. Include independent and collaborative interventions.
   b. Are used by nurses in all settings.
   c. Include illness treatment, illness prevention, and health promotion.
   d. The fifth edition includes 542 research-based interventions (Bulechek et al., 2008).
   e. Updated every 4 years.
   f. Linked to NANDA nursing diagnoses.
3. Medically directed interventions include:
   a. Administering medications.
   b. Administering IV solutions.
   c. Providing wound care or other procedures.
   d. Carrying out other orders as directed by a physician, physician's assistant, advanced practice nurse, or other person authorized to write orders.

4. Prior to performing a procedure, the nurse:
   a. Reviews the procedure, intervention, protocol, or guideline.
   b. Educates the patient and family.
   c. Allows time for questions.
   d. Documents understanding through "teach back" technique.
   e. Ensures the safety of the patient.

H. Evaluation: the nurse analyzes the patient outcomes. The nurse assesses the patient's response to the plan of care by determining the effectiveness of the actions and the degree of goal attainment. If the patient is not satisfied, the plan is revised. Critical thinking questions at this time would be: "Have the patient's goals been met?" "Did the status of the problem change with the interventions?" "What else can be done to assist the patient?"

1. Collect assessment data.
   a. Compare the patient's actual outcome with expected outcomes to determine to what extent the goals have been met.
   b. Include the patient, family, and other health care team members in the evaluation.
   c. Identify alterations that need to be made in the goals and in the nursing plan of care.
   d. RN in CCTM may collect data during face-to-face encounters or during telephonic encounters.
2. Nursing outcomes may employ one of the 12 ANA-recognized terminologies that support nursing practice such as the Nursing Outcomes Classifications, a standardized classification for patient outcomes to evaluate the effects of nursing interventions (Donahue & Brighton, 1998).
   a. Developed for use in all settings and with all patient populations.
   b. Provide a list of indicators to evaluate patient status in relation to outcomes.
   c. Yield more information than just whether or not a goal was achieved.
   d. Linked to NANDA.
   e. Continually updated based on new research and published in a 4-year cycle.
3. Evaluation is an ongoing process. The professional nurse will continue all steps of the nursing process until all patient goals and outcomes are met to the nurse's and patient's satisfaction.
   a. The RN in CCTM will utilize structured monitoring to measure both patient and health care team performance, and communicate performance to both the patient and health care team.

**Table 1.**
**Nursing Process: Knowledge, Skills, and Attitudes for Competency**

| **Evidence-Based Practice (EBP)** | | | |
|---|---|---|---|
| Integrate best current evidence with clinical expertise and patient/family preferences and values for delivery of optimal health care (Cronenwett et al., 2007). | | | |
| **Knowledge** | **Skills** | **Attitudes** | **Sources** |
| Demonstrate knowledge of basic scientific methods and processes.<br>Describe EBP to include the components of research evidence, clinical expertise, and patient/family values. | Participate effectively in appropriate data collection and other research activities.<br>Adhere to institutional review board (IRB) guidelines.<br>Base individualized care plan on patient values, clinical expertise, and evidence. | Appreciate strengths and weaknesses of scientific bases for practice.<br>Value the need for ethical conduct of research and quality improvement.<br>Value the concept of EBP as integral to determining best clinical practice. | Cronenwett et al., 2007 |
| Differentiate clinical opinion from research and evidence summaries.<br>Describe reliable sources for locating evidence reports and clinical practice guidelines. | Read original research and evidence reports related to area of practice.<br>Locate evidence reports related to clinical practice topics and guidelines. | Appreciate the importance of regularly reading relevant professional journals. | Cronenwett et al., 2007 |
| Explain the role of evidence in determining best clinical practice.<br>Describe how the strength and relevance of available evidence influences the choice of interventions in provision of patient-centered care. | Participate in structuring the work environment to facilitate integration of new evidence into standards of practice.<br>Question rationale for routine approaches to care that result in less-than-desired outcomes or adverse events. | Value the need for continuous improvement in clinical practice based on new knowledge. | Cronenwett et al., 2007 |
| Discriminate between valid and invalid reasons for modifying evidence-based clinical practice based on clinical expertise or patient/family preferences. | Consult with clinical experts before deciding to deviate from evidence-based protocols. | Acknowledge own limitations in knowledge and clinical expertise before determining when to deviate from evidence-based best practices. | Cronenwett et al., 2007 |
| **Quality Improvement** | | | |
| Use data to monitor the outcomes of care processes and use improvement methods to design and test changes to continuously improve the quality and safety of health care systems (Cronenwett et al., 2007). | | | |
| **Knowledge** | **Skills** | **Attitudes** | **Sources** |
| Describe approaches for changing processes of care. | "Design a small test of change in daily work (using an experiential learning method such as Plan-Do-Study-Act).<br>Practice aligning the aims, measures, and changes involved in improving care.<br>Use measures to evaluate the effect of change." | Value local change (in individual practice or team practice on a unit) and its role in creating joy in work.<br>Appreciate the value of what individuals and teams can do to improve care. | Cronenwett et al., 2007 |

*continued on next page*

**Source Note:** Cronenwett et al. (2007) reprinted from *Nursing Outlook, 55*(3), 122-131, with permission from Elsevier.

**Table 1. (continued)**
**Nursing Process: Knowledge, Skills, and Attitudes for Competency**

| Safety | | | |
|---|---|---|---|
| Minimize risk of harm to patients and providers through both system effectiveness and individual performance (Cronenwett et al., 2007). | | | |
| **Knowledge** | **Skills** | **Attitudes** | **Sources** |
| Delineate general categories of errors and hazards in care.<br>Describe factors that create a culture of safety (such as open communication strategies and organizational error-reporting systems). | Communicate observations or concerns related to hazards and errors to patients, families, and the health care team.<br>Use organizational error-reporting systems for near-miss and error reporting. | Value own role in preventing errors. | Cronenwett et al., 2007 |
| Describe processes used in understanding causes of error and allocation of responsibility and accountability (such as root cause analysis and failure mode effects analysis). | Actively participates in analyzing errors and designing system improvements.<br>Engage in root cause analysis rather than blaming when errors or near misses occur. | Value vigilance and monitoring (even of own performance of care activities) by patients, families, and other members of the health care team. | Cronenwett et al., 2007 |
| Discuss potential and actual impact of national patient safety resources, initiatives, and regulations. | Use national patient safety resources for own professional development and to focus attention on safety in care settings. | Value relationship between national safety campaigns and implementation in local practices and practice settings. | Cronenwett et al., 2007 |
| **Patient-Centered Care** | | | |
| Recognize the patient or designee as the source of control and full partner in providing compassionate and coordinated care based on respect for patient's preferences, values, and needs (Cronenwett et al., 2007). | | | |
| **Knowledge** | **Skills** | **Attitudes** | **Sources** |
| Demonstrate comprehensive understanding of the concepts of pain and suffering, including physiologic models of pain and comfort. | Assess presence and extent of pain and suffering.<br>Assess levels of physical and emotional comfort.<br>Elicit expectations of patient and family for relief of pain, discomfort, or suffering.<br>Initiate effective treatments to relieve pain and suffering in light of patient values, preferences, and expressed needs. | Recognize personally held values and beliefs about the management of pain or suffering.<br>Appreciate the role of the nurse in relief of all types and sources of pain or suffering.<br>Recognize patient expectations influence outcomes in management of pain or suffering. | Cronenwett et al., 2007 |

*continued on next page*

**Table 1. (continued)**
**Nursing Process: Knowledge, Skills, and Attitudes for Competency**

| Patient-Centered Care (continued) | | | |
|---|---|---|---|
| **Knowledge** | **Skills** | **Attitudes** | **Sources** |
| Integrate understanding of multiple dimensions of patient-centered care:<br>• Patient/family/community preferences, values.<br>• Coordination and integration of care.<br>• Information, communication, and education.<br>• Physical comfort and emotional support.<br>• Involvement of family and friends.<br>• Transition and continuity.<br>Describe how diverse cultural, ethnic, and social backgrounds function as sources of patient, family, and community values. | Elicit patient values, preferences, and expressed needs as part of clinical interview, implementation of care plan, and evaluation of care.<br>Communicate patient values, preferences, and expressed needs to other members of health care team.<br>Provide patient-centered care with sensitivity and respect for the diversity of human experience. | Value seeing health care situations 'through patients' eyes.<br>Respect and encourage individual expression of patient values, preferences, and expressed needs.<br>Value the patient's expertise with own health and symptoms.<br>Seek learning opportunities with patients who represent all aspects of human diversity.<br>Recognize personally held attitudes about working with patients from different ethnic, cultural, and social backgrounds.<br>Willingly support patient-centered care for individuals and groups whose values differ from own. | Cronenwett et al., 2007 |
| Examine how the safety, quality, and cost effectiveness of health care can be improved through the active involvement of patients and families.<br>Examine common barriers to active involvement of patients in their own health care processes.<br>Describe strategies to empower patients or families in all aspects of the health care process. | Remove barriers to presence of families and other designated surrogates based on patient preferences.<br>Assess level of patient's decisional conflict and provide access to resources.<br>Engage patients or designated surrogates in active partnerships that promote health, safety and well-being, and self-care management. | Value active partnership with patients or designated surrogates in planning, implementation, and evaluation of care.<br>Respect patient preferences for degree of active engagement in care process.<br>Respect patient's right to access to personal health records. | Cronenwett et al., 2007 |
| **Nursing Process** | | | |
| **Knowledge** | **Skills** | **Attitudes** | **Sources** |
| Know questions to ask and cues to look for regarding physical, psychological, and social readiness to learn. (Assessment)<br>Identify questions to ask to holistically design an integrated care plan that encompasses a variety of care methods to provide patients with complex care needs with the resources needed to maintain the highest level of function. (Assessment and Diagnosis)<br>Have awareness of known risk factors that place a patient at risk for rehospitalization or exacerbation and utilizes knowledge and critical thinking to identify actions to mitigate risk. (Diagnosis and Plan) | Use techniques that invite/engage patient and significant others in learning.<br>Use techniques to assess learning such as "teach back."<br>Identify full range of medical, functional, social, and emotional problems that increase patient's risk of adverse health events.<br>Monitor patients for progress and early signs of problems.<br>Utilize data collection and analysis to design interventions to improve patient outcomes. | Demonstrate creativity in planning appropriate learning experiences for patients and significant others.<br>Value the services available to patients by delivering services that facilitate beneficial, efficient, safe, and high-quality patient experiences and improve patient health care outcomes. | Boult et al., 2008 |

*continued on next page*

**Table 1. (continued)**
**Nursing Process: Knowledge, Skills, and Attitudes for Competency**

| Nursing Process (continued) | | | |
|---|---|---|---|
| **Knowledge** | **Skills** | **Attitudes** | **Sources** |
| Understand the importance of instilling confidence in patients and caregivers regarding their ability to manage future transitions. (Plan and Implementation) | Competence in medication review and reconciliation, experience in helping patients communicate their needs to different health care professionals, and ability to shift from doing things for patients to encouraging them to do as much as possible independently.<br>Ability to impart skills to patients and caregivers for effectively communicating care needs during subsequent encounters. | Value the importance of empowering patients with knowledge and self-confidence to self-manage safely through care transitions. | Coleman et al., 2006 |
| Know the information and clinical skills needed to support and teach the patient in his or her process of self-management. (Implementation) | Use evidence-based clinical guidelines to direct a patient's care.<br>Use effective communication within the context of a trusting, therapeutic relationship.<br>Can assess the cognition/aptitude of a patient and readiness to learn.<br>Able to set clear expectations, goals, and boundaries from the beginning. | Require flexibility, creativity, and an understanding all patients learn differently.<br>Require the ability to stick with a patient over the "long haul," as this could be a relationship that needs to be in place for years. | Epping-Jordan et al., 2004 |
| Understand illness and chronic care management of specific disease. (Plan and Implementation)<br>Understanding of and ability to utilize community resources effectively. (Implementation) | Effective communication and leadership.<br>Be able to provide patient with skills to overcome barriers and cope with chronic illness. | Ability to be a confident and compassionate leader in a patient's health care experience.<br>Commitment and longevity. | Glasgow et al., 2002 |
| Understand the goals of patient-centered care and community resources that are available and appropriate. (Plan and Implementation) | Ability to link people with resources and other team members. | Holistic team approach is necessary. | Grumbach et al., 2009 |

*continued on next page*

Table 1. (continued)
Nursing Process: Knowledge, Skills, and Attitudes for Competency

| Nursing Process (continued) | | | |
|---|---|---|---|
| **Knowledge** | **Skills** | **Attitudes** | **Sources** |
| Knowledge of teaching and coaching strategies to support patient and caregiver self-management skills "in areas of medication management, condition management, and patient confidence about what was required of them during the transition" (p. 1826). (Implementation and Evaluation)<br>Knowledge of personal health record tool. (Implementation and Evaluation) | Teach patients how to utilize and update personal health record tool.<br>Teach and coaches patient and caregiver self-management skills.<br>Teach so "patient schedules and completes follow-up visit with primary care provider or specialist and is prepared to be an active participant in interactions" (p. 1824). | "Recognizing and supporting the key roles that patients and their caregivers play in improving care transitions…" (p. 1826).<br>Value greater involvement of patient and families in care transitions to improve outcomes/decrease re-admissions. | Coleman et al., 2006 |
| Knowledge in use of nursing process in home setting.<br>Understand sources of evidence-based nursing interventions. (Implementation) | Perform comprehensive nursing assessment.<br>Create care plan/care guide. | Value evidence-based practice and lifelong learning. | Leff et al., 2009 |
| Demonstrate awareness of effective team communication methods and nursing role within team. (Implementation and Evaluation) | Utilize effective communication methods.<br>Function competently within own scope of practice as a member of the health care team. | Value nurse role and scope of practice as part of multidisciplinary team. | Manderson et al., 2011 |
| Demonstrate understanding of various electronic medical record features and use, including personal health records. (Assessment, Diagnosis, Plan, Implementation, Evaluation) | Navigate the electronic health record and document and plan patient care in an electronic health record.<br>Employ communication technologies to coordinate care for patients and communicate with patients. | Value technologies that support clinical decision making, communication with patients, and care coordination.<br>Protect confidentiality of protected health information in electronic health records. | Manderson et al., 2011 |
| Knowledge of evidence-based coaching and shared decision making methods. (Plan, Implementation, and Evaluation) | Intervene in effective method (some face-to-face) and setting to provide self-management support. | Value involvement of patient and families in shared decision making.<br>Recognize value of face-to-face patient interactions in developing a therapeutic relationship. | Motheral, 2011 |
| Knowledge of structured assessment tools. (Assessment) | Utilize evidence-based tools for assessment and care planning. | | Muender et al., 2000 |
| Describe methods to incorporate patients and family caregiver beliefs, values, and needs into care planning. (Plan, Implementation, and Evaluation) | Develop patient and family caregiver-centered care plan. | Belief patient and family perspectives and participation are important in developing an effective care plan. | Naylor et al., 2011 |

*continued on next page*

**Table 1. (continued)**
**Nursing Process: Knowledge, Skills, and Attitudes for Competency**

| Nursing Process (continued) | | | |
|---|---|---|---|
| **Knowledge** | **Skills** | **Attitudes** | **Sources** |
| Know all aspects of the patient's disease, treatment, and support. (Assessment, Diagnosis, Plan, Implementation, Evaluation) | Critical thinking.<br>Manages the care process.<br>Development and communication of the care plan.<br>Timely needs assessment.<br>Assessment for symptoms and provision of interventions or other required management.<br>Information provision.<br>Ability to develop therapeutic relationships. | Belief it is the nurses' responsibility to navigate the health care system for the patient. | Nutt & Hungerford, 2010 |
| Knowledge of chronic illness and needs of transitional care.<br>Knowledge regarding patient education and adult learning theory (assessing patients and teaching what patients need; involving them in their plan of care).<br>Knowledge of motivational interviewing skills to foster behavior change. | Ability to assess patients and caregivers to determine learning needs; build upon strengths. | Open and accepting attitude toward patients; coaching. | Coleman et al., 2007<br>Coleman & Berenson, 2004 |
| Evidence-based, clinical guidelines of care for defined chronic conditions.<br>Interdependence of clinical conditions.<br>Medication indications, interactions, side effects, refill management, and safe administration.<br>"Six domains of practice activity that are critical to the quality of care in a medical home:<br>1. organizational capacity,<br>2. chronic condition management,<br>3. care coordination,<br>4. community outreach,<br>5. data management,<br>6. quality improvement" (p. 783). | Advocate for patient and family needs.<br>Communication, teaching.<br>Use of survey instruments for data collection and data analysis. | Holistic, family-centered philosophy.<br>Patient as partner.<br>Adaptable to changing patient needs and complexity. | Berry et al., 2011 |

 

## References


Alfaro-LeFevre, R. (2005). *Applying nursing process a tool for critical thinking* (6th ed.). Philadelphia, PA: Lippincott, Williams & Wilkins

American Nurses Association (ANA). (2014a). *What is nursing?* Retrieved from http://www.nursingworld.org/EspeciallyForYou/What-is-Nursing

American Nurses Association (ANA). (2014b). *The nursing process.* Retrieved from http://www.nursingworld.org/EspeciallyForYou/What-is-Nursing/Tools-You-Need/Thenursingprocess.html

Benner, P., Hughes, R., & Sutphen, M. (2008). Clinical reasoning, decision-making, and action: Thinking critically and clinically. In R. Hughes (Ed.), *Patient safety and quality: An evidence-based handbook for nurses.* Retrieved from http://www.ahrq.gov/professionals/clinicians-providers/resources/nursing/resources/nurseshdbk/nurseshdbk.pdf

Benner, P., Sutphen, M., Leonard, V., & Day, L. (2010). *Educating nurses: A call for radical transformation.* Stanford, CA: Jossey-Bass.

Berry, S., Soltau, E., Richmond, N.E., Kieltyka, R.L., Tran, T., & Wiliams, A. (2011). Care coordination in a medical home in post-Katrina New Orleans: Lessons learned. *Maternal and Child Health Journal, 15*(6), 782-793.

Bittner, N., & Tobin, E. (1998). Critical thinking: Strategies for clinical practice. *Journal of Nursing Staff Development, 14,* 267-272.

Boult, C., Reider, L., Frey, K., Leff, B., Boyd, C.M., Wolff, J.L., ... Scharfstein, D. (2008). Early effects of "guided care" on the quality of health care for multimorbid older persons: A cluster-randomized controlled trial. *The Journals of Gerontology. Series A, Biological Sciences and Medical Sciencies, 63*(3), 321-327.

Bulechek, G.M., Butcher, H.K., & Dochterman, J.M. (Eds.). (2008). *Nursing interventions classification* (5th ed.). St. Louis, MO: Mosby.

Coleman, E.A., & Berenson, R. (2004). Lost in transition: Challenges and opportunities for improving the quality of transitional care. *Annals of Internal Medicine, 141,* 533-536.

Coleman, E.A., Parry, C., Chalmers, S., Chugh, A., & Mahoney, E. (2007). The central role of performance improvement in improving the quality of transitional care. *Home Health Care Service Quarterly, 26*(4), 93-104.

Coleman, E.A., Parry, C., Chalmers, S., & Min, S.J. (2006). The care transitions intervention: Results of a randomized controlled trial. *Archives of Internal Medicine, 166*(17), 1822-1828.

Cronenwett, L., Sherwood, G., Barnsteiner, J., Disch J., Johnson, J., Mitchell, P., ... Warren, J. (2007). Quality and safety education for nurses. *Nursing Outlook, 55*(3), 122-131.

Donahue, M.P., & Brighton, V. (1998). Nursing outcome classification: Development and implementation. *Journal of Nursing Care Quality, 12*(5).

Epping-Jordan, J.E., Pruitt, S.D., Bengoa, R., & Wagner, E.H. (2004). Improving the quality of health care for chronic conditions. *Quality & Safety in Health Care, 13*(4), 299-305.

Glasgow, R.E., Funnell, M.M., Bonomi, A.E., Davis, C., Beckham, V., & Wagner, E.H. (2002). Self-management aspects of the improving chronic illness care breakthrough series: Implementation with diabetes and heart failure teams. *Annals of Behavioral Medicine, 24*(2), 80-87

Grumbach, K., Bodenheimer, T., & Grundy, P. (2009). *The outcomes of implementing patient-centered medical home interventions: A review of the evidence on quality, access and costs from recent prospective evaluation studies.* San Francisco, CA: UCSF Center for Excellence in Primary Care. Retrieved from http://familymedicine.medschool.ucsf.edu/cepc/pdf/outcomes%20of%20pcmh%20for%20White%20House%20Aug%202009.pdf

Healthcare Information and Management Systems. (2012). *Nursing informatics.* Retrieved from http://www.himss.org/library/nursing-informatics/?navItemNumber=16520

Institute of Medicine. (2010). *The future of nursing: Leading change, advancing health* (1st ed.). Washington, DC: National Academies Press.

Kesner, K., & Mayo, W. (2013). Application of the nursing process in ambulatory care. In C.B. Laughlin (Ed.), *Core curriculum for ambulatory care nursing* (3rd ed., pp. 191-215). Pitman, NJ: American Academy of Ambulatory Care Nursing.

Leff, B., Reider, L., Frick, K.D., Scharfstein, D.O., Boyd, C.M., Frey, K., ... Boult, C. (2009). Guided care and the cost of complex healthcare: A preliminary report. The *American Journal of Managed Care, 15*(8), 555-559.

Maiocco, G. (2010). *Nursing process.* Retrieved from http://www.scribd.com/doc/58356419/Bedside-Nursing-Process-Notes

Manderson, B., McMurray, J., Piraino, E., & Stolee, P. (2011). Navigation roles support chronically ill older adults through healthcare transitions: A systematic review of the literature. *Health & Social Care in the Community, 20*(12), 113-127. doi:10.1111/j.1365-2524.2011.01032.x.

Motheral, B.R. (2011). Telephone-based disease management: Why it does not save money. *American Journal of Managed Care, 17*(1), e10-16.

Muender, M.M., Moore, M.L., Chen, G.J., & Sevick, M.A. (2000). Cost-benefit of a nursing telephone intervention to reduce preterm and low-birth weight births in an African American clinic population. *Preventive Medicine,* 30(4), 271-276.

National League for Nursing Accreditation Commission. (2002). *Accreditation manual.* Retrieved from http://www.nlnac.org/Manual%20&%20IG/2003_manual_TOC.htm

Naylor, M.D., Aiken, L.H., Kurtzman, E.T., Olds, D.M., & Hirschman, K.B. (2011). The care span: The importance of transitional care in achieving health reform. *Health Affairs* (Millwood), *30*(4), 746-754.

Nettina, S.M. (Ed.) (2006). *Lippincott manual of nursing practice* (8th ed.). New York, NY: Lippincott, Williams & Wilkins.

North American Nursing Diagnosis Association (NANDA). (2009). *Nursing diagnoses: Definitions and classification 2009-2011.* Philadelphia, PA: Author.

Nutt, M., & Hungerford, C. (2010). Nurse care coordinators: Definitions and scope of practice. *Contemporary Nurse, 36*(1-2), 71-81.

Patient Protection and Affordable Care Act. (2010). Public Law 111-1148, §2702, 124 Stat. 119, 318-319.

Scheffer, B.K., & Rubenfeld, M.G. (2000). A consensus statement on critical thinking in nursing. *Journal of Nursing Education, 39*(8), 352-359.

Smith, S., Duell, D., & Martin, B. (2008). *Clinical nursing skills: Basic to advanced skills* (6th ed.). Upper Saddle River, NJ: Prentice Hall Health.

Toth-Lewis, J.M., Sheehan, K.T., & Jessie, A.T. (2014). Patient-centered care planning. In S. Haas, B.A. Swan, & T. Haynes (Eds.), *Care coordination and transition management core curriculum* (pp. 47-63). Pitman, NJ: American Academy of Ambulatory Care Nursing.


## Additional Readings


Heaslip, P. (2008). *Critical thinking: To think like a nurse.* Retrieved from http://www.criticalthinking.org/pages/critical-thinking-and-nursing/834

Neuspiel, D.R. (2011). *Peak flow rate measurement.* Retrieved from http://emedicine.medscape.com/article/1413347-overview

# CHAPTER 8

# Teamwork and Collaboration

*Denise Hannagan, MSN, MHA, RN-BC*
*Mary Anne Bord-Hoffman, MN, RN-BC*
*Kathy Mertens, MN, MPH, RN*

## Learning Outcome Statement

The purpose of this chapter is to enable the reader to integrate the American Academy of Ambulatory Care Nursing professional practice standards to the registered nurse (RN) in the Care Coordination and Transition Management (CCTM) role in ambulatory care by applying effective teamwork and collaboration skills and overcoming barriers to produce quality and effective patient outcomes.

## Learning Objectives

After reading the chapter, the RN working in the CCTM role will be able to:

- Define teamwork and collaboration.
- Integrate the American Academy of Ambulatory Care Nursing Professional Practice Standards with the RN in CCTM role.
- Identify the importance of teamwork and collaboration and the effects on patient care processes and outcomes.
- Describe evidence-based strategies that support teamwork including overcoming common barriers.
- Describe the role of the RN in CCTM within a team.
- Demonstrate how the RN in CCTM practices the knowledge, skills, and attitudes required for teamwork and collaboration (see Table 1).

## Competency Definitions

The terms *teamwork* and *collaboration* are often used interchangeably though there can be significant differences in the meaning of each term. Collaboration, for example, can occur between strangers who may be combining their labors for different and even conflicting ends. Teamwork implies a structure among people who know something about each other and their competencies. Teamwork also implies members are working toward a common end, though each team member has distinct roles in reaching that end. Notwithstanding the potential differences in these terms, we will treat the terms interchangeably and will use the following definition. Teamwork in health care is a "dynamic process involving two or more health professionals with complementary backgrounds and skills, sharing common health goals and exercising concerted physical and mental effort in assessing, planning, or evaluating patient care. This is accomplished through interdependent collaboration, open communication and shared decision-making. This in turn generates value-added patient, organizational and staff outcomes" (Xyrichis & Ream, 2007, p. 238).

The Institute of Medicine (IOM, 2000; 2001) has noted the American health care system is not yet adequately equipped to deliver chronic care with consistently positive effect, in part because there has been a focus on acute illness. Effective care of those with chronic conditions and diseases, the IOM notes, requires careful attention not only to *what* care is delivered but also to *how* it is delivered. Moreover, it is necessary to appreciate that care is given not just to the patient, but also to caregivers and families. To make the necessary changes, the IOM says professionals need to use skills that build relationships with patients and their peers. The most critical way in which the *what* and *how* of care coordination and transition management will be carried out effectively is through the building of strong inter-professional teams (Interprofessional Education Collaborative [IPEC], 2011). While there is a general need to deploy effective teams to serve those with chronic conditions and diseases, recent legislation has added to the urgency with which professionals in the ambulatory and other settings across the care continuum must acquire the knowledge, skills, and values associated with highly effective teams. Both the American Recovery and Reinvestment Act of 2009 and the Patient Protection and Affordable Care Act of 2010 are stimulating new approaches to providing care. A common element of these new approaches, of which the "medical home" model is just one example, is that they depend on inter-professional teamwork and on team-based care. Furthermore, legislation from Washington is pressuring the reconsideration of the concept of health and the relationship of primary care to that concept. The centrality of community is a theme across nearly all of the major health care reform laws that have emerged in recent years. Accountability in primary care for population health management of chronic disease goes beyond individuals and extends to the health care community in its entirety. There is a sharing of roles and responsibilities between health care delivery professionals and public health professionals across several domains, including health promotion, primary prevention, care, and behavioral change. Members of these two groups must work in a coordinated manner on behalf of patients, families, and communities. The responsibilities of such teams extend to maintaining healthy environments and responding to public health emergencies, not just to provision of primary care. Health care reform requires health care professionals connect within the community to work for the good of patients, families, and communities as responsible members of inter-professional teams (IPEC, 2011). Responding to the emerging changes in the structure of health care in the context of community, the IOM, in its report *The Future of Nursing* (2010), emphasized nurses must play a key role not just as members of inter-professional teams, but also as leaders within those teams. The role of collaboration and coordination of care across a variety of settings is part of the role of nurses and are needed to prepare nurses for coordination and collaboration (IOM, 2010). The knowledge, skills, and attitudes (KSAs) needed for nurses to undertake and participate in their role on inter-professional teams are described in Table 1. The KSAs are dependent upon one's own competence as a nurse and the ability to work with others, realizing team members all have differing levels of competencies. Team members, who exhibit qualities of open and honest communication, create an environment of mutual respect that supports shared decision making. Quality patient care will be the result.

Recent work by Mitchell and colleagues (2012) described basic principles and values to guide and accelerate team-based care effectiveness. As part of a Best Practices Innovation Collaborative, Mitchell and associates synthesized previous work, developed the team-based principles and values, and then conducted interviews of team-based health care practices to further develop and validate efforts. This set of principles of team-based care is among their work products (see Figure 1).

Additionally, five personal values identifying and characterizing the most effective members of well-functioning teams included honesty, discipline, creativity, humility, and curiosity (Mitchell et al., 2012). Among examples were putting a high value on effective communication and transparency, carrying out duties even when inconvenient, excitement in tackling problems creatively, reliance on others to help recognize and avoid failures regardless of hierarchy, and dedication to using insights for continuous improvement (Mitchell et al., 2012).

**Figure 1.**
**Principles of Team-Based Health Care**

| **Shared Goals** |
|---|
| The team – including the patient and, where appropriate, family members or other support persons – works to establish shared goals that reflect patient and family priorities, and can be clearly articulated, understood, and supported by all team members. |
| **Clear Roles** |
| There are clear expectations for each team member's functions, responsibilities, and accountabilities, which optimize the team's efficiency and often make it possible for the team to take advantage of division of labor, thereby accomplishing more than the sum of its parts. |
| **Mutual Trust** |
| Team members earn each other's trust, creating strong norms of reciprocity and greater opportunities for shared achievement. |
| **Effective Communication** |
| The team prioritizes and continuously refines its communication skills. It has consistent channels for candid and complete communication, which are accessed and used by all team members across all settings. |
| **Measurable Processes and Outcomes** |
| The team agrees on and implements reliable and timely feedback on successes and failures in both the functioning of the team and achievement of the team's goals. These are used to track and improve performance immediately and over time. |

**Source:** Mitchell et al. (2012). Reprinted with permission.

## I. Collaboration and Teamwork and Professional Practice Standards

The discussion of the scope of practice for professional ambulatory care nursing included collaboration as one of the main characteristics: "ambulatory care nurses address, in partnership and collaboration with other health care professionals, patients' wellness, acute illness, chronic disease, disability and end-of-life needs" (American Academy of Ambulatory Care Nursing [AAACN, 2010, p. 6). From this, the standards flow and the components of teamwork and collaboration can be seen throughout the individual standards themselves.

A. Application of professional standards to the RN in CCTM dimension of Teamwork and Collaboration Standard 11: Collaboration (AAACN, 2010, p. 31).

1. Communicate openly with patients, caregivers, and other health care professionals regarding patient care and the nurse's role in the provision of care.
2. Partner with patients, caregivers, and appropriate health care providers and resource agencies to develop a documented plan of nursing care that is focused on outcomes and decisions related to treatment modalities and the delivery of services.
3. Unite the colleagues to achieve positive clinical and other changes that improve patient and organizational outcomes.
4. Use effective professional communication skills and tools to acquire and disseminate relevant information to patients, caregivers, and health care providers across the care continuum.

B. Application of Standard 10: Collegiality (AAACN, 2010, p. 30).
1. Participate in systematic peer review as appropriate.
2. Share knowledge and skills with peers and colleagues from such activities as patient care conference or presentation at formal or informal meetings.
3. Serve as mentors for new staff, colleagues, and students.
4. Provide peers with constructive feedback regarding their practice and/or role performance.
5. Interact with peers and colleagues to enhance one's own professional nursing practice and/or role performance.
6. Maintain compassionate and caring relationships with peers and work colleagues.
7. Proactively recognize the needs of others, using positive interactions and creative solutions to achieve effective outcomes.
8. Contribute to a positive, supportive, and healthy nursing work environment that is conducive to the education and professional growth of nursing staff and other health care providers.
9. Use effective professional communication skills and tools to acquire and disseminate relevant information to patients, caregivers, and health care providers across the care continuum.

C. Application of Standard 12: Ethics (AAACN, 2010, p. 32).
1. Participate in the identification and resolution of ethical concerns, utilizing professional codes of ethics within professional parameters.
2. Actively engage in identifying and resolving the ethical concerns of patients, colleagues, or system.
3. Utilize the principles contained in the American Nurses Association Social Policy Statement and Code of Ethics.
4. Preserve patients' rights to confidentiality, privacy, and self-determination within legal, regulatory, and ethical parameters.
5. Ensure that patient care reflects the cultural, spiritual, intellectual, age, educational, and psychosocial differences of individual patients, families, groups, and communities.
6. Disclose to supervisory personnel any observed illegal or incompetent practice and decision made by real or potentially impaired health care personnel.
7. Advocate for informed decision making by the patient or legally designated representative.
8. Ensure that patients have opportunities to voice opinions regarding care and services received and have these issues reviewed and resolved, without fear of recrimination.
9. Educate and support patients in developing skills for self-efficacy.
10. Project a therapeutic, professional approach to patients, colleagues, and staff, maintaining appropriate role boundaries.

D. Application of Standard 14: Environment (AAACN, 2010, p. 35).
1. Ensure there is an effective match between nurse self-competencies and patient care needs.
2. Supervise, counsel, and evaluate the practice of non-professional nursing staff.
3. Ensure the space accommodates the delivery of nursing care and the administrative activities associated with the patient encounter and that age-specific, disability-specific, and diverse population needs are considered and accommodated.

## II. Importance of Teamwork and Collaboration and How They Affect Patient Care Processes and Outcomes

TeamSTEPPS™ is an evidence-based teamwork system aimed at optimizing patient outcomes through improving communication and teamwork skills among team members across the health care delivery system. It was developed by the Department of Defense's (DoD) Patient Safety Program in collaboration with the Agency for Healthcare Research and Quality (AHRQ). The evidence upon which TeamSTEPPS is based demonstrates that effective teamwork and collaboration result in (AHRQ, 2013):

A. Improved patient safety, fewer errors.
B. Improved patient outcomes.
C. Improved process outcomes.
D. Improved patient satisfaction.
E. Improved satisfaction among team members.

## III. Key Elements for Effective Teamwork and Evidence-Based Strategies that Support it, Including Methods to Overcome Common Barriers

A. Characteristics of high-performing teams (AHRQ, 2013; Mitchell et al., 2012; Salas, Sims, & Burke, 2005).
   1. Clear roles and responsibilities.
      a. Patient as key member of team.
      b. "There are clear expectations for each team member's functions, responsibilities, and accountabilities which optimize the team's efficiency and often make it possible for the team to take advantage of division of labor, thereby accomplish more than sum of its parts" (Mitchell et al., 2012, p. 9).
         (1) Members of different backgrounds.
         (2) Discipline-specific knowledge and skills.
         (3) Influenced by cultural and organizational norms.
      c. Best utilization of resources, staff skills, and interests.
         (1) Interdependent actions needed, including coordination of steps and hand-offs (Edmonson, 2012).
         (2) Decrease unnecessary redundancy.
         (3) Consider assignments (e.g., assigning all physician's patients to same care coordinator, attributed to physician willingness to work with care coordinators) (Brown, Peikes, & Peterson, 2013).
      d. Focus all practice personnel to work at their highest education and potential (Bodenheimer & Laing, 2007). Performing duties that are permitted by the license and/or education and allowing other team members to concentrate or delegate other duties.
   2. Clear, valued, and shared vision.
      a. Common purpose.
      b. High-functioning teams work to establish shared goals that reflect patient, family, caregiver priorities that can be understood and supported by all team members (Mitchell et al., 2012).
   3. Shared mental models.
      a. Provide information (e.g., provide information before being asked).
      b. Provide support (e.g., provide assistance before being asked).
      c. Team initiative (e.g., provide guidance or makes suggestions to team members).
      d. Communicate situational awareness (e.g., provide situation updates) (Westli, Johnsen, Eid, Rasten, & Brattebo, 2010).
   4. Shared training and meetings across organizations or departments.
      a. Local and collaborative learning meetings (between hospitals and primary care staff help to increase understanding of each other's competencies and how each other's actions impact quality and safety at transitions (Hesselink et al., 2013).
   5. Mutual trust and confidence.
      a. Manage conflict.
      b. Strong team orientation.
      c. Team's collective ability to succeed.
      d. Team member's psychological safety and willingness to take interpersonal risks (Edmonson, 2012).
   6. Strong team leadership.
      a. Two types of leaders (AHRQ, 2013).
         (1) Designated: the person assigned to lead and organize a designated core team, establish clear goals and facilitate open communication and teamwork among team members.
         (2) Situational: any team member who has the skills to manage the situation at hand.
            (a) Recognize when team communication is not functioning well and act as facilitator (Mitchell et al., 2012).
      b. Behaviors of effective team leaders (AHRQ, 2013).
         (1) Organize the team.
         (2) Articulate clear goals.
         (3) Empower members to speak up and challenge, when appropriate.
         (4) Actively promote and facilitate good teamwork.
         (5) Skillful at conflict resolution.
         (6) Project positive role model behaviors.
      c. Effective communication, regular feedback.
         (1) Set high standard for consistent, clear professional communication.
         (2) Communicate often and at right time.
         (3) "Speaks up:" candid communication that includes asking questions, seeking feedback, talking about errors, asking for help, offering suggestions, sharing ideas, and discussing problems and concerns (Edmonson, 2012).
      d. Training on skills for effective communication.
         (1) Conflict resolution.
         (2) Use active listening and closed-loop communication.
      e. Continually strive to learn.
      f. Multiple methods for team communication and coordination (AHRQ, 2013; Bodenheimer & Laing, 2007; O'Malley, Tynan, Cohen, Kemper, & Davis, 2009).

(1) Huddles, briefings, and team meetings.
(a) Routine and ad hoc.
(b) Happens on a consistent basis, whether daily, weekly or other project-specific timing (Edmonson, 2012).
(c) Reflection that includes use of explicit observations, questions, and discussions of processes and outcomes (Edmondson, 2012).
(2) Weekly caseload reviews to assess new cases and patient progress (RN care manager with caseload consultant physicians) (McGregor, Lin, & Katon, 2011).
(3) Remote teams – virtual communication methods.
(4) Electronic medical record standards.
(5) Patient portals for RN in CCTM and patient communication.
(6) Enlisting patient assistance with information transfer.

g. Optimize resources available to the team and patients. Listing, maintaining, and accessing resources available at all times and considering:
(1) Community-based, state, national, and institutional resources.
(2) Access, dependent on location and cost.

h. Measurable processes and outcomes.
(1) Have the communication and resources assisted or placed a barrier in the process and producing a positive patient outcome.

7. Barriers and methods to overcome.

a. Unclear or blurred roles and responsibilities of team, variation in communication styles and practices, different levels of experience and training (Kelly & Penney, 2011) multiple team members and duplication of services (inefficiency). Role transitions, both self-identity and group identity (Cadmus, Reis, & Turner, 2013).
(1) Documentation of team roles at each transition setting and member responsibilities; clarify new roles upfront.
(2) Create new interdisciplinary workflows (Cadmus et al., 2013).
(3) Conduct orientation for team members.
(4) Develop orientation materials; conduct training and document attendance.
(5) Establish forums and methods for ongoing communication and follow-up.
(6) Develop buddy system for new team members.

b. Team development processes are forming, storming, norming, and performing (Scholtes, Joiner, & Streibel, 2003).
(1) Team forming can include participants of different expertise, cultures, and ethics and defining and establishing roles and objectives.
(2) Storming occurs when members are establishing their position within the team, which can cause conflict and the need for clarification.
(3) The norming stage is where a clear agreement as to the roles and goals of the team, and collaboration and group interaction, is more apparent.
(4) A performing team shares the vision, team members identify areas for continued refinement and goals are achieved. This process allows for:
(a) Set clear objectives for team.
(b) Establish process and structure.
(c) Build good relationships among team members.
(d) Develop conflict-resolution skills.
(e) Celebrate successes.

c. Communication challenges between team members or across care sites.
(1) Act as a facilitator to resolve.
(2) Act as coach for patients and families not accustomed to or comfortable with active team membership and communication (Mitchell et al., 2012).
(3) Establish cross-site meetings or collaborative trainings to improve mutual understanding (Hesselink et al., 2013).

d. Resources change or are not available.
(1) Team members change, inconsistency of members.
(a) Nurses can perform many roles of other health care team members "in the event that these team members are not available, such as nutrition education, medication education, psychosocial support, and clerical duties" (Paschke, 2013, p. 36).
(b) Change management and adaptability of the members to interact with multiple roles, disciplines, incoming, and outgoing members are required to maintain an ongoing productive flow of work being done by the team.
(c) Maintaining a log, minutes, examples, and communications that have occurred will provide an overview to assist new members joining at any time in the process.
(2) Community resources change.

e. Unclear processes.
    (1) Establish guidelines, timeframes, and deadlines to provide clear guidance.
    (2) Utilize tools such as guidelines, protocols, workflow documents, or checklists.
    (3) If unavailable, initiate/develop a guideline/workflow to provide clear direction, especially in tasks that are complex.

f. Lack of information, coordination, sharing, and follow-up.
    (1) Establish standardized methods of sharing information that best allows team members to participate.
        (a) Huddles.
        (b) Briefs and debriefs.
        (c) Case conferencing-telephone, other virtual method or in-person face-to-face.
        (d) Webinars.

g. Collaborative behaviors required when working in teams create tensions and conflict.
    (1) Leaders should identify the nature of the conflict, model good communications, identify shared goals, and encourage difficult conversations (Edmonson, 2012).
    (2) Give timely and constructive feedback, providing examples as applicable.
    (3) May be instances of "productive conflict" which, while must be moderated, may encourage climate of discussion and innovation (Edmonson, 2012).

h. Team member fear of being seen as ignorant, incompetent, negative, or disruptive.
    (1) Methods to create climate of psychological safety among team members (Edmonson, 2012).
        (a) Develop trust and respect; if a mistake is made or someone asks for help, others will not penalize.
        (b) Emphasize group tasks and what is needed to perform well.
        (c) Team leaders should be accessible and approachable, invite participation, use direct language, acknowledge limits of current knowledge, be willing to display fallibility, set boundaries and hold people accountable, and highlight failures as learning opportunities.
    (2) Benefits of psychological safety: encourages speaking up, enables clarity of thought, supports productive conflict, promotes innovation, and increases accountability (Edmonson, 2012).

## IV. How the RN in CCTM Participates as a Member or Leader of a Team

A. Assumes leadership role and displays positive and patient-focused care.

B. Articulates RN in CCTM role as part of interdisciplinary team.

C. Facilitates role transitions by participating in creation of new interdisciplinary workflows for team (Cadmus et al., 2013).

D. Encourages teamwork from all members; builds relationships.

E. Includes and engages the patient, family, caregivers, or others as participants in the design and delivery of service or care.

F. Facilitates communication and trust between team members.
    1. Meeting with providers in person, talking with providers when accompanying patients on visits, and serving as a communication hub between visits, making sure providers have key information (Brown et al., 2013). Takes time to become familiar with each other's roles, responsibilities, expectations, practices, and backgrounds (transitions across settings) (Hesselink et al., 2013; Kelly & Penney, 2011).

G. Mentors team members.

H. Practices and monitors accountability of all team members (Registered Nurses' Association of Ontario, 2006).

I. Provides other key domains of RN in CCTM practice: population health management, nursing process, patient-centered care planning, education and engagement of patient and family, coaching and counseling of patients and families, support for self-management, advocacy, and care setting communication and transitions (Haas et al., 2013).

**Table 1.**
**Teamwork and Collaboration: Knowledge, Skills, and Attitudes for Competency**

"Function effectively within nursing and inter-professional teams, fostering open communication, mutual respect and shared decision-making to achieve quality patient care" (Cronenwett et al., 2007, p. 122).

Teamwork and collaboration, has been identified as one of the dimensions of professional nursing care coordination and transition management (Haas, Swan, & Haynes, 2013). The development of knowledge, skills, and attitudes (KSAs) needed to incorporate teamwork and collaboration into practice can be guided by the table below.

| Knowledge | Skills | Attitudes | Sources |
|---|---|---|---|
| | **Team Development** | | |
| "Describe the process of team development and the roles and practices of effective teams" (p. 25). | "Communicate consistently the importance of teamwork in patient-centered and community-focused care" (p. 23).<br><br>Use practices "that support collaborative practice and team effectiveness" (p. 25).<br><br>"Contribute to the development of consensus on the ethical principles for guiding patient care and teamwork" (p. 25).<br><br>"Demonstrate high standards of ethical conduct in own contributions to team-based care" (p. 19).<br><br>"Act with honesty and integrity in relationships with patients, families, and other team members" (p. 19). | | Interprofessional Education Collaborative (IPEC), 2011 |
| Describe own strengths, limitations, and values in functioning as a member of a team. | Demonstrate awareness of own strengths and limitations as a team member.<br><br>Initiate plan for self-development as a team member.<br><br>Act with integrity, consistency, and respect for differing views. | Acknowledge own potential to contribute to effective team functioning.<br><br>Appreciate importance of intra- and inter-professional collaboration. | Cronenwett et al., 2007 |

*continued on next page*

**Source Note:** Cronenwett et al. (2007) reprinted from *Nursing Outlook, 55*(3), 122-131, with permission from Elsevier.

**Table 1. (continued)**
**Teamwork and Collaboration: Knowledge, Skills, and Attitudes for Competency**

| Knowledge | Skills | Attitudes | Sources |
|---|---|---|---|
| **Team Development** | | | |
| "Describe the impact of team-based practice" (p. 9). | | "Value the team approach to providing high quality care" (p. 9).<br><br>"Commit to being an effective team member" (p. 9).<br><br>"Commit to interprofessional and intraprofessional collaboration" (p. 10).<br><br>"Respect the boundaries of therapeutic relationships" (p. 12). | American Association of Colleges of Nursing (AACN), QSEN Education Consortium, 2012 |
| Describe ethics as a standard for professional ambulatory care nursing practice. | | | American Academy of Ambulatory Care Nursing AAACN, 2010 |
| **Knowledge** | **Skills** | **Attitudes** | **Sources** |
| **Team Roles** | | | |
| Describe scopes of practice and roles of health care team members.<br><br>Describe strategies for identifying and managing overlaps in team member roles and accountabilities.<br><br>Recognize contributions of other individuals and groups in helping patient/family achieve health goals. | Function competently within own scope of practice as a member of the health care team.<br><br>Assume role of team member or leader based on the situation.<br><br>Initiate requests for help when appropriate to situation.<br><br>Clarify roles and accountabilities under conditions of potential overlap in team member functioning.<br><br>Integrate the contributions of others who play a role in helping patient/family achieve health goals. | Value the perspectives and expertise of all health team members.<br><br>Respect the unique attributes that members bring to a team, including variations in professional orientations and accountabilities.<br><br>Respect the centrality of the patient/family as core members of any health care team. | Cronenwett et al., 2007 |

*continued on next page*

**Table 1. (continued)**
**Teamwork and Collaboration: Knowledge, Skills, and Attitudes for Competency**

| Knowledge | Skills | Attitudes | Sources |
|---|---|---|---|
| **Team Roles (continued)** | | | |
| | "Engage other health professionals – appropriate to the specific care situation – in shared patient-centered problem-solving" (p. 25).<br><br>"Communicate information with patients, families and healthcare team members in a form that is understandable, avoiding discipline-specific terminology when possible" (p. 23).<br><br>"Communicate one's roles and responsibilities clearly to patients, families and other professionals" (p. 21).<br><br>"Explain the roles and responsibilities of other care providers and how the team works together to provide care" (p. 21). | "Share accountability with other professions, patients, and communities for outcomes relevant to prevention and health care" (p. 25). | IPEC, 2011 |
| | "Partners effectively with key stakeholders and groups in care delivery to individuals, families and groups" (p. 531). | | Swider, Krothe, Reyes, & Cravetz, 2013 |
| "Describe strategies to integrate patients/families as primary members of the health team" (p. 10). | "Use patient engagement strategies to involve patients/families in the healthcare team" (p. 10).<br><br>"Work with team members to identify goals for individual patients and populations" (p. 9).<br><br>"Ensure inclusion of patients and family members as part of the team based on their preferences to be included" (p. 9). | "Value patients/families as the source of control for their health" (p. 10). | AACN, QSEN Education Consortium, 2012 |

*continued on next page*

**Table 1.**
**Teamwork and Collaboration: Knowledge, Skills, and Attitudes for Competency**

| Knowledge | Skills | Attitudes | Sources |
|---|---|---|---|
| **Communication** | | | |
| Analyze differences in communication style preferences among patients and families, nurses and other members of the health team.<br><br>Describe impact of own communication style on others.<br><br>Discuss effective strategies for communicating and resolving conflict. | Communicate with team members, adapting own style of communicating to needs of the team and situation.<br><br>Demonstrate commitment to team goals.<br><br>Solicit input from other team members to improve individual, and team performance. | Value teamwork and the relationships upon which it is based.<br><br>Value different styles of communication used by patients, families, and health care providers. | Cronenwett et al., 2007 |
| | | "Support the development of a safe team environment where issues can be addressed between team members and conflict can be resolved."<br><br>"Value conflict resolution as a means to improve team functioning." | AACN, QSEN Education Consortium, 2012, p. 9 |
| | "Give timely, sensitive, and instructive feedback to others about their performance on the team, responding respectfully as a team member to feedback from others."<br><br>"Listen actively, and encourage ideas and opinions of other team members."<br><br>Use "effective communication tools and techniques, including information systems and communication technologies, to facilitate discussions and interactions that enhance team function."<br><br>"Use respectful language appropriate for a given difficult situation, crucial conversation, or interprofessional conflict." | | IPEC, 2011, p. 23 |
| | Initiate actions to resolve conflict.<br><br>Contribute to resolution of conflict and disagreement. | | Cronenwett et al., 2007 |

*continued on next page*

**Table 1.**
**Teamwork and Collaboration: Knowledge, Skills, and Attitudes for Competency**

| Knowledge | Skills | Attitudes | Sources |
|---|---|---|---|
| **Impact of Team on Safety and Quality of Care** | | | |
| Describe examples of the impact of team functioning on safety and quality of care.<br><br>Explain how authority gradients influence teamwork and patient safety. | Follow communication practices that minimize risks associated with handoffs among providers and across transitions in care.<br><br>Assert own position/perspective in discussions about patient care.<br><br>Choose communication styles that diminish the risks associated with authority gradients among team members. | Appreciate the risks associated with handoffs among providers and across transitions in care. | Cronenwett et al., 2007 |
| Describe "the risks associated with handoffs among providers and across transitions of care." | | | AACN, QSEN Education Consortium, 2012, p. 10 |
| | Use process improvement strategies to increase the effectiveness of the interprofessional teamwork and team based care. | | IPEC, 2011, p. 25 |
| **Impact of Team on Systems** | | | |
| Identify system barriers and facilitators of effective team functioning.<br><br>Examine strategies for improving systems to support team functioning. | Lead or participate in the design and implementation of systems that support effective teamwork.<br><br>Engage in state and national policy initiatives aimed at improving teamwork and collaboration. | Value the influence of system solutions in achieving team functioning. | Cronenwett et al., 2007 |

## References


Agency for Healthcare Research and Quality (AHRQ). (2013). *TeamSTEPPS®: National implementation.* Retrieved from http://teamstepps.ahrq.gov/aboutnationalIP.htm

American Academy of Ambulatory Care Nursing (AAACN). (2010). *Scope and standards of practice for professional ambulatory care nursing.* Pitman, NJ: Author.

American Association of Colleges of Nursing (AACN), QSEN Education Consortium. (2012). *Graduate-level QSEN competencies, knowledge, skills and attitudes.* Retrieved from http://www.aacn.nche.edu/faculty/qsen/competencies.pdf

American Recovery and Reinvestment Act of 2009. (2009). Retrieved from http://www.fcc.gov/encyclopedia/american-recovery-and-reinvestment-act-2009

Bodenheimer, T., & Laing, B.Y. (2007). The teamlet model of primary care. *Annals of Family Medicine, 5*(5), 457-461.

Brown, R., Peikes, D., & Peterson, G.J. (2013). Six features of Medicare coordinated care demonstration programs that cut hospital admissions of high-risk patients. *Health Affairs, 31*(6), 1156-1166.

Cadmus, E., Reis, L., & Turner, B. (2013). Ever-evolving: Population care coordinators. *Nursing Management, 44*(12), 9-11.

Cronenwett, L., Sherwood, G., Barnsteiner, J., Disch, J., Johnson, J., Mitchell, P., … Warren, J. (2007). Quality and safety education of nurses. *Nursing Outlook, 55*(3), 122-131.

Edmonson, A. (2012). *Teaming: How organizations learn, innovate, and compete in the knowledge economy.* San Francisco, CA: Jossey-Bass.

Haas, S., Swan, B., & Haynes, T. (2013). Developing ambulatory care registered nurses competencies for care coordination. *Nursing Economic$, 31*(1), 43.

Hesselink, G., Vernooig-Dassen, M., Pijnenborg, L., Barach, P., Gademan, P., Dudzik-Urbaniak, E., … European HANDOVER Research Collaborative. (2013). Organizational culture an important context for addressing and improving hospital to community patient discharge. *Medical Care, 51*(1), 90-98.

Institute of Medicine (IOM). (2000). *To err is human: Building a safer health system.* Washington, DC: National Academies Press.

Institute of Medicine (IOM). (2001). *Crossing the quality chasm.* Washington, DC: National Academies Press.

Institute of Medicine (IOM). (2003). *Health professions education.* Washington, DC: National Academies Press.

Institute of Medicine (IOM). (2010). *The future of nursing: Leading change, advancing health.* Washington, DC: National Academies Press.

Interprofessional Education Collaborative (IPEC). (2011). *Core competencies for interporfessional collaborative practice.* Retrieved from www.aacn.nche.edu/education-resources/ipecreport.pdf

Kelly, N.M., & Penney, E.D. (2011). Collaboration of hospital case managers and home care liaisons when transitioning patients. *Professional Case Management, 16*(3), 128-136.

McGregor, M., Lin, E., & Katon, W. (2011). TEAMcare: An integrated multicondition collaborative care program for chronic illnesses and depression. *Journal of Ambulatory Care Management, 34*(2), 152-162.

Mitchell, P., Wynia, M., Golden, R., McNellis, B., Okun, S., Webb, C., … Von Kohorn, I. (2012). *Core principles and values of effective team-based health care.* Retrieved from http://www.iom.edu/Global/Perspectives/2012/TeamBasedCare.aspx

O'Malley, O., Tynan, A., Cohen, G., Kemper, N., & Davis, M. (2009). *Coordination of care by primary care physicians: Strategies, lessons and implications.* HSC Research Brief No. 12. Retrieved from http://www.hschange.com/CONTENT/1058/

Patient Protection and Affordable Care Act, 42 U.S.C. § 18001. (2010). Retrieved from https://www.healthcare.gov/

Paschke, S.M. (2013). Ambulatory care operations. In C.B. Laughlin (Ed.), *Core curriculum for ambulatory care nursing* (3rd ed., pp. 35-47). Pitman, NJ: American Academy of Ambulatory Care Nursing.

Registered Nurses' Association of Ontario. (2006). *Collaborative practice among nursing teams.* Toronto, Canada: Author.

Salas, E., Sims, D., & Burke, C. (2005). Is there a "Big Five" in teamwork? *Small Group Research, 36*(5), 555-599.

Scholtes, P., Joiner, B., & Streibel, B. (2003). *The team handbook.* Madison, WI: Oriel.

Swider, S.M., Krothe, K., Reyes, D., & Cravetz, M. (2013). The Quad council practice for competencies for public health nursing. *Public Health Nursing, 30*(6), 519-536.

Westli, H.K., Johnsen, B.H., Eid, J., Rasten, I., & Brattebo, G. (2010). Teamwork skillls, shared mental models, and performance in simulated trauma teams: An independent group design. *Scandinavian Journal of Trauma, Resuscitation and Emergency Medicine, 18,* 47.

Xyrichis, A., & Ream, E. (2007). Teamwork: A concept analysis. *Journal of Advanced Nursing, 62*(2), 232-241.


## Additional Reading


Manderson, B., McMurray, J., Piraino, E., & Stolee, P. (2011). Navigation roles support chronically ill older adults through healthcare transition: A systematic review of the literature. *Health and Social Care in the Community, 20*(2), 113-127.

# CHAPTER 9

# Cross-Setting Communications and Care Transitions

*Deborah E. Aylard, MSN, RN*
*Janet Fuchs, MBA, MSN, RN, NEA-BC*
*Stefanie Coffey, DNP, MBA, FNP-BC, RN-BC*

## Learning Outcome Statement

The purpose of this chapter is to enable the reader to demonstrate the knowledge, skills, and attitudes required for Cross-Setting Communication and Transitions in Care.

## Learning Objectives

Upon completion of this chapter, the registered nurse (RN) working in the Care Coordination and Transition Management (CCTM) role will be able to:

- Explain the concept of care transitions.
- Explain the communication deficiencies that commonly occur with care transitions.
- Define the role of the ambulatory care RN in CCTM in cross-setting communication and care transition.
- Identify key characteristics of effective communication for care transitions.
- Design and implement processes to provide sufficient, timely, and useful information necessary to achieve the successful patient care transitions.
- Analyze processes and identify improvement opportunities in cross-setting communication.
- Evaluate evidence and do small tests of change to improve cross-setting communication during care transitions.
- Demonstrate the knowledge, skills, and attitudes required for Cross-Setting Communication and Transitions in Care (see Table 1).

## Competency Definition

Effective utilization of communication skills to gain and transmit information, encourage team participation, leverage electronic medical record and other standard communication tools, and design and implement processes to provide sufficient, timely, and useful information necessary to achieve successful patient care transitions (Cronenwett et al., 2007).

Effective care transition communication is a basic expectation of quality patient care, yet negative events and risk exposures continue to occur due to poor communication during care transitions.

- Ineffective communication is the most frequently reported cause of sentinel events in U.S. hospitals (Dufault et al., 2010).
- The Institute of Medicine reported upwards of 80% of mistakes occur because of ineffective or absent communication (IOM, 2001).
- Poor communication among health care providers and the lack of shared information about patients are common causes of under-treatment, suboptimal therapy, adverse drug events, and hospital admissions or re-admissions (Carter et al., 2008).
- The potential for medical errors increases when more than one health care provider or site of care is involved in providing services to a patient (Clancy, 2008).
- 1 in 5 Medicare patients discharged from hospitals are re-admitted within 30 days (Robert Wood Johnson Foundation, 2013a, 2013b).
- 4 out of 5 patients are discharged from hospitals without direct communication with primary care provider (PCP) (Robert Wood Johnson, 2013a, 2013b).
- The Medicare Payment Advisory Committee (MedPac) estimated that up to 76% of rehospitalizations occurring within 30 days in the Medicare population are potentially avoidable (Institute for Healthcare Improvement [IHI], 2013a, 2013b).

Given the potential for adverse events and possible rehospitalization, cross-setting communication becomes a critical intervention to improve patient care quality and decrease cost (Cibulskis, Giardino, & Moyer, 2011). The need for cross-setting communication is further compounded by patient acuity, co-morbidities, decreasing lengths of stay, and increasing financial pressures.

The impact of nursing during care transitions is not fully understood or recognized. Effective communication during care transitions is not likely to be transformational until a culture and system is in place that supports bidirectional, interactive communication (Cibulskis et al., 2011). However, research into care transitions is intense and there are several models in practice that can provide guidance on standards and best practices for improving cross-setting communication.

An example of an effective cross-setting communication system occurs through contractual agreements between the Veterans Health Administration outpatient clinics (VAOPC) and selected Hospital Corporation of America (HCA) hospitals. This is accomplished by coordinating care through a Patient Aligned Care Team (PACT) Coordinator (PACTCC) at a VAOPC and the Veteran's Navigator/Case Manager at the HCA facility. The PACT model in the Veteran's Administration (VA) is analogous to the Patient-Centered Medical Home model utilized in non-VA settings. The VAOPC daily census report is sent securely to the PACTCCs who access patient information through the secure virtual HCA portal to retrieve hospital records. This access facilitates a timely, efficient method to enhance information sharing between the providers who provide care in the hospital and the PACT members (provider, nursing personnel, and clerical personnel) at the VA. Follow-up care is arranged through a post-hospital visit (face-to-face or virtual) for the veteran and immediate availability of medications is prioritized. With "real-time" accessibility of discharge medication lists, the pharmacy is able to perform medication reconciliation before medication errors can occur. In addition, the availability of care coordination between the navigator and PACTCC enables immediate home health consult and approval (Coffey, 2014).

## I. Transition of Care

A. A care transition is defined as a change in the level of service or location of providers of care as patients move within the health system (Kim & Flanders, 2013).

B. The care necessary during a transition is "a set of actions designed to ensure the coordination and continuity of healthcare as patients transfer between different levels of care and among a diverse range of providers, services and settings" (Gray et al., 2012, p. 1).

C. There may be multiple care transitions in the process of a patient's journey from, and return to, his or her home setting. Each one of these transitions requires communication among and across caregivers.

D. Care transitions require the effective transfer of information between settings and thus are highly dependent on effective communication for success (Cibulskis et al., 2011).

## II. Communication and Care Coordination

A. Definition.
   1. Donabedian (1982) describes care coordination as the "process by which the elements and relationships of medical care during any one sequence of care are fitted together in the overall design" (Wenger & Young, 2007, p. 285).
   2. This process is largely achieved through the use of communication.
   3. "Transitional care is defined as a broad range of time-limited services designed to ensure health care continuity, avoid preventable poor outcomes among at-risk populations, and promote the safe and timely transfer of patients from one level of care to another or from one type of setting to another" (Kim & Flanders, 2013, p. IT3-2).
      a. The hallmarks of transitional care are the focus on highly vulnerable, chronically ill patients throughout critical transitions in health and health care, and the emphasis on educating patients and family caregivers to address root causes of poor outcomes and avoid preventable rehospitalizations (Coleman & Boult, 2003).
   4. The core features of transitional care as defined by Naylor and Sochalski (2010) include:
      a. Comprehensive assessment of an individual's health goals and preferences; physical, emotional, cognitive, and functional capacities and needs; and social and environmental considerations.
      b. Implementation of an evidence-based plan of transitional care.
      c. Care that is initiated at hospital admission, but extends beyond discharge through home and telephone visits.
      d. Mechanisms to gather and share information across sites of care.
      e. Engagement of patients and family caregivers in planning and executing the plan of care.
      f. Coordinated services during and following the hospitalization by a health care professional with special preparation in the care of chronically ill people, often a master's-prepared nurse (Naylor & Sochalski, 2010).

B. Cross-setting communication challenges. The Center for Transforming Healthcare and others have identified a number of risk factors related to inadequate communication.
   1. Differing expectations between senders and receivers of information.
   2. Lack of teamwork and respect.
   3. Inadequate amount of time devoted to the hand-off.
   4. Lack of standardized process or procedure for a successful hand-off, such as the SBAR tool (The Joint Commission, 2013).

5. Direct involvement of primary care physicians during hospitalization has become less common and the involvement of multiple specialist providers more common (Cibulskis et al., 2011).
6. Failure to produce a timely discharge summary or transition document.
7. Lack of integrated or accessible electronic medical records (EMRs) (Bonner, Schneider, & Weissman, 2010).
8. Lack of longitudinal responsibility across setting (Bonner et al., 2010).
9. Failure to complete diagnostic testing, specialty visits, therapy (Kim & Flanders, 2013).
10. Lack of team-based approach to care across settings (Bonner et al., 2010).
11. Failure to re-engage primary care through a post-discharge office visit (Kim & Flanders, 2013).

## III. Communication and Continuity of Care

A. Needed care is uninterrupted and the success is dependent on the relatedness between the sequences (Wenger & Young, 2007).

B. Continuity of care has been defined as, "Care over time by a single individual or a team of health professionals" including "effective and timely communication of health care communication" (Donaldson, Yordy, Lohr, & Vanselow, 1996, p. 49).

## IV. Cross-Setting Communication Methods

A. Verbal.
   1. Pros.
      a. Direct.
      b. Allows for bidirectional conversation in real time.
   2. Cons.
      a. Inconsistent content.
      b. Varying communication styles and skill levels.
      c. Variable skill mix (RN, licensed practical nurse, medical assistant).

B. Written.
   1. Chart summaries.
   2. Health Information Exchange documents.
   3. Discharge summaries.
   4. Pros.
      a. Content can be standardized.
   5. Cons.
      a. Timeliness.
      b. Content may vary, be insufficient, or be overwhelming.
      c. Lack opportunity for bidirectional communication.

C. Electronic health record (American Academy of Family Physicians, 2014).
   1. Pros.
      a. Customizable and able to achieve standard format and content.
      b. Patient information easily shared across continuum of care if access available.
      c. Up-to-date medication and allergy lists.
      d. Order entry available on-site or remotely.
      e. Standardized order sets.
      f. Ability to develop and share patient plan of care and patient goals.
      g. Ability to identify team members and contact information.
      h. Able to trend data for patient monitoring and population management.
      i. Create patient-specific problem lists.
   2. Cons.
      a. Lack of universal design and access within and across systems.
      b. Content can be overwhelming (information overload) decreasing usefulness.
      c. Cost.
      d. Time required for training.

## V. Principles of Communication with Patients and Caregivers

A. Should begin prior to discharge from one setting to another.
   1. Considerations.
      a. Patient may be medicated.
      b. Disjointed instructions from multiple team members.
      c. Health literacy of patient and family.
      d. Lack of printed information to support verbal instructions.

B. Should be team based with members of health care team and patient, family, and significant others.

## VI. Communication Failures

A. Prospective cohort study published in 2003 found 19% of patients discharged from a single U.S. academic medical center had an adverse event within 2 weeks of hospital discharge; one-third could have been prevented and another third minimized (Kim & Flanders, 2013).

B. Ineffective transitions of care can lead to adverse outcomes and risk for patients as well as higher hospital re-admission rates and cost (Medicare Payment Advisory Commission, 2008).

C. Contributing problems.
   1. Medication injuries most prevalent.
      a. Polypharmacy.
      b. Nonfamiliar provider admits patient to hospital but does not provide post-hospital care.
      c. Medication reconciliation may be done, but patient/family does not know which prior drugs should be continued post discharge.
   2. Procedure related complications.
   3. Falls.

4. Re-admissions.
   a. Most undesired by patient, family, and hospital.
      (1) Frustration.
      (2) Increased cost.
      (3) Increased mortality and morbidity.
      (4) Loss of potential earnings.

## VII. Interventions

A. Assess current care transition process.
B. Evaluate existing evidence-based programs for adoption.
C. Build a coordinated acute care enterprise from admission to discharge to home or transfer to post-acute facility to post-discharge follow-up (Advisory Board, 2013).
   1. Multidisciplinary communication and collaboration from admission through discharge or transition.
D. Involvement of a consistent care team member who oversees all care transitions.
E. Structured hand-off reports with consistent content.
   1. Discharge checklist (Robert Wood Johnson Foundation, 2013a, 2013b).
   2. Engagement of all team members including patient and family.
F. Improved access to EMR systems or products.
   1. Standardized documentation.
   2. Simple, Health Insurance Portability and Accountability Act (HIPAA) compliant process, for obtaining appropriate use access.
G. Notification of PCP when patient experiences a care transition.
   1. Admission and discharge.
   2. Early and consistent primary care involvement.
H. Clear assignment of longitudinal responsibility for follow-up care and testing; shared accountability along continuum of care.
I. Building a culture of communication and team-based approach to patient care across disciplines.
J. Building capacity and process to achieve timely primary care re-engagement post-discharge.

## VIII. Care Transition Models

A. Care Transitions Intervention.
   1. Developed by Eric Coleman, MD, MPH.
   2. Looked at promoting effective and practical care transitions for vulnerable adults.
   3. Forged partnerships between hospitals and community-based organizations to facilitate seamless discharges.
   4. Provided patients with transition coaches who taught patients how to manage their complex medical conditions including medication management, maintenance of personal health records, importance of seeing their PCP post-discharge, and knowledgeable regarding red flags for their conditions.
B. Better Outcomes for Older Adults through Safe Transitions (Project BOOST).
   1. Developed by Society of Hospital Medicine (2010).
   2. Utilizes multidisciplinary mentors to work with patients and care providers as they transition from hospital to home.
   3. Identifies essential elements for discharge process, communication with PCP prior to discharge, telephone contact within 72 hours post-discharge, assess patients for discharge plan comprehension and adherence ("teach back") citation.
   4. BOOST tool incorporating the 8 Ps that are evidence-based predictors of unsuccessful transitions and can be used as a guide for information sharing in the transition process. These 8 Ps include:
      a. Problem medications (e.g., anticoagulants, insulin).
      b. Psychological concerns (e.g., depression).
      c. Principle diagnosis (e.g., cancer, stroke, diabetes).
      d. Polypharmacy (five or more routine medications).
      e. Patient support (absence of caregiver to assist post discharge).
      f. Poor health literacy (inability to demonstrate "teach back").
      g. Prior hospitalization (nonelective) within last 6 months.
      h. Palliative care (would you be surprised if the patient died within the next year?).
C. The Bridge Model (Illinois Transitional Care Consortium, n.d.).
   1. Developed and refined by Rush University Medical Center Older Adult Programs and Aging Care Connections.
   2. Utilizes master's-prepared social workers.
   3. Provides transitional care through intensive care coordination that starts in the hospital and continues after discharge.
   4. Bridge consists of three intervention phases.
      a. Pre-discharge: an in-hospital assessment to identify unmet needs and to set up community-based services (including medical provider linkages) prior to discharge.
      b. Post-discharge: secondary assessment made via phone call 2 days after discharge to identify and intervene on additional identified needs.
      c. Follow-up: conducted 30 days post-discharge to track participant's progress, address any emerging needs, and provide stable connection to services.
D. Guided Care (Boult, Karm, & Groves, 2008).
   1. Developed at the Johns Hopkins Bloomberg School of Public Health.

2. Focuses on coordinated, multidisciplinary, patient-centered, cost-effective teams.
3. Includes in-home nursing assessments, care planning, patient self-management, smooth transitions, access to community resources.

E. Geriatric Resources for Assessment and Care of Elders (GRACE) (Counsell, Callahan, Buttar, Clark, & Frank, 2006).
1. Includes a certified registered nurse practitioner and social worker to address health care needs of low-income seniors.
2. Develops individualized care plan, including GRACE-based protocols for care of the elderly.
3. Utilizes EMR and ongoing tracking system to monitor longitudinal progress.

F. Re-Engineered Discharge (Project RED).
1. Developed by Dr. Brian Jack of Boston University Medical Center and funded by the Agency for Healthcare Research and Quality.
2. A patient-centered, standardized approach to discharge planning.
3. Developed strategies to improve the hospital discharge process to promote patient safety and decrease re-admission rates.
4. Identified 12 discrete interventions or practices that reduce re-admissions.

G. State Action on Avoidable Rehospitalizations (IHI, 2013a).
1. Identified key changes in ideal transition to clinical office practice.
   a. Provide timely access to care following hospitalization.
   b. Develop standardized processes outlining expected content of communication, format, preferred method of communication, responsibility.
   c. Review anticipated discharges on a daily basis. Risk-stratify hospitalized patients into high-risk, moderate, low-risk categories.
   d. Adjust post-discharge care based upon risk.
   e. Complete post-discharge phone calls focusing on medication management, self-care, worsening symptoms; and action plan, date, and time for follow-up appointment.
   f. Schedule regular follow-up with hospitalist and PCP.
   g. Develop standardized process for communication between hospitalist and PCP.
   h. Prepare patient and clinical team prior to post-hospital visit.
      (1) Assure access for post-hospital appointments (carve outs, group visits for medium or low-risk patients).
      (2) Place reminder call to patient prior to post-hospital visit to remind patient of visit, need to bring medications, patient knowledge of available resources.
      (3) Communicate with home-care providers and case managers as appropriate prior to visit.
   i. Assess patient and review or revise plan of care.
      (1) Ask patient about health-related goals, medication reconciliation, instruct patient in self-management, explain warning signs, and how to contact help; hospitalist to compare admission medications to discharge medications.
      (2) Discuss end-of-life wishes as applicable.
      (3) Instruct patient in self-care management using "teach back."
   j. At conclusion of visit, communicate and coordinate ongoing plan of care.
      (1) Print reconciled dated medication list and provide a copy to patient and caregiver.
      (2) Ensure next visit is scheduled.

**Table 1.**
**Cross-Setting Communications and Transitions: Knowledge, Skills, and Attitudes for Competency**

| Communication | | | |
|---|---|---|---|
| "Understand and utilize communication skills with patients, team members, and across care transition settings to communicate effectively and build consensus" (Cronenwett et al., 2009, p. 341). | | | |
| **Knowledge** | **Skills** | **Attitudes** | **Sources** |
| Analyze own communication style.<br>Describe impact of own communication style on others.<br>Analyze differences in communication style preferences among patients and families, advanced practice nurses and other members of the health team. | Reflect, solicit feedback, and utilize assessment tools to gain insight into personal communication skills, areas for improvement, and techniques to bridge communication styles.<br>Initiate actions to resolve conflict.<br>Communicate respect for team member competence in communication. | Appreciate your impact on communication success.<br>Value different styles of communication. | Cronenwett et al., 2009 |
| Discuss principles of effective.<br>Describe basic principles of consensus building and conflict resolution.<br>Examine nursing roles in assuring coordination, integration, and continuity of care. | Assess own level of communication skill in encounters with patients and families through reflection and feedback.<br>Participate in building consensus or resolving conflict in the context of patient care.<br>Communicate care provided and needed at each transition in care. | Value continuous improvement of own communication and conflict resolution skills. | Cronenwett et al., 2007 |
| **Team Building and Collaboration** | | | |
| "Build, support and participate effectively within nursing and inter-professional teams, fostering open communication, mutual respect, and shared decision-making to achieve quality patient care during care transitions" (Cronenwett et al., 2007, p. 125). | | | |
| **Knowledge** | **Skills** | **Attitudes** | **Sources** |
| Describe examples of the impact of team functioning on safety and quality of care.<br>Analyze authority gradients and their influence on teamwork and patient safety. | Follow communication practices that minimize risks associated with handoffs among providers, and across transitions in care. | Appreciate the risks associated with handoffs among providers and across transitions in care. | Cronenwett et al., 2007 |

*continued on next page*

**Source Notes:** Cronenwett et al. (2007) reprinted from *Nursing Outlook, 55*(3), 122-131, with permission from Elsevier. Cronenwett et al. (2009) reprinted from *Nursing Outlook, 57*(6), 338-348, with permission from the author.

**Table 1. (continued)**
**Cross-Setting Communications and Transitions: Knowledge, Skills, and Attitudes for Competency**

| Team Building and Collaboration (continued) | | | |
|---|---|---|---|
| **Knowledge** | **Skills** | **Attitudes** | **Sources** |
| | Choose communication styles that diminish the risks associated with authority gradients among team members. Assert own position/ perspective and supporting evidence in discussions about patient care. | | |
| | Communicate regularly with patient, support teams, and providers to discuss plan of care. Demonstrate awareness of the complex patient with multi-specialty involvement.<br><br>Identify relationships and systems to provide an organized communication pathway between team members, Patient-Centered Medical Home (PCMH), patient, and caregivers.<br><br>Establish regular gathering of stakeholders to evaluate processes and design improvements. | Value the solutions obtained through systematic, inter professional collaborative efforts. | Cronenwett et al., 2009 |
| Analyze own strengths, limitations and values as a member of a team.<br><br>Describe scopes of practice and roles of all health care team members. | Demonstrate awareness of own strengths and limitations as a team member.<br><br>Continuously plan for improvement in use of self in effective team development and functioning.<br><br>Act with integrity, consistency and respect for differing views.<br><br>Function competently within own scope of practice as a member of the health care team.<br><br>Assume role of team member or leader based on the situation. | Acknowledge own contributions to effective or ineffective team functioning.<br><br>Respect the unique attributes that members bring to a team, including variation in professional orientations, competencies and accountabilities.<br><br>Respect the centrality of the patient/family as core members of any health care team. | Cronenwett et al., 2007 |

*continued on next page*

Table 1. (continued)
Cross-Setting Communications and Transitions: Knowledge, Skills, and Attitudes for Competency

| Team Building and Collaboration (continued) | | | |
|---|---|---|---|
| **Knowledge** | **Skills** | **Attitudes** | **Sources** |
| Analyze strategies for identifying and managing overlaps in team member roles and accountabilities. | Function as the primary point-of-contact for care coordination for the patient and the team, PCMH stakeholders, and other team leaders.<br><br>Guide the team in managing areas of overlap in team member functioning.<br><br>Solicit input from other team members to improve individual, as well as team performance.<br><br>Facilitate multi-disciplinary team meetings for care coordination and transitions of care.<br><br>Empower contributions of others who play a role in helping patients/ families achieve health goals. | | Cronenwett et al., 2009 |
| Identify system barriers and facilitators of effective team functioning.<br><br>Examine strategies for improving systems to support team functioning. | | Value the influence of system solutions in achieving team functioning. | Cronenwett et al., 2007 |
| Analyze strategies that influence the ability to initiate and sustain effective partnerships with members of nursing and inter-professional teams.<br><br>Analyze impact of cultural diversity on team functioning. | Initiate and sustain effective health care teams.<br><br>Communicate with team members, adapting own style of communicating to needs of the team and situation.<br><br>Lead or participate in the design and implementation of systems that support effective teamwork.<br><br>Engage in state and national policy initiatives aimed at improving teamwork and collaboration. | Appreciate importance of inter-professional collaboration.<br><br>Value collaboration with nurses and other members of the nursing team. | Cronenwett et al., 2009 |

continued on next page

**Table 1. (continued)**
**Cross-Setting Communications and Transitions: Knowledge, Skills, and Attitudes for Competency**

| Quality Improvement Using Evidence-Based Practice | | | |
|---|---|---|---|
| "Evaluate practice evidence and research, and use data to monitor the outcomes of care processes and improvement methods to design and test changes to continuously improve the quality and safety of health care systems" (Cronenwett et al., 2007, p. 126). | | | |
| **Knowledge** | **Skills** | **Attitudes** | **Sources** |
| Differentiate clinical opinion from research and evidence summaries<br><br>Describe reliable sources for locating evidence reports and clinical practice guidelines. | Read original research and evidence reports related to area of practice.<br><br>Locate evidence reports related to clinical practice topics and guidelines. | Appreciate the importance of regularly reading relevant professional journals. | Cronenwett et al., 2007 |
| Identify principles that comprise the critical appraisal of research evidence.<br><br>Summarize current evidence regarding major diagnostic and treatment actions within the practice specialty.<br><br>Determine evidence gaps within the practice specialty.<br><br>Describe strategies for learning about the outcomes of care in the setting in which one is engaged in clinical practice. | Critically appraise original research and evidence summaries related to area of practice.<br><br>Exhibit contemporary knowledge of best evidence related to practice specialty.<br><br>Promote research agenda for evidence that is needed in practice specialty.<br><br>Initiate changes in approaches to care when new evidence warrants evaluation of other options for improving outcomes or decreasing adverse events.<br><br>Seek information about outcomes of care for populations served in care setting.<br><br>Seek information about quality improvement projects in the care setting. | Value knowing the evidence base for practice specialty.<br><br>Value public policies that support evidence-based practice.<br><br>Appreciate that continuous quality improvement is an essential part of the daily work of all health professionals. | Cronenwett et al., 2009 |

*continued on next page*

 

**Table 1. (continued)**
**Cross-Setting Communications and Transitions: Knowledge, Skills, and Attitudes for Competency**

| Quality Improvement Using Evidence-Based Practice (continued) | | | |
|---|---|---|---|
| **Knowledge** | **Skills** | **Attitudes** | **Sources** |
| Describe the benefits and limitations of quality improvement data sources, and measurement and data analysis strategies. | Design and use databases as sources of information for improving patient care.<br>Select and use relevant benchmarks. | Appreciate the importance of data that allows one to estimate the quality of local care. | Cronenwett et al., 2009 |
| Describe processes used in understanding causes of error and allocation of responsibility and accountability (such as root cause analysis and failure mode effects analysis). | Participate appropriately in analyzing errors and designing system improvements.<br>Engage in root cause analysis rather than blame when errors or near misses occur. | Value vigilance and monitoring (even of own performance of care activities) by patients, families, and other members of the health care team. | Cronenwett et al., 2007 |
| Analyze the differences between micro-system and macro-system change (p. 344).<br>Understand principles of change management (p. 344).<br>Analyze the strengths and limitations of common quality improvement methods (p. 344).<br>Analyze potential and actual impact of national patient safety resources, initiatives and regulations" on care transitions. (p. 346). | Use principles of change management to implement and evaluate care processes at the micro-system level (p. 344).<br>Design, implement and evaluate tests of change in daily work (using an experiential learning method such as Plan-Do-Study-Act) (p. 344).<br>Align the aims, measures and changes involved in improving care (p. 344).<br>Use measures to evaluate the effect of change.<br>Use national patient safety resources to design and implement improvements in practice. | Appreciate the value of what individuals and teams can to do to improve care (p. 344).<br>Value local systems improvement (in individual practice, team practice on a unit, or in the macro-system) and its role in professional job satisfaction (p. 344).<br>Appreciate that all improvement is change but not all change is improvement (p. 344).<br>Value relationship between national patient safety campaigns and implementation in local practice and practice settings (p. 346). | Cronenwett et al., 2009 |

*continued on next page*

**Table 1. (continued)**
**Cross-Setting Communications and Transitions: Knowledge, Skills, and Attitudes for Competency**

| Informatics | | | |
|---|---|---|---|
| "Use and support the use of information and technology to communicate, manage knowledge, mitigate error, and support decision making" (Cronenwett et al, 2007, p. 129). | | | |
| **Knowledge** | **Skills** | **Attitudes** | **Sources** |
| Contrast benefits and limitations of common information technology strategies used in the delivery of patient care.<br>Evaluate the strengths and weaknesses of information systems used in patient care. | Participate in the selection, design, implementation and evaluation of information systems.<br>Communicate the integral role of information technology in nurses' work.<br>Model behaviors that support implementation and appropriate use of electronic health records.<br>Assist team members to adopt information technology by piloting and evaluating proposed technologies. | Value the use of information and communication technologies in patient care. | Cronenwett et al., 2009 |
| Formulate essential information that must be available in a common database to support patient care in the practice specialty.<br>Evaluate benefits and limitations of different communication technologies and their impact on safety and quality. | Promote access to patient care information for all professionals who provide care to patients.<br>Serve as a resource for how to document nursing care at basic and advanced levels.<br>Develop and utilize standard communication tools for care transitions based on evidence and available technology.<br>Develop safeguards for protected health information.<br>Champion communication technologies that support clinical decision-making, error prevention, care coordination, and protection of patient privacy.<br>Develop order sets, alerts and tools to aid in care transitions.<br>Advocate for a central documentation location, format and exchange process to improve care transitions. | Appreciate the need for consensus and collaboration in developing systems to manage information for patient care.<br>Value the confidentiality and security of all patient records. | Cronenwett et al., 2009 |

*continued on next page*

 

**Table 1. (continued)**
**Cross-Setting Communications and Transitions: Knowledge, Skills, and Attitudes for Competency**

| Informatics | | | |
|---|---|---|---|
| **Knowledge** | **Skills** | **Attitudes** | **Sources** |
| Describe and critique taxonomic and terminology systems used in national efforts to enhance interoperability of information systems and knowledge management systems. | Access and evaluate high quality electronic sources of healthcare information.<br>Participate in the design of clinical decision-making supports and alerts.<br>Search, retrieve, and manage data to make decisions using information and knowledge management systems.<br>Anticipate unintended consequences of new technology. | Value the importance of standardized terminologies in conducting searches for patient information.<br>Appreciate the contribution of technological alert systems.<br>Appreciate the time, effort, and skill required for computers, databases and other technologies to become reliable and effective tools for patient care. | Cronenwett et al., 2009 |

## References


Advisory Board Company, The. (2013). *Building the coordinated acute care enterprise: Critical transition points in the continuum of care.* Washington, DC: Author.

American Academy of Family Physicians. (2014). *Understanding features & functions of an EHR.* Retrieved from http://www.aafp.org/practice-management/health-it/product/features-functions.html

Bonner, A., Schneider, C.D., & Weissman, J.S. (2010). *Massachusetts strategic plan for care transitions.* Boston, MA: Massachusetts Executive Office of Health and Human Services.

Boult, C., Karm, L., & Groves, C. (2008). Improving chronic care: The "guided care" model. *Permanente Journal, 12*(1), 50-54.

Carter, B.L., Bergus, G.R., Dawson, J.D., Farris, K.B., Doucette, W.R., Chrischilles, E.A., & Hartz, A.J. (2008). A cluster randomized trial to evaluate physician/pharmacist collaboration to improve blood pressure control. *The Journal of Clinical Hypertension, 10*(4), 260-271.

Cibulskis, C.C., Giardino, A.P., & Moyer, V.A. (2011). Care transitions from inpatient to outpatient settings: Ongoing challenges and emerging best practices. *Hospital Practice, 39*(3), 128-139.

Clancy, C.M. (2008). Improving the safety and quality of care transitions. *AORN Journal, 88*(1), 111-113.

Coffey, S. (2013). *The Veterans Health Administration PCMH model: An ambulatory care pact.* Paper presented at the American Academy of Ambulatory Care Nursing Annual Conference, Las Vegas, NV.

Coleman, E., & Boult, C. (2003). Improving the quality of transitional care for persons with complex care needs. *Journal of the American Geriatrics Society, 51*(4), 556-557.

Counsell, S.R., Callahan, C.M. Buttar, A.B., Clark , D.O., & Frank, K.I. (2006). Geriatric resources for assessment and care of elders (GRACE): A new model of primary care for low income seniors. *Journal of American Geriatrics Society, 54*(7), 1136-1141.

Cronenwett, L., Sherwood, G., Barnsteiner, J., Disch, J., Johnson, J., … Warren, J. (2007). Quality and safety education for nurses. *Nursing Outlook, 55*(3), 122-131.

Cronenwett, L., Sherwood, G., Pohl, J., Barnsteiner, J., Moore, S., Sullivan, D., … Warren, J. (2009). Quality and safety education for advanced nursing practice. *Nursing Outlook, 57*(6), 338-348.

Donabedian, A. (1982). *The criteria and standards of quality.* Ann Arbor, MI: Health Administration Press.

Donaldson, M.S., Yordy, K.D., Lohr, K.N., & Vanselow, N.A. (1996) Primary care: America's health in a new era. Washington, DC: Institute of Medicine.

Dufault, M., Duquette, C.E., Ehmann, J., Hehl, R., Lavin, M., Martin, V., … Willey, C. (2010). Translating an evidence based protocol for nurse-to-nurse shift handoffs. *Worldviews on Evidence-Based Nursing, 7*(2), 59-75.

Gray, L.C., Peel, N.M., Crotty, M., Kurrle, S.E., Giles, L.C., & Cameron, I.D. (2012). How effective are programs at managing transition from hospital to home? A case study of the Australian transition care program. *BMC Geriatrics, 12,* 6.

Illinois Transitional Care Consortium. (n.d.). *The bridge model.* Retrieved from http://www.transitionalcare.org/the-bridge-model

Institute for Healthcare Improvement (IHI). (2013a). *How-to guide: Improving transitions from the hospital to community settings to reduce avoidable rehospitalizations.* Cambridge, MA: Author.

Institute for Healthcare Improvement (IHI). (2013b). *State action on avoidable rehospitalizations: How-to-guide: Improving transitions from hospital to community settings.* Cambridge, MA: Author.

Institute of Medicine (IOM). (2001). *Crossing the quality chasm: A new health system for the 21st century.* Washington, DC: National Academies Press.

Joint Commission,The. (2013). *Improving transitions of care: Hand off communications.* Retrieved from http://www.centerfortransforminghealthcare.org/assets/4/6/CTH_Hand-off_commun_set_final_2010.pdf

Kim, C.S., & Flanders, S.A. (2013). Transitions of care. *Annals of Internal Medicine, 158*(5, Part 1), ITC3-1.

Medicare Payment Advisory Commission. (2008). *Report to the Congress: Redefining the delivery system.* Washington, DC: Author.

Naylor, M.D., & Sochalski, J.A. (2010). *Scaling up: Bringing the transitional care model into the mainstream.* The Commonwealth Fund. Retrieved from http://www.wapatientsafety.org/downloads/TCM_Forefront.pdf

Robert Wood Johnson Foundation. (2013a). *Reducing avoidable readmissions through better care transitions.* Retrieved from http://www.rwjf.org/content/dam/farm/toolkits/toolkits/2013/rwjf404051

Robert Wood Johnson Foundation. (2013b). *The revolving door: A report on U.S. hospital readmissions.* Princeton, NJ: Author.

Society of Hospital Medicine. (2010). *Project BOOST — Better outcomes for older adults through safe transitions. Implementation guide to improve care transitions.* Philadelphia, PA: Author.

Wenger, N.S., & Young, R.T. (2007). Quality indicators for continuity and coordination of care in vulnerable elders. *Journal of the American Geriatrics Society, 5*(s2), s285-s292.

# CHAPTER 10

# Population Health Management

*Anne Talbott Jessie, MSN, RN*
*Sheila A. Johnson, MBA, RN*
*Barbara Ellis Trehearne, PhD, RN*

## Learning Outcome Statement

The purpose of this chapter is to enable the reader to describe population management principles and key elements and how they apply to the registered nurse (RN) in the Care Coordination and Transition Management (CCTM) role.

## Learning Objectives

After reading this chapter, the RN working in the CCTM role will be able to:

- Explain the purpose of population health management (PHM) and how it applies to the RN in the CCTM role in ambulatory care.
- Define and describe key elements of PHM.
- Apply key elements of PHM to the RN in CCTM practice.
- Describe the benefits of having data for managing a population.
- Discuss methods organizations employ for storage and management of data.
- Describe the value of stratification of risk within a population.
- Identify the value of closing gaps in care.
- Identify key members of the interdisciplinary care team and discuss how they contribute to discipline-based interventions that are a part of PHM.
- Discuss methods to engage and activate patients and their caregivers in partnering in care management.
- Define and identify wraparound services that are essential for ongoing care and support for populations.
- Discuss how informatics and decision-support tools are utilized in the provision of PHM.
- Describe elements for measuring PHM from an individual and group perspective.
- Interpret evolving health care policy development and appropriately comply with quality monitoring, and regulatory and payer expectations in the provision of care to defined populations.
- Demonstrate how the RN in CCTM practices the knowledge, skills, and attitudes required for PHM (see Tables 1 and 2).

## Competency Definition

The Association of American Medical Colleges defines *population health* in this way: "A population health perspective encompasses the ability to assess the health needs of a specific population; implement and evaluate interventions to improve the health of that population; and provide care for individual patients in the context of the culture, health status, and health needs of the populations of which that patient is a member" (Halpern & Boulter, 2000, p. 1).

Population health management (PHM) is critical to the RN in CCTM role. It goes beyond traditional disease management and incorporates both preventive, wellness, and chronic care needs. The RN in CCTM uses PHM as a means to organize systems of care for populations, identify and implement evidence-based interventions, and measure both short and long-term outcomes for both the individual and the population. Patient-centered care as well as patient engagement and activation are necessary to engage in PHM.

The goal of population health management is to keep a patient population as healthy as possible, minimizing the need for expensive interventions such as emergency department (ED) visits, hospitalizations, imaging tests, and procedures. This not only lowers costs, but also redefines health care as an activity that encompasses far more than sick care. While PHM focuses partly on the high-risk patients who generate the majority of health costs, it systematically addresses the preventive and chronic care needs of every patient. Because the distribution of health risks changes over time, the objective is to modify the factors that make people sick or exacerbate their illnesses (Hodach, 2011).

In addition, practice-based population health is described as "an approach to care that uses information on a group of patients within a primary care practice or group of practices to improve the care and clinical outcomes of patients within that practice" (Cusack, Knudsen, Kronstadt, Singer, & Brown, 2010, p. 4).

Among the key characteristics of health organizations that implement PHM are an organized system of care; the use of multidisciplinary care teams; coordination across care settings; enhanced access to primary care; centralized resource planning; continuous care, both in and outside of office visits; patient self-management education; a focus on health behavior and lifestyle changes; and the use of health

**Figure 1.**
**Population Health Process Model**

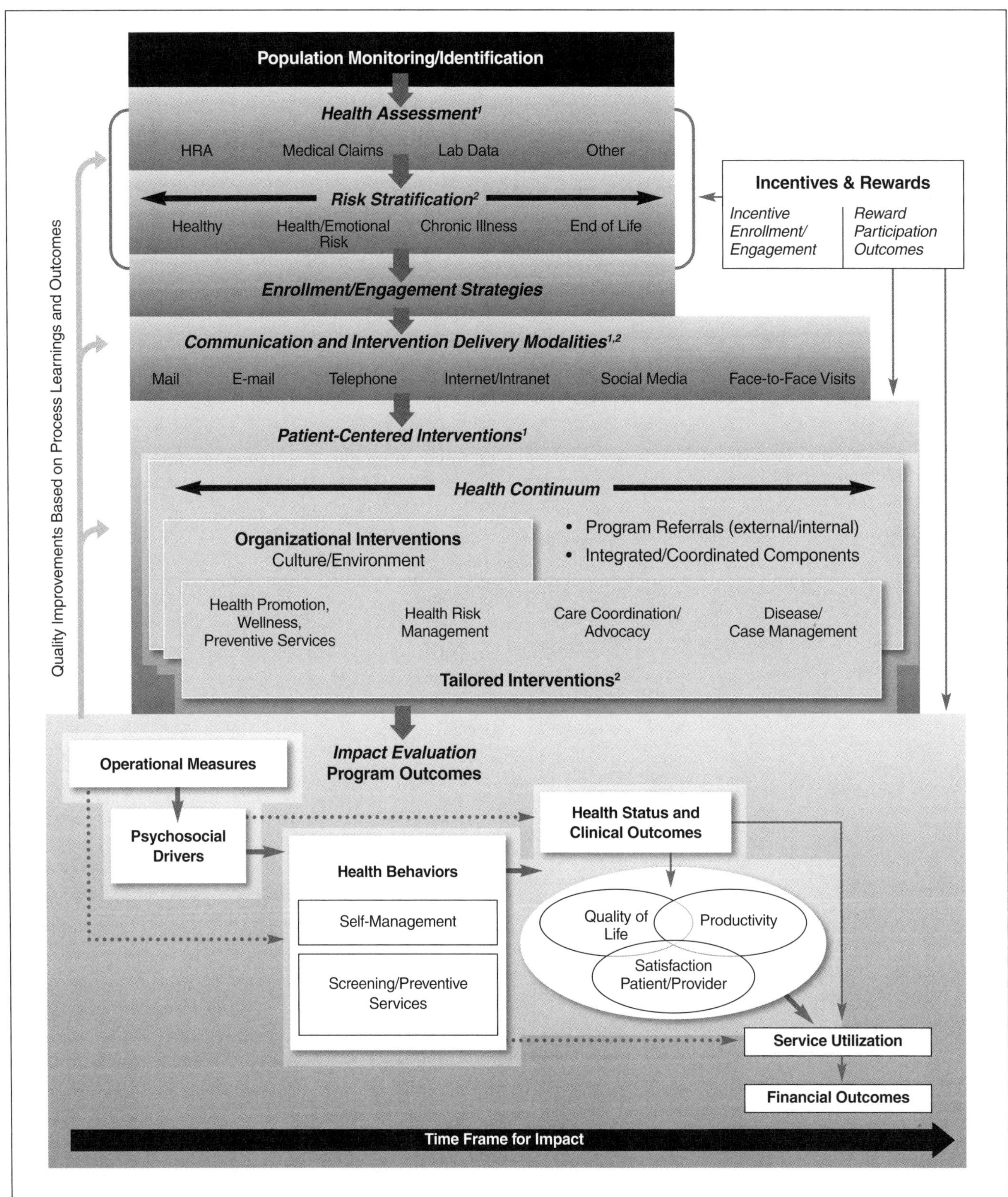


[1] Represents example components of each essential element. Does not necessarily reflect the universe of components.
[2] Communication may utilize one or more touch points within the delivery system.

**Source:** Care Continuum Alliance, Inc. Reprinted with permission.

Figure 2.
The Chronic Care Model

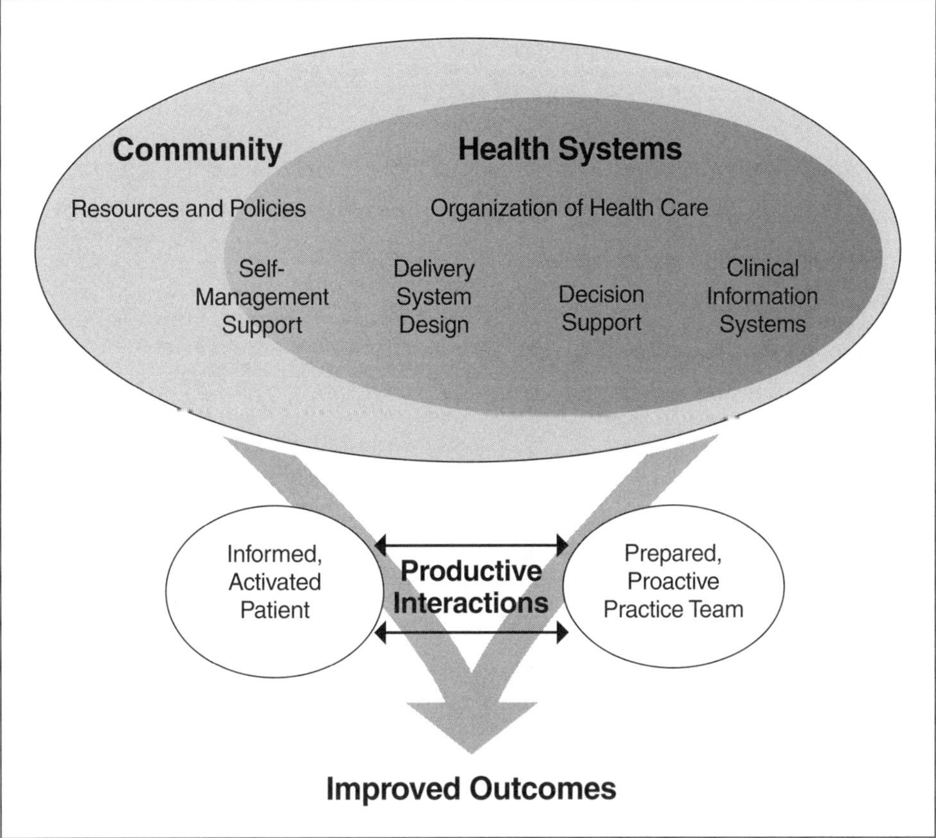


Developed by The MacColl Institute.
® ACP-ASIM Journals and Books. Reprinted with permission.

information technology for data access and reporting for communication among providers and between providers and patients (Hodach, 2011).

The Population Health Management Process Model (see Figure 1) depicts the steps in the process beginning with population identification, continues with enrollment and engagement, delivery modalities, patient-centered interventions, and ends with evaluation. This framework is useful to organize the work that needs to occur in population health.

In addition to the Population Health Process Model, Wagner's Chronic Care Model (see Figure 2) was developed to improve chronic illness care, a significant part of population management. The model identifies several elements that support the patient-provider interactions and can result in improved outcomes. These elements include:

- Well-developed processes and incentives for making changes in the care delivery system.
- Behaviorally sophisticated self-management support that gives priority to increasing patients' confidence and skills so they can be the ultimate manager of their illness (Von Korff, Gruman, Schaefer, Curry, & Wagner, 1997).
- Reorganized team function and practice systems (e.g., appointments and follow-up) to meet the needs of chronically ill patients.
- Evidence-based guidelines and support for those guidelines through provider education, reminders, and increased interaction between generalists and specialists.
- Enhanced information systems to facilitate the development of disease registries, tracking systems, and reminders and to give feedback on performance (Wagner, 1998).

The RN in CCTM needs to be a master of the use of population management tools (e.g., registries, analytic tools) to track and monitor select population characteristics, and to work with automated reminder and appointment systems for preventive services/chronic disease care/reminders (Cusack et al., 2010).

## I. Population Identification

To manage population health effectively, an organization must be able to track and monitor the health of individual patients. Providers must be able to identify subpopulations of patients who might benefit from additional services. Examples of these groups include: patients needing reminders for preventive care or tests; patients overdue for care or not meeting management goals; patients who have failed to receive follow-up after being sent reminders; and patients who might benefit from discussion of risk reduction (Gulley, Rasch, & Chan, 2011). To identify patient populations for outreach and intervention, tools and data sets are utilized.

A. While there is commitment to implement population health management in practice, there is a "need for guidance and assistance in putting the necessary tools into practice" (Moorehead, May, Ganda, & Jarm, 2012, p. 12).
   1. At the practice setting level, health plan eligibility and administrative data are used to identify the assigned population. Assignment to a practice setting occurs through health plan assignment or from health plan and government payers using claims usage patterns to attribute patients.
      a. Practice management systems within the practice setting are then used to assign patients to an individual clinician (physician or advanced practice nurse or physician assistant) (Care Continuum Alliance, 2012).
      b. Patients in the population may be identified to the clinician through an alert in the practice management system or through a patient registry.
   2. From a population health management perspective, clinicians are responsible for the totality of the population in their assignment, including those patients who do not seek care at the practice setting.
      a. RNs in CCTM, as members of the patient-centered care team, play a pivotal role in understanding the population as they assist the clinician with the management of the population.
   3. Population health management looks beyond the traditional practice of only caring for patients who contact the health care delivery system through phone calls and office visits to the practice setting.
   4. Population health management includes patients lost to care outside of the primary care practice setting.

B. "To aid in understanding the characteristics of population, a health assessment of patient-reported information provides information related to patient demographics, values and special needs" (Care Continuum Alliance, 2012, p.14). Other characteristics include self-identified health risks, care preferences, patient activation, and readiness for change.
   1. The results of the health assessment combined with claims data, clinical data from the electronic health record, diagnostic results, pharmacy usage, hospital activity data (admissions, ED usage), and evidence-based medicine parameters provide a registry of patient-specific information that can be used to understand the population at the practice level and at the individual patient level.
   2. The registry, combined with the use of analytic tools, provides the clinicians and nurses with the information they need to manage the individual patient.

## II. Data Collection, Storage, and Management

Clinical data from the electronic health record (EHR), billing data, claims data, and patient self-reported data are all stored in a data warehouse. Predictive analytics blend these data sources, stratifying patients at risk using defined data elements, prioritizing patients for outreach and interventions.

   1. Electronic health records are not the complete source of information.
   2. Registries, health information exchanges, and other types of electronic applications fill the void.

A. Organizations store multiple sources of data in a data warehouse that information technology professionals use to produce registries for clinicians and ambulatory care nurses to use.

B. Registries should not be limited to patients with specific diseases. Registries must cover the entire population and are used for improvements in preventive and chronic care.

C. Health information exchanges (HIE) allow for the storage and sharing of information across payers, practice settings, and tracking systems.
   1. Laboratory results, medications, health problems, and procedures are housed within HIEs.

D. Population health management requires new functional capabilities of health information technology including:
   1. A master identifier is needed to be able to link patients with clinicians and for linking the various datasets together.
   2. The ability for multiple member access and permissions.
      a. "Efficient systematic data collection, storage and management drive automation, quality measurement, and performance analysis; and comprehensive, timely, relevant information is essential to high-quality patient care" (Institute for Health Technology Transformation, 2012, p. 11).

E. Examples of unique populations include:
   1. Patients with chronic medical conditions and multiple co-morbidities.
   2. Homeless adults and families.

3. Patients who reside in short-term care facilities or long-term care facilities.
4. Mentally ill and those with chronic substance abuse.
5. Patients undergoing a surgery or procedure that requires targeted/intensive care management for a defined period of time (e.g., bariatric surgery, total joint replacement, spine surgery, high-risk pregnancy).

## III. Stratification

To manage population health effectively, an organization must be able to track and monitor the health of individual patients. The organization must stratify its population into subgroups that require particular services at specified intervals. Patients are stratified into risk categories using tools, including registries with decision-support algorithms built in, to allow identification of patients who could benefit from proactive outreach, pre-visit planning, care coordination, and identification of gaps in care.

A. Patients should be grouped by their risk of getting sick or sicker, and stratified into subgroups that require particular services at specified intervals.
   1. Grouping patients into categories by condition has been the traditional approach of disease management programs.
   2. In contrast, care management stratification focuses on whether patients are ill enough to require ongoing support from a care manager, have less serious chronic conditions that warrant interventions to prevent them from worsening, or are fairly healthy and just need preventive care and education (Katon et al., 2010).

B. Agency for Healthcare Research and Quality (AHRQ, 2012) describes one method of segmenting patients.
   1. Providers must be able to identify subpopulations of patients who might benefit from additional services.

C. Stratification can be done using proprietary mathematical algorithms to predict risk, or by using a count of risks to prioritize patients (Care Continuum Alliance, 2012).
   1. Additional considerations such as socioeconomic factors, physical and mental issues should also be included as part of risk stratification.

D. Risk stratification allows:
   1. The clinician and RN in CCTM to access information to enrich the patient-clinician conversation.
   2. The clinician and RN in CCTM to decide which patients to focus efforts.
   3. The clinician to know which interventions are appropriate.
   4. The clinician to align patients with assistance (Care Continuum Alliance, 2012).

E. When stratification and evidence-based clinical protocols are applied to registries, the resulting output guides action in the form of appointment reminders for chronic care and preventive care, and to remind providers and the RN in CCTM of their patient's care gaps.

F. The registry is used to allocate resources for identified patients, provides real-time information to use at the point of care, provides key clinical diagnoses, diagnostic tests, and adherence to evidence-based medicine (Care Continuum Alliance, 2012).
   1. Practices that have a population with a higher stratification of healthy people would focus their care efforts on prevention and wellness.
   2. Practices with a higher stratification of chronically ill people would focus their care efforts on chronic condition management.
      a. An example of allocating resources based on risk stratification is providing nutrition education for patients with diabetes and obesity instead of providing nutritional education for all patients in a practice.
   3. Stratification reveals cost drivers and at-risk individuals within the patient population.
      a. RN in CCTM tailors interventions for the at-risk individuals and offers appropriate support to improve health and decrease risk.
   4. Stratification illuminates "frequent flier" status patients for the RN in CCTM and clinicians to work with personalized interventions.
   5. Condition severity from stratification provides the opportunity for understanding how behaviors impact risks and conditions. Resources are offered specific to identified needs (Care Continuum Alliance, 2012).
      a. Typically, 20% of the population represents those patients with highest complexity of chronic conditions and/or catastrophic injuries.
   6. A variety of electronic predictive modeling techniques provide proactive identification of at-risk individuals and subpopulations to use patient-specific action plans to implement timely interventions (Rich, Lipson, Libersky, & Parchman, 2012).
   7. Modified LACE: an assessment tool that incorporates length of stay, acuity of admission, co-morbidity, ED to identify patients with a high predicted risk for re-admission or death (Kim & Flanders, 2013).
   8. Project Boost's "8Ps" Risk Assessment Tool identifies patient factors linked to high rates of adverse events after discharge (Kim & Flanders, 2013).
      a. The tool is completed on admission, identifying patients at risk for adverse events post-hospitalization.
      b. For the duration of the admission, the tool is utilized to mitigate post-discharge risks. Interventions initiated to address identified risks are communicated with the patient's post-hospitalization providers.

c. Specific areas assessed in the tool are:
   (1) "Problem" medications (e.g., warfarin, insulin, digoxin).
   (2) Polypharmacy.
   (3) Psychological condition (e.g., depression).
   (4) Principle diagnosis (e.g., cancer, stroke, diabetes, chronic obstructive pulmonary disease [COPD], congestive heart failure [CHF]).
   (5) Poor health literacy.
   (6) Patient support (the absence of social support, either formal or informal).
   (7) Prior hospitalizations (in the past 6 months).
   (8) Palliative care.
   (9) Other: lack of primary care or public support (Kim & Flanders, 2013).

d. Additional risk re-admission tools that can also be used in the ambulatory setting are:
   (1) PARR 30: Patients at Risk for Re-hospitalization (Billings et al., 2012).
   (2) Philbin Tool to predict re-admission for patients with congestive heart failure (Philbin & DiSalvo, 1999).

## IV. Identification of Gaps in Care

A. A cornerstone of population health management is the ability to be proactive in closing gaps in care for preventive services and chronic condition management.

B. A registry provides the RN in CCTM with information related to potential gaps in care.
   1. An example of a gap in a preventive service is influenza vaccination.
   2. The registry highlights gaps related to evidence-based measures for chronic conditions (e.g., HbA1c test performed and result identifying the level of control for a patient with diabetes).
   3. Medication non-adherence is often included in the registry. Outreach can then be made to patients who are exhibiting non-adherence.

C. Transitions in care across continuum points require closure in gaps in care.
   1. Ensure follow-up care post-hospital discharge is in place including medication reconciliation and provider appointment scheduling.
   2. Wrap community services around patient and family to prevent re-admissions.
   3. Reminders for preventive and chronic care specific to patients' health conditions and status are facilitated through the use of electronic health records and integrated software applications (Grundy, Davis, & Fisher, 2011).
   4. Gap closure through patient engagement and activation provide an enhanced patient experience and supports development of a more transparent relationship between providers and patients built on trust (Grundy et al., 2011).

## V. Patient Education and Counseling

A. Goals of education in ambulatory care (Laughlin, 2013).
   1. Self-management.
   2. Health promotion.
   3. Disease prevention.
   4. Appropriate patient/significant other involvement in treatment, care, and service decisions.

B. Education approaches for population health management.
   1. One-to-one teaching based on the patient's main concerns.
   2. Provide resources based on health literacy and learning preferences.
   3. Link patient/family with community resources.
   4. Consider various forms of visual aids including patient education videos developed by professional organizations and often placed on YouTube.
   5. Consider lay led groups for chronic conditions such as Living Well with Chronic Conditions (Lorig et al., 2012).

C. Cultural diversity and population health: as of 2008, minority populations make up approximately one-third of the United States population (U.S. Census Bureau, 2010), and are expected to be the majority by 2042 (Chambers & Laughlin, 2013). To effectively manage culturally diverse populations, the RN in CCTM must develop a knowledge and understanding of cultural factors and disparities in health care, and the impact on patient/caregiver activation in the design and implementation interventions. To be culturally competent, the RN in CCTM must be educated in the following areas.
   1. Cultural disparities in health and health care: racial and ethnic minorities experience a lower quality of health services and are less likely to receive even routine medical procedures than Caucasians. Perceptions of illness, disease, and their causes vary by culture (Chambers & Laughlin, 2013).
   2. Cultural competency: "An ongoing process in which the health care professional continually strives to work within the cultural context of the patient, individual, family and community" (Chambers & Laughlin, 2013, p. 221).
   3. Cultural safety: "Providing culturally safe care requires the nurse to be respectful of nationality, culture, age, sex and political and religious beliefs" (Chambers & Laughlin, 2013, p. 222).
   4. Strategies to improve cultural knowledge and skills: the RN in CCTM learns basic information about the predominant cultural groups served within the care setting of responsibility and influence; learns and understands culturally influenced health behaviors; and develops culture-specific assessment skills.

5. Cultural differences in disease incidence and management: the RN in CCTM needs to identify disease prevalence that commonly occurs within given ethnic populations and design screening and care interventions that meet the needs and unique characteristics of the populations served.

## VI. Team-Based Interventions

Successful population-based care requires staff and resources beyond what individual primary care physicians (PCPs) can provide. It involves planning and implementing care for groups, working with patients outside of the office visit, and monitoring effectiveness.

A. "Multidisciplinary teams should develop patient-centered care plans and implement protocols and systems for maintaining health of all population members and for treating subgroups afflicted with various conditions" (Halpern & Boulter, 2000, p. 3).
   1. Organizations dedicated to PHM provide care between as well as during encounters.
   2. Care teams must strive to deliver appropriate, evidence-based care during patient visits but they must also ensure care gaps are addressed when patients do not come into the office.
   3. Care teams must also find ways to help patients understand their care plans and the importance of complying with recommended guidelines (Chen & Bodenheimer, 2011).
   4. Teams proactively track care activities and interventions, and transparently share clinical information across the continuum with providers and patients.
   5. The PCP and the health care team, in full partnership with the patient and caregiver, provide "compassionate and coordinated care based on respect for patient's preferences, values, and needs" (Cronenwett et al., 2007, p. 123).

B. Primary care is at the heart of PHM with PCPs supplying the continuity required to ensure patients receive appropriate preventive and chronic care.
   1. PCPs are in short supply, and will be stretched even further when health care reform increases the number of insured patients and the demand for primary care.
      a. It has been estimated that a PCP would have to work 18 hours a day to deliver all of the care that his or her population needs.
      b. Other clinicians can perform much of this work, enabling physicians to focus on areas where their expertise is required.
      c. Care teams led by physicians, nurse practitioners, or other professionals can manage more patients and address more of their needs than the current primary care model.
      d. Team-based care supports effective and efficient care delivery as an extension of the PCP, providing critical resources to ensure improved outcomes (Grundy et al., 2011).

C. Team-based care redefines continuity as continuity with a team rather than continuity with just the provider (Gupta & Bodenheimer, 2013).
   1. Regular communication and collaboration within the team enhances clinical and social expertise of the team, provides peer support, and allows for sharing of best practices.
   2. Patient panels or populations are assigned to teams or "teamlets" consisting of a provider and clinical support staff such as RNs, licensed practical nurses, medical assistants, health coach, and receptionist.
   3. Smaller teams comprise a provider, clinical support staff, and a receptionist, while larger teams can have additional members such as health coaches, pharmacists, and therapists.
      a. Provider: designs and directs the medical plan of care.
      b. Other members of the team: pharmacists, social workers, behavioral health experts, dieticians, therapists.

D. Characteristics of an effective team (The Advisory Board Company, 2012).
   1. Wide range of clinical skills.
   2. Strong critical-thinking skills: promote resolution of complex care problems.
   3. Ability to engage and partner with patients and caregivers: activate and form meaningful relationships; patient advocate.
   4. Communication skills.
   5. Experience in linking services.

E. Navigation activities performed by the RN in CCTM (The Advisory Board Company, 2012) include:
   1. Coordinates care across sites.
      a. Facilitates access to services.
      b. Develops care plan with PCP.
      c. Oversees disease education and wellness coaching.
      d. Provides face-to-face and telephone patient care.
      e. Accountable for identifying gaps in care; communicate concerns to physicians.
      f. Embedded in the PCP practice or can work centrally.
   2. Manages referrals.
      a. To internal payer-based formalized disease management programs.
      b. To specialists.
      c. To pharmacy: medication management support.
      d. To behavioral health, psychosocial support.

3. Tracks patient activity.
   a. Uses information technology system alerts/registries to identify inpatient, ED utilization.

F. Team patient activation.
   1. Provides education.
      a. Coaches patients on disease management goals, monitors progress, offers encouragement, ensures understanding of necessary skills.
      b. Supports symptom management.
   2. Supports self-management.
      a. Encourages adherence to care plan, improvement through patient-centric goal setting.
      b. Fosters patient and caregiver activation, offers education.
      c. Patient portable health record.
   3. Encourages frequent communication.
      a. Promotes open communication through consistent monitoring, feedback, and follow-up.
      b. Forges one-on-one relationship with patient to promote two-way communication.

G. Team caseload: the ratio of the RN in CCTM to the volume of patients (or patient panel) they are responsible for managing.
   1. Panel size or caseload can vary based on the complexity and acuity of the patient population served, payer contracting, and health care organization mission.
   2. Examples of caseloads one RN in CCTM can typically manage include:
      a. One RN in CCTM: 10,000 commercial plan patients using a team-based care model.
      b. One RN in CCTM: 5,000 Medicare patients.
      c. Low risk: prevention focus with one or fewer chronic disease condition; one RN in CCTM: 500-1,000 patients.
      d. Moderate risk: one or more chronic disease conditions; one RN-CCTM: 300-500 patients.
      e. High risk: multiple co-morbid conditions, frequent hospital and ED utilization; one RN in CCTM: 200-250 (The Advisory Board Company, 2012).

H. Team communication.
   1. Pre-visit preparation: chart review prior to the office visit, identifying preventive measures or interventions to be addressed at the time of the visit. Items are documented in the EHR for ease of communication.
   2. Decision-support alerts in the EHR notify team members of actions needed for health maintenance or chronic disease monitoring (vaccinations, lab work, preventive screenings, referrals).
   3. Daily huddles: team gathers briefly the day of the office visit to communicate patient interventions to be addressed, delegate tasks, and to ensure comprehensive care delivery.
   4. Unified care plan: mode of documentation in the EHR that allows members of the care team across all care settings to view and edit the plan of care.

I. Electronic messaging to patients and care team: use of the EHR to send messages to patients via a secure patient portal and for team members to message each other electronically with key communication regarding the plan of care.

J. Interdisciplinary team members (Butcher, 2012).
   1. Primary care physician: provides medical oversight of treatments and interventions.
   2. Mid-level or advanced clinical practitioner (nurse practitioner or physician's assistant): designs and modifies the plan of care. RN in CCTM coordinates all aspects of the plan of care across transitions and care settings.
   3. Pharmacist: consultant in medication management, medication reconciliation, medication assistance programs. Ensures the quality and accuracy of medication management.
   4. Social worker: identifies and coordinates essential nonclinical services such as housing, food, transportation.
   5. Caregiver: family member, significant other or person identified by the patient to participate in or provide direct patient care (biological family member, legal partner, case worker, patient care aide, church member, neighbor).
   6. Health coach: nonclinical.
      a. Meets with patient before/after physician, explains care plan component.
      b. Manages progress via phone, web-based communication.
      c. Coordinates holistic patient needs, follow-up, monitors medication regimen adherence.
   7. RN in CCTM.
   8. Health plan management.
   9. Other team members can include medical assistants; practice nurses; hospital-based case managers; dieticians; physical and occupational therapists; community resource specialists; community care agencies; hospitalist, home care staff, palliative care and hospice nurses; skilled nursing facility nurses and discharge planners; homeless shelter staff; nonprofit community agencies; lay workers.

## VII. Patient Engagement

There is a growing body of evidence that demonstrates patients who are more engaged in their care are more likely to be adherent to the plan of care and achieve better outcomes (Hibbard, Greene, & Overton, 2013). Organizations dedicated to PHM require providers to care for patients between as well as during encounters. Care teams must strive to deliver appropriate, evidence-based care during and between patient visits. That requires motivating, collaborating,

**Figure 3.**
**Patient Engagement Pyramid**

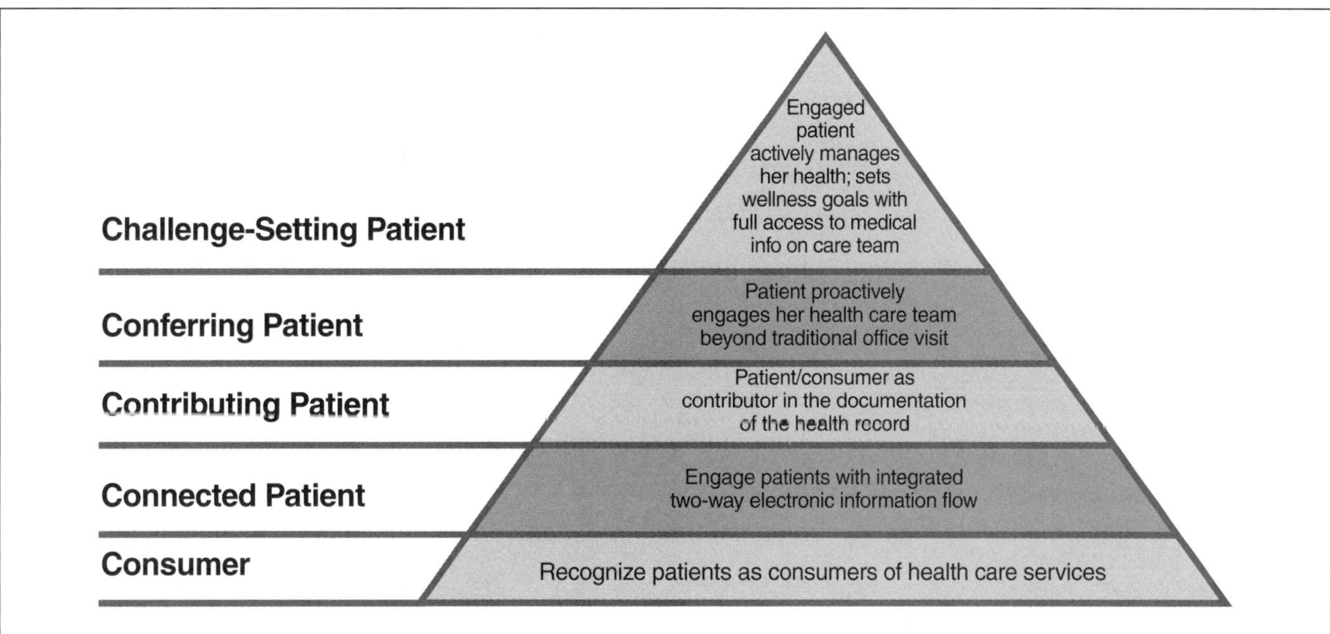
Challenge-Setting Patient
Engaged patient actively manages her health; sets wellness goals with full access to medical info on care team
Conferring Patient
Patient proactively engages her health care team beyond traditional office visit
Contributing Patient
Patient/consumer as contributor in the documentation of the health record
Connected Patient
Engage patients with integrated two-way electronic information flow
Consumer
Recognize patients as consumers of health care services

**Source:** Hello Health, Inc. Reprinted with permission.

and partnering with patients and families to help them take care of themselves. Care teams must also find ways to help patients understand their conditions, plans of care, and the importance of adhering to the treatment plan (see Figure 3).

A. Definition.
   1. Support active patient and public health involvement in securing appropriate, effective, and safe health care decisions at both the individual and collective levels (Coulter & Ellins, 2006).
   2. Engagement includes "actions people take for their health and to benefit from health care" (Center for Advancing Health, 2010, p. 2).
   3. Patient and family engagement includes patients, families, and other caregivers working with health professionals across the health care system to improve care.

B. Framework.
   1. Impact of engagement on health outcomes (Hibbard, Stockard, Mahoney, & Tusler, 2004).
      a. Patients demonstrate better outcomes when they:
         (1) Self-manage symptoms/problems.
         (2) Engage in activities that maintain function and reduce health decline.
         (3) Are involved in treatment and diagnostic choices.
         (4) Collaborate with providers.
         (5) Select providers and provider organizations based on performance or quality.
         (6) Navigate the health care system.
   2. Continuum of engagement/levels of engagement (Carman et al., 2013).
      a. Consultation: patients receive information about a diagnosis.
      b. Involvement: patients are asked about their preferences in treatment plan.
      c. Partnership: treatment decisions are made based on patient preferences, medical evidence, and clinical judgment.
   3. Level of engagement depends on multiple factors.
      a. Patient values, experiences, perspectives.
      b. Health literacy.
      c. Patients ability to engage with clinicians or with groups, self-management/community support groups.

C. Patient activation.
   1. Patient activation measure (PAM) is a valid and reliable scale that reflects a model of activation (Hibbard et al., 2004). The PAM measure quantifies the patient's level of engagement or activation in their care.
   2. PAM includes four stages (Hibbard et al., 2004).
      a. Believing the patient role is important.
      b. Having the confidence and knowledge necessary to take action including:
         (1) Knowledge of medications and lifestyle changes.
         (2) Confidence in talking to health provider.
         (3) Knowing when to seek help.
         (4) Confidence in following through on recommendations.

(5) Knowing the nature and causes of the health condition and different medical options.

c. Actually taking action to maintain and improve one's health.
   (1) Taking actions including maintaining lifestyle changes.
   (2) Handling symptoms on one's own.
d. Staying the course even under stress.
   (1) Handling problems at home on one's own.
   (2) Keep problems from interfering with one's life.

3. Use PAM at individual/group level to tailor interventions and assess change.
4. Strategies for patient activation.
   a. Motivational interviewing.
   b. Tailored coaching.
   c. Self-management programs (collaborative assessment, goal setting, action planning, and problem solving).
   d. Decision support.
   e. Education and counseling.
   f. Care protocols.
5. Skills for activating patients (Hibbard & Lorig, 2012).
   a. Help patient learn to formulate questions for the visit.
   b. Encourage patient to build on current strengths.
   c. Base teaching on patient's main concern.
   d. Screen for depression.
   e. Consistent positive feedback.
   f. Listen to break down problems into manageable parts.
   g. Listen to what patient describes.
   h. Establish mutually agreed-upon goals.
   i. Acknowledge barriers and difficulties.
   j. Share community resources.
   k. Be available to the patient.
6. Consider relationship between patient activation measure and disease burden (Hibbard et al., 2013).
   a. Patients with high PAM and low disease burden may not require RN-level resource.
   b. Patients with low PAM and high disease burden may require RN and physician-level resources.

## VIII. Care Coordination and Case Management

System-wide care transformation requires care management that is "coordinated across sites of care and prioritized to meet the needs of a range of patient populations" (The Advisory Board Company, 2012, p. 9).

A. The goal is to partner patient populations with care managers capable of coordinating resources across the continuum; and to engage patients in ongoing care plans and proactively manage CCTM utilization.
   1. Patients are matched with appropriate care management staff based on:
      a. Identified clinical and psychosocial needs.
      b. Improving patient management and engagement.
      c. Impacting quality.
      d. Reducing avoidable costs.
   2. Care management infrastructures target populations of patients in the following manner.
      a. Intensive care management (catastrophic care): comprehensive care for the highest risk patients with multiple co-morbid conditions, on six or more chronic medications, requiring integration of services, advanced illness planning (palliative care and hospice), and intensive management.
      b. The focus is patient centric with the goals of optimizing quality of life and reducing cost. Requires an interdisciplinary team with the RN in CCTM at the center coordinating care and services.
      c. Examples of populations managed:
         (1) End-stage renal disease patients requiring dialysis.
         (2) Advanced stages of cancer.
         (3) Stages 3 and 4 COPD and CHF.
         (4) Advanced neurological diseases: Parkinson's, multiple sclerosis, Lou Gehrig disease.
         (5) Patients with three or more co-morbid conditions, regardless of age.
   3. Chronic care management: targeted management of specific chronic conditions or episodes of care for moderate risk patients (The Advisory Board Company, 2012). Patients typically have one to three chronic medical conditions.

B. Care delivery can consist of a blend of automated reminders for routine testing and follow-up appointments, as well as care coordinated by the RN in CCTM. The RN in CCTM prioritizes and implements interventions, mitigates re-admission risk, and addresses quality measures tied to reimbursement. Examples of populations managed:
   1. Patients with one to three medial conditions who utilize hospital and ED services regularly (e.g., pain management, substance abuse, mental health).
   2. Patients with a medical condition who experience an acute exacerbation of disease or experience an acute illness that worsens control of their underlying condition (e.g., pneumonia, stroke).
      a. At-risk care management: uses automated reminders and health coaching for patients at risk for developing a chronic disease.
         (1) The RN in CCTM provides in-person or telephonic health coaching, medication compliance support, connects patients with community-based services, partners with the patient in setting mutually agreed upon goals, and tracks progress and outcomes.

(2) The RN in CCTM proactively communicates with the patient to identify minor or progressing symptoms before they escalate to the need for higher-acuity care or utilization.

3. Examples of populations managed:
   a. Obese patients.
   b. Patients with abnormal lab results (e.g., metabolic syndrome, elevated blood pressure or blood sugar without a chronic disease diagnosis).
      (1) Patients with predisposing risk factors for developing a chronic disease (familial or genetic history).

## IX. Preventive Care Management

Utilizes automated outreach and reminders to ensure patients are reminded to receive preventive tests and screenings, adhere with annual wellness exams, and receive immunizations appropriate to their age and medical condition.

A. Examples include:
   1. Immunizations for flu and pneumonia prevention, pediatric immunizations.
   2. Mammogram and colonoscopy screening.
   3. Maintenance tests for HbA1c, spirometry, metabolic lab monitoring.
   4. Medicare wellness visits, well-child checks.

## X. Wraparound Services

Wraparound services refer to an intensive, individualized care planning and management process. The goal is to "achieve positive outcomes by providing a structured, creative and individualized team planning process that results in plans that are more effective and more relevant to the patient and family" (National Wraparound Initiative, 2014, para. 2).

A. Wraparound plans are more holistic than traditional care plans in that they are designed to meet the identified needs of caregivers and family unit to address a range of life areas (National Wraparound Initiative, 2014).
   1. The team-based planning and implementation process aims to develop the problem-solving skills, coping skills, and self-efficacy of patients and family members.
   2. The wraparound plan typically includes formal services and interventions, together with community services and interpersonal support and assistance provided by friends, families, and case workers.
   3. Examples of wraparound services include but are not limited to:
      a. Community or school-based programs (e.g., League of Older Americans, school lunch programs, Meals on Wheels, parish nurses).
      b. Public health nurses.
      c. Pharmacy services.
         (1) Provides prescription recommendations to consolidate medications on regimen, suggest appropriate/affordable medications, reduce the risk of medication errors, educate patients on medications/side effects/interactions.
         (2) Performs medication reconciliation across the continuum (admission/discharge).
         (3) Post-hospital discharge medication follow-up.

B. Behavioral health: psychiatrist available for consultation in-person or by phone, suggest treatment options/modifications (medication and behavioral therapy). Assigned community case worker.

C. Palliative care, hospice.

D. Nonclinical services "fill" prescriptions for food and fuel assistance, housing, transportation (can be volunteers).

E. Community education and involvement in promoting healthy lifestyle behaviors.

## XI. Informatics and Decision-Support Systems

"Nursing informatics is a specialty that integrates nursing science, computer science, and information science to manage and communicate data, information, knowledge, and wisdom in nursing practice. The goal is to improve the health of populations, communities, families, and individuals by optimizing information management and communication" (American Nurses Association, 2008, p. 1).

A. Electronic health records enable teams to record and share information across systems to facilitate accurate and timely access to patient information.
   1. "Results from needs assessments for different domains (health, medications, home environment, social support, family/caregiver)" (AHRQ, 2012, p. 19).
   2. Referrals and results from lab and radiologic tests, specialty consults, home health, and community-based care.
   3. Real-time monitoring of hospital admissions and ED visits that trigger the need for follow-up.
   4. Prompts reminders regarding visits and preventive care.
   5. Decision-support tools for complex patient care (clinical pathways and guidelines).
   6. Community resource lists.
   7. Standardized evidence-based education.
   8. Support for primary care.

B. Registries are a critical tool used to prioritize patients with high-risk clinical conditions, serious unmet clinical needs for outreach, and intervention to manage outcomes. Can include metrics for identifying multiple co-morbid chronic conditions, hospital and ED utilization, and gaps in care such as unfilled prescriptions, missed preventive screenings, and lack of post-discharge follow-up after hospitalization.

1. Prevention.
   a. Identifies patients needing preventive screening/interventions/ongoing disease surveillance.
2. At-risk patients.
   a. Identifies patients at risk for chronic disease exacerbation based on lack of disease control.
      (1) Blood pressure monitoring indicates that hypertension is not controlled.
      (2) Elevated hemoglobin A1C levels indicate diabetes is not controlled.
3. High-risk patients.
   a. Patients with multiple co-morbid conditions at risk for catastrophic health event, adverse disease outcome, or death.
4. Hospital admissions/re-admissions and ED visits.
   a. Frequency of utilization of high-cost health care services.

C. Decision-support tools.
   1. Clinical alerts.
      a. Prevention: automated reminders and appointment systems for preventive disease care.
      b. Safety: high clinical values, potential drug interactions, allergies.
      c. Utilization: ED/hospital/missed follow-up appointment/no discharge appointment, prescriptions unfilled.

D. Analytics.
   1. Predictive models: identify patients at increased risk early for proactive intervention; combination of clinical data and paid medical and pharmacy claims information for a comprehensive patient snapshot. Based on predictive algorithms that rank patients by risk profile that predicts future utilization.
   2. Risk assessment: scoring modified LACE, psychosocial plus clinical status. Identifies patients most likely to benefit from care management.
   3. Determines population performance against quality/service/cost goals and seeks opportunity for improvement.
   4. Uses information technology (portals and health information exchanges) to communicate data related to care of individuals and populations.

## XII. Telehealth

"The delivery, management, and coordination of care and services that integrate electronic information and telecommunication technologies to increase access, improve outcomes, and contain or reduce costs of health care" (Rutenberg & Greenberg, 2012, p. 5).

A. An interactive process that occurs between the nurse and patient that serves as a method to extend care telephonically to where the patient resides.

B. Implications for the RN in CCTM and population health management:
   1. Telephone triage: centralized triage of symptoms by experienced RNs who utilize the nursing process to assess patients and determine the most appropriate care setting for treatment and intervention.
   2. Health information exchanges mobilize health care information electronically across organizations within a region, community, or hospital system.
   3. Telehealth/remote monitoring: extends population health management into the patient's home using biometric monitoring units and branching logic to identify worsening symptoms or disease exacerbation for nursing or medical intervention. The monitoring tool can be interfaced with the EHR and leveraged to control hospital and ED utilization.

## XIII. Measuring Outcomes

To describe population health at any given time, organizations can use a variety of measures, including those that describe processes (e.g., how many patients with diabetes received an appropriate HbA1c test?), intermediate outcomes (e.g., HbA1c or blood pressure levels), and long-term outcomes (e.g., quality of life). The latter requires a combination of clinical data and patient-reported data, such as functional status and self-perceived health. It is important to consistently measure for patient experience, quality standards, quality of care, and cost effectiveness.

A. Patient experience.
   1. Self-perceived.
   2. Productivity (disability, absenteeism).

B. Quality of life and well-being.
   1. Functional status assessments should be performed regularly by the RN in CCTM for chronically ill patients to determine progression/improvement.
   2. Psychosocial assessment is necessary especially for patients with chronic conditions. The PHQ2, a patient health questionnaire assessment for depression in the past 2 weeks, should be done at every visit or routinely to determine need for further assessment.
   3. Economic status assessment to determine patient's ability to self-manage, purchase medications and supplies.

C. Health care utilization.
   1. Re-admissions at 30 days is the key measure for conditions in which re-admission is preventable.
   2. ED visits is an indicator of the patient's ability to understand what to do when the condition is worsening.

3. Primary care visits (face-to-face and/or telephonic).
4. Claims cost.
5. Other resource utilization: lab, imaging.

D. Health behaviors.
1. Self-management.
2. Engagement: initial and sustained can be measured with the PAM.
3. Treatment adherence to the plan including medications, visits, lifestyle changes, diet modification.
4. Behavior change can be measured via many tools including PAM.
5. Screening and prevention.

E. Measurement of impact on population health disparities is needed to assure equitable care across racial and ethnic groups.

F. Clinical/health status indicators can be used to measure progress both short and long term for individuals and groups.
1. Process indicators (e.g., blood pressure, hemoglobin A1C levels for patients with diabetes, etc.).
2. Intermediate (blood pressure, hemoglobin A1C and lipid blood levels, etc).
3. Long term.
4. Morbidity and mortality.
5. Coded interventions embedded in routine documentation.

G. Displaying data using patient dashboards or reports can be done in a variety of ways depending on the need.
1. Payer requirements.
2. Patient care activities.
3. By provider.
4. By health condition.
5. Identified care gap.

## XIV. Population Health and Policy Development

Health care policy development is a dynamic process influenced by legislation, governmental agencies, health care organizations, payer entities, academia, and public opinion. The RN in CCTM must stay current with emerging trends, new legislation, and payment and reimbursement models in the provision of care design and delivery in the populations managed. Examples of areas influence by health care policy development:

1. Health care quality measures.
   a. HEDIS measure.
   b. Centers for Medicare & Medicaid Services (CMS) 5 star quality ratings.
2. Required compliance activities: Occupational Safety and Health Administration, The Joint Commission, CMS, and Core Measures.
   a. National Patient Safety Goals.
3. Emerging reimbursement models that recognize the value of the role of the RN in CCTM.
4. Regulations regarding EHR utilization and security.
   a. HIPAA (Health Insurance Portability and Accountability Act).
   b. HITECH (Health Information Technology for Economic and Clinical Health Act).
5. Disease certification programs and quality designations.
   a. National Committee for Quality Assurance Patient-Centered Medical Home recognition.
   b. The Joint Commission Disease Management Recognition Programs.
   c. Magnet® designation for nursing excellence.

**Table 1.**
**Definitions of Competencies**

| |
|---|
| **Patient-Centered Care** |
| "Recognize the patient or designee as the source of control and full partner in providing compassionate and coordinated care based on respect for the patient's preferences, values, and needs" (American Association of Colleges of Nursing [AACN], 2012, p. 4). |
| **Teamwork and Collaboration** |
| "Function effectively within nursing and interdisciplinary teams, fostering open communication, mutual respect, and shared decision making to achieve quality patient care" (AACN, 2012, p. 4). |
| **Evidence-Based Practice** |
| "Integrate best current evidence with clinical expertise and patient/family preferences and values for delivery of optimal care" (AACN, 2012, p. 4). |
| **Quality Improvement** |
| "Use data to monitor the outcomes of care processes and use improvement methods to design and test changes to continuously improve the quality and safety of healthcare systems" (AACN, 2012, p. 4). |
| **Safety** |
| "Minimize risk of harm to patients and providers through both systems effectiveness and individual performance" (AACN, 2012, p. 4). |
| **Informatics** |
| "Use information and technology to communicate, manage knowledge, mitigate error, and support decision making" (AACN, 2012, p. 4). |

"The overall goal for the Quality and Safety Education for Nurses (QSEN) project is to meet the challenge of preparing future nurses who will have the knowledge, skills and attitudes (KSAs) necessary to continuously improve the quality and safety of the healthcare systems within which they work" (QSEN Institute, 2014, p. 1).

**Table 2.**
**Population Health Management: Knowledge, Skills, and Attitudes for Competency**

| Patient/Population-Centered Care | | | |
|---|---|---|---|
| **Knowledge** | **Skills** | **Attitudes** | **Sources** |
| Analyze and integrate multiple dimensions of patient-centered care and the care needs of identified patient populations:<br>• patient/family/community preferences, values<br>• coordination and integration of care<br>• information, communication, and education<br>• physical comfort and emotional support<br>• involvement of family and friends<br>• transition and continuity | Elicit patient values, preferences, and expressed needs as part of clinical interview, diagnosis, implementation of care plan, and evaluation of care.<br><br>Communicate patient and group values, preferences, and expressed needs to other members of health care team.<br><br>Provide patient-centered care with sensitivity, empathy, and respect for the diversity of human experience. | Value seeing health care situations "through patients' eyes."<br><br>Respect and encourage individual expression of patient values, preferences, and expressed needs.<br><br>Honor learning opportunities with patients and populations who represent all aspects of human diversity.<br><br>Seek to understand one's personally held attitudes about working with patients from different ethnic, cultural, and social backgrounds.<br><br>Willingly support patient-centered care for individuals and groups whose values differ from own. | Cronenwett et al., 2007 |
| Analyze how diverse cultural, ethnic, spiritual, and social backgrounds of both individual patients and populations function as sources of patient, family, and community values.<br><br>Analyze social, political, economic, and historical dimensions of patient care processes and the implications for patient-centered care and the care of populations. | Ensure the systems within which one practices support patient-centered care for individuals and populations whose values differ from the majority or one's own. | | Cronenwett et al., 2009 |
| Analyze ethical and legal implications of caring for populations of patients.<br><br>Describe the limits and boundaries of therapeutic patient-centered care. | Respect the boundaries of therapeutic relationships. | Value shared decision making with empowered patients, families, and communities even when conflicts occur. | Cronenwett et al., 2007 |
| | Acknowledge the tension that may exist between patient and population preferences and organizational and professional responsibilities for ethical care.<br><br>Facilitate informed patient consent for care. | | Cronenwett et al., 2009 |

*continued on next page*

**Source Notes:** Cronenwett et al. (2007) reprinted from *Nursing Outlook, 55*(3), 122-131, with permission from Elsevier. Cronenwett et al. (2009) reprinted from *Nursing Outlook, 57*(6), 338-348, with permission from the author.
**Editors' Note:** Population Health Management is so new there are not always full KSA statements; therefore, the chapter authors, as experts, developed needed skills and attitudes.

 

**Table 2. (continued)**
**Population Health Management: Knowledge, Skills, and Attitudes for Competency**

| Patient/Population-Centered Care (continued) | | | |
|---|---|---|---|
| **Knowledge** | **Skills** | **Attitu** | **Sources** |
| Analyze strategies that empower patients, families, or communities in all aspects of the health care process.<br><br>Analyze reasons for common barriers to active involvement of patients, families, and groups in their own health care processes. | Engage patients, designated surrogates, or groups in active partnerships along the health illness continuum. | Respect patient preferences for degree of active engagement in care process.<br><br>Honor active partnerships with patients, designated surrogates or groups in planning, implementation, and evaluation of care.<br><br>Respect patient's right to access to personal health records. | Cronenwett et al., 2007 |
| Analyze features of physical facilities that support or pose barriers to patient-centered care. | Create or change organizational cultures so that patient, family, and community preferences are assessed and supported. | | Cronenwett et al., 2009 |
| | Assess level of patient's decisional conflict and provide access to resources.<br><br>Eliminate barriers to presence of families and other designated surrogates based on patient preferences. | | Cronenwett et al., 2007 |
| | | Value system changes that support patient-centered and population-based care. | Cronenwett et al., 2009 |
| Analyze principles of consensus building and conflict resolution.<br><br>Describe nursing's role in assuring coordination, integration, and continuity of care. | Communicate care provided and needed at each transition in care. | Value continuous improvement of own communication and conflict-resolution skills. | Cronenwett et al., 2007 |
| Integrate principles of effective communication with knowledge of quality and safety competencies. | Continuously analyze and improve own level of communication skill in encounters with patients, families, and teams.<br><br>Provide leadership in building consensus or resolving conflict in the context of patient care. | Value consensus. | Cronenwett et al., 2009 |

*continued on next page*

 

Table 2. (continued)
Population Health Management: Knowledge, Skills, and Attitudes for Competency

| Patient/Population-Centered Care (continued) | | | |
|---|---|---|---|
| **Knowledge** | **Skills** | **Attitu** | **Sources** |
| "Describe the characteristics of a population-based health problem (e.g., health care equity, social determinants, environmental barriers)." | | Appreciate the impact of social determinants on patient engagement in self-care and outcomes of care interventions. | Council on Linkages Between Academia and Public Health Practice, 2010, p. 7 |
| | Identify population characteristics that influence the effective-ness of care delivery, such as age, demo-graphics, ethnicity, financial status, psycho-social challenges. | | Jessie, Johnson, & Trehearne, 2014 |
| "Identify the health literacy of populations served." | | | Council on Linkages Between Academia and Public Health Practice, 2010, p. 11 |
| | Demonstrate the ability to determine levels of individual and population health literacy.<br><br>Ensure sensitivity to unique characteristics of populations in the evaluation of health literacy. | Value the diversity in population education levels, experiences, and backgrounds that influence health literacy. | Jessie et al., 2014 |
| "Incorporate strategies for interacting with persons from diverse backgrounds (e.g., cultural, socioeconomic, educational, racial, gender, age, ethnic, sexual orientation, professional, religious affiliation, mental and physical capabilities)." | "Describe the role of cultural, social, and behavioral factors in the accessibility, availability, acceptability, and delivery of health care."<br><br>"Respond to diverse needs that are the result of cultural differences." | | Council on Linkages Between Academia and Public Health Practice, 2010, p. 12 |
| | | Value the diversity of individuals and populations.<br><br>Seek to understand one's personally held attitudes about working with patients from different ethnic, cultural, and social backgrounds. | Jessie et al., 2014 |

*continued on next page*

Table 2. (continued)
Population Health Management: Knowledge, Skills, and Attitudes for Competency

| Teamwork and Collaboration | | | |
|---|---|---|---|
| **Knowledge** | **Skills** | **Attitudes** | **Sources** |
| Analyze own strengths, limitations, and values as a member of a team. | Demonstrate awareness of own strengths and limitations as a team member. | Acknowledge own contributions to effective or ineffective team functioning. | Cronenwett et al., 2007 |
| Analyze impact of own nursing practice role and its contributions to team functioning. | Continuously plan for improvement in use of self in effective team development and functioning. | | Cronenwett et al., 2009 |
| Analyze strategies for identifying and managing overlaps in team member roles and accountabilities. | Function competently within own scope of practice as a member of the health care team.<br><br>Solicit input from other team members to improve individual, as well as team, performance.<br><br>Assume role of team member or leader based on the situation. | Respect the unique attributes that members bring to a team, including variation in professional orientations, competencies, and accountabilities.<br><br>Respect the centrality of the patient/family as core members of any health care team. | Cronenwett et al., 2007 |
| | Guide the team in managing areas of overlap in team member functioning. | | Cronenwett et al., 2009 |
| "Describe the process of team development and scopes of practice and roles of all health care team members."<br><br>"Share accountability with other professions, patients, and communities for outcomes relevant to prevention and health care."<br><br>"Apply leadership practices that support collaborative practice and team effectiveness." | Empower "contributions of others who play a role in helping patients/families achieve health goals." | | Interprofessional Education Collaborative (IPEC), 2011, p. 25 |
| | | Value the contributions of all members of the care team in population care planning and health care management. | Jessie et al., 2014 |

*continued on next page*

 

Table 2. (continued)
Population Health Management: Knowledge, Skills, and Attitudes for Competency

| Teamwork and Collaboration (continued) | | | |
|---|---|---|---|
| **Knowledge** | **Skills** | **Attitudes** | **Sources** |
| | Communicate with team members, adapting own style of communicating to needs of the team and situation. | | Cronenwett et al., 2007 |
| Analyze strategies that influence the ability to initiate and sustain effective partnerships with members of nursing and interprofessional teams.<br><br>Analyze impact of cultural diversity on team functioning.<br><br>Engage diverse health care professionals who complement one's own professional expertise, as well as associated resources, to develop strategies to meet specific patient care needs. | Initiate and sustain effective health care teams. | Appreciate importance of interprofessional collaboration.<br><br>Value collaboration with nurses and other members of the nursing team. | Cronenwett et al., 2009 |
| Analyze differences in communication style preferences among patients and families, care coordinators, and other members of the health team. | | Value different styles of communication. | Cronenwett et al., 2007 |
| Describe impact of own communication style on others. | Communicate respect for team member competence in communication. | | Cronenwett et al., 2009 |

*continued on next page*

**Table 2. (continued)**
**Population Health Management: Knowledge, Skills, and Attitudes for Competency**

| Teamwork and Collaboration (continued) | | | |
|---|---|---|---|
| **Knowledge** | **Skills** | **Attitudes** | **Sources** |
| "Apply communication and group dynamic strategies (e.g., principled negotiation, conflict resolution, active listening, risk communication) in interactions with individuals and groups." | | | Council on Linkages Between Academia and Public Health Practice, 2010, p. 11 |
| "Organize and communicate information with patients, families, and health care team members in a form that is understandable, avoiding discipline-specific terminology when possible." | "Engage self and others to constructively manage disagreements about values, roles, goals, and actions that arise among health care professionals and with patients and families." | | IPEC, 2011, p. 23 |
| Describe examples of the impact of team functioning on safety and quality of care. | Follow communication practices that minimize risks associated with hand-offs among providers and across transitions in care.<br><br>Choose communication styles that diminish the risks associated with authority gradients among team members.<br><br>Initiate actions to resolve conflict.<br><br>Assert own position/perspective and supporting evidence in discussions about patient care.<br><br>Act with integrity, consistency, and respect for differing views. | Appreciate the risks associated with hand-offs among providers and across transitions in care. | Cronenwett et al., 2007 |
| | | Value the solutions obtained through systematic, interprofessional collaborative efforts. | Cronenwett et al., 2009 |
| | | Appreciate and value the effectiveness of diverse communication techniques. | Jessie et al., 2014 |

*continued on next page*

Table 2. (continued)
Population Health Management: Knowledge, Skills, and Attitudes for Competency

| Teamwork and Collaboration (continued) | | | |
|---|---|---|---|
| **Knowledge** | **Skills** | **Attitudes** | **Sources** |
| Identify system barriers and facilitators of effective team functioning.<br><br>Examine strategies for improving systems to support team functioning. | | | Cronenwett et al., 2007 |
| | Lead or participate in the design and implementation of systems that support effective teamwork.<br><br>Engage in state and national policy initiatives aimed at improving teamwork and collaboration. | Value the influence of system solutions in achieving team functioning. | Cronenwett et al., 2009 |
| | "Use the full scope of knowledge, skills, and abilities of available health professionals and health care workers to provide care that is safe, timely, efficient, effective, and equitable." | | IPEC, 2011, p. 21 |
| **Evidence-Based Practice** | | | |
| **Knowledge** | **Skills** | **Attitudes** | **Sources** |
| Demonstrate knowledge of basic scientific methods and processes.<br><br>Describe evidence-based practice to include the components of research evidence, clinical expertise, and patient/family values. | | Appreciate strengths and weaknesses of scientific bases for practice.<br><br>Value the need for ethical conduct of research and quality improvement. | Cronenwett et al., 2007 |
| | Use health research methods and processes, alone or in partnership with scientists, to generate new knowledge for practice. | Value all components of evidence-based practice. | Cronenwett et al., 2009 |
| | Base evidence-based interventions on individualized care plan based on patient/population values and nursing expertise. | | Jessie et al., 2014 |
| Identify efficient and effective search strategies to locate reliable sources of evidence. | Employ efficient and effective search strategies to answer focused clinical questions. | Value development of search skills for locating evidence for best practice. | Cronenwett et al., 2009 |

*continued on next page*

**Table 2. (continued)**
**Population Health Management: Knowledge, Skills, and Attitudes for Competency**

| Evidence-Based Practice (continued) | | | |
|---|---|---|---|
| **Knowledge** | **Skills** | **Attitudes** | **Sources** |
| Differentiate clinical opinion for research and evidence and identify sources for locating evidence-based reports and clinical practice guidelines. | Locate evidence-based reports and clinical practice guidelines. | Appreciate the importance of regularly reading professional journals and attending educational conferences. | Cronenwett et al., 2007 |
| Summarize current evidence regarding major diagnostic and treatment actions within the practice specialty.<br><br>Determine evidence gaps within the practice specialty. | Exhibit contemporary knowledge of best evidence related to practice specialty.<br><br>Promote research agenda for evidence that is needed in practice specialty.<br><br>Initiate changes in approaches to care when new evidence warrants evaluation of other options for improving outcomes or decreasing adverse events. | Value knowing the evidence-base for practice specialty.<br><br>Value public policies that support evidence-based practice. | Cronenwett et al., 2009 |
| | | Acknowledge own limitations in knowledge and clinical expertise before determining when to deviate from evidence-based best practices.<br><br>Value the need for continuous improvement in clinical practice based on new knowledge. | Cronenwett et al., 2007 |
| Analyze how the strength of available evidence influences the provision of care (assessment, diagnosis, treatment, and evaluation).<br><br>Evaluate organizational cultures and structures that promote evidence-based practice. | Develop guidelines for clinical decision making regarding departure from established protocols/ standards of care.<br><br>Participate in designing systems that support evidence-based practice. | | Cronenwett et al., 2009 |

*continued on next page*

**Table 2. (continued)**
**Population Health Management: Knowledge, Skills, and Attitudes for Competency**

| Quality Improvement | | | |
|---|---|---|---|
| **Knowledge** | **Skills** | **Attitudes** | **Sources** |
| | Use a variety of sources of information to review outcomes of care and identify potential areas for improvement.<br><br>Propose appropriate goals for quality improvement activities. | | Cronenwett et al., 2009 |
| Describe strategies for improving outcomes of care for identified patient populations.<br><br>Analyze the impact of context and social determinants (e.g., access, cost, team functioning, age, demographics) on improvement efforts. | | Appreciate that continuous quality improvement is an essential role of the RN in CCTM. | Jessie et al., 2014 |
| Analyze ethical issues associated with quality improvement. | Assure ethical oversight of quality improvement projects. | Value the need for ethical conduct of quality improvement. | Cronenwett et al., 2009 |
| | Use databases as sources of information for improving patient care. | Appreciate the importance of data as a tool to measure and/or estimate the quality of care. | Cronenwett et al., 2009 |
| Understand the benefits and limitations of quality improvement data sources and measurement. | Select and use population-relevant benchmarks. | | Jessie et al., 2014 |
| Explain common causes of variation in outcomes. | Select and use tools (such as control charts and run charts) that are helpful for understanding variation.<br><br>Identify gaps between local and best practice. | Appreciate how unexpected variation affects outcomes of care processes. | Cronenwett et al., 2009 |

*continued on next page*

Table 2. (continued)
Population Health Management: Knowledge, Skills, and Attitudes for Competency

| Quality Improvement (continued) | | | |
|---|---|---|---|
| **Knowledge** | **Skills** | **Attitudes** | **Sources** |
| | Use measures to evaluate the effect of change.<br><br>Design, implement, and evaluate tests of change in daily work (using an experiential learning method such as Plan-Do-Study-Act). | Appreciate the value of what individuals and teams can to do to improve care. | Cronenwett et al., 2007 |
| Analyze the differences between micro-system and macro-system change.<br><br>Understand principles of change management.<br><br>Analyze the strengths and limitations of common quality improvement methods. | Use principles of change management to implement and evaluate care processes at the micro-system level.<br><br>Align the aims, measures, and changes involved in improving care. | Value local systems improvement (in individual practice, team practice on a unit, or in the macro-system) and its role in professional job satisfaction.<br><br>Appreciate that all improvement is change but not all change is improvement. | Cronenwett et al., 2009 |
| "Identify mechanisms to monitor and evaluate programs for their effectiveness and quality and apply strategies for continuous improvement." | | | Council on Linkages Between Academia and Public Health Practice, 2010, p. 10 |

*continued on next page*

 

**Table 2. (continued)**
**Population Health Management: Knowledge, Skills, and Attitudes for Competency**

| Safety | | | |
|---|---|---|---|
| **Knowledge** | **Skills** | **Attitudes** | **Sources** |
| Describe the benefits and limitations of selected safety-enhancing technologies (health maintenance alerts, patient reminder systems, computer provider order entry, and electronic prescribing). | | Value the contributions of standardization and reliability to safety. | Cronenwett et al., 2007 |
| Describe human factors and other basic safety design principles as well as commonly used unsafe practices (such as work-arounds, lack of consistent communication across care delivery settings, and in complete follow-up). | Participate in the design, promotion, and effective use of technology and standardized practices that support safety and quality.<br><br>Participate as a team member to design, promote, and model effective use of strategies to reduce risk of harm to self and others.<br><br>Promote a practice culture conducive to highly reliable processes.<br><br>Utilize automated reminder systems to prompt future actions required. | Appreciate the importance of safety consciousness both in the provision of care and in the work environment. | Cronenwett et al., 2009 |
| Describe factors that create a just culture and culture of safety. | Communicate observations or concerns related to hazards and errors to patients, families, and the health care team. | Value own role in reporting and preventing errors. | Cronenwett et al., 2007 |
| Describe best practices that promote patient and provider safety in the practice specialty. | | Value systems approaches to improving patient safety in lieu of blaming individuals.<br><br>Value the use of organizational error-reporting systems. | Cronenwett et al., 2009 |
| Identify categories of potential errors and hazards in care delivery.<br><br>Identify best practices for organizational responses to error. | Participate in identifying and correcting system failures and hazards in care.<br><br>Engage in systems-focused problem solving. | Value an organizational just culture. | Jessie et al., 2014 |

*continued on next page*

**Table 2. (continued)**
**Population Health Management: Knowledge, Skills, and Attitudes for Competency**

| Informatics | | | |
|---|---|---|---|
| **Knowledge** | **Skills** | **Attitudes** | **Sources** |
| Evaluate the strengths and weaknesses of information systems used in patient care and population management. | Communicate the integral role of information technology in nurses' work.<br><br>Assist team members to adopt information technology by piloting and evaluating proposed workflows and technologies. | Value the use of information and communication technologies in patient, population care, and transition management. | Cronenwett et al., 2009 |
| | Demonstrate the appropriate use of electronic health records and technology in the care of patients and populations. | | Jessie et al., 2014 |
| | Promote access to patient care information through use of standardized documentation tools for all professionals who provide care to patients and populations.<br><br>Serve as a resource for how to document nursing care at basic and advanced levels.<br><br>Develop safeguards for protected health information.<br><br>Champion communication technologies that support clinical decision making, error prevention, care coordination, and protection of patient privacy. | Appreciate the need for consensus and collaboration in developing systems to manage information for patient and population-based care.<br><br>Value the confidentiality and security of all patient records. | Cronenwett et al., 2007 |
| Identify essential information that must be available in a common database to support patient and population care delivery."<br><br>Evaluate benefits and limitations of different communication technologies and their impact on safety, quality, and effective care management. | | | Cronenwett et al., 2009 |

*continued on next page*

 

Table 2. (continued)
Population Health Management: Knowledge, Skills, and Attitudes for Competency

| Informatics (continued) | | | |
|---|---|---|---|
| **Knowledge** | **Skills** | **Attitudes** | **Sources** |
| Identify the health status of populations and their related determinants of health and illness using electronic decision-support tools (e.g., factors contributing to health promotion and disease prevention; the quality, availability, and use of health services). | | | Council on Linkages Between Academia and Public Health Practice, 2010, p. 7 |
| | Use basic statistical analysis and quality improvement techniques to review population characteristics, variation, health risks.<br><br>Using decision-support tools, demonstrate the ability to identify factors that facilitate or impede care coordination at both a systems and individual level depending on the complexity of specific circumstances (resources available, payment structure, patient complexity, capacity). | Value the use of decision-support tools in identifying patients and populations for interventions, preventive services, chronic disease management, and health care delivery design. | Jessie et al., 2014 |

*continued on next page*

Table 2. (continued)
Population Health Management: Knowledge, Skills, and Attitudes for Competency

| Informatics (continued) | | | |
|---|---|---|---|
| **Knowledge** | **Skills** | **Attitudes** | **Sources** |
| | Navigate the electronic health record.<br><br>Seek education about how information is managed in care settings before providing care.<br><br>Apply technology and information management tools to support safe processes of care.<br><br>Respond appropriately to clinical decision-making supports and alerts.<br><br>Use information management tools to monitor outcomes of care processes.<br><br>Use high-quality electronic sources of health care information | Value technologies that support clinical decision making, error prevention, and care coordination.<br><br>Appreciate the necessity for all health professionals to seek lifelong, continuous learning of information technology skills.<br><br>Value nurses' involvement in design, selection, implementation, and evaluation of information technologies to support patient care. | Cronenwett et al., 2007 |
| "Use information technology to collect, store, and retrieve data." | | | Council on Linkages Between Academia and Public Health Practice, 2010, p. 8 |
| Use electronic reporting to identify variables that measure public health conditions, gaps in care.<br><br>Choose effective communication tools and techniques, including information systems and communication technologies, to facilitate discussions and interactions that enhance team function. | | | Jessie et al., 2014 |

 

## References


Advisory Board, The. (2012). *High-risk patient care management.* Washington, DC; Author.

Agency for Healthcare Research and Quality (AHRQ). (2012). *Coordinating care for adults with complex care needs in the patient-centered medical home: Challenges and solutions.* Rockville, MD: Author.

American Association of Colleges of Nursing [AACN] QSEN Education Consortium. (2012). *Graduate-level QSEN competencies.* Retrieved from http://www.aacn.nche.edu/faculty/qsen/competencies.pdf

American Nurses Association. (2008*). Nursing informatics: Scope & standards of practice.* Silver Spring, MD: Author.

Billings, J., Blunt, I., Steventon, A., Georghiou, T., Lewis, G., & Bardsley, M. (2012). Development of a predictive model to identify inpatients at risk of re-admission within 30 days of discharge (PARR-30). *British Medical Journal, 2*(4). doi:10.1136/bmjopen-2012-001667

Butcher, L. (2012). Making care teams work. *Trustee, 65*(5), 13-16.

Care Continuum Alliance. (2012). *Implementation and evaluation: A population health guide for primary care models.* Retrieved from http://www.carecontinuumalliance.org/pdf/I-E-Document.pdf

Carman, K.L., Dardess, P., Maurer, M., Sofaer, S., Adams, K., Bechtel, C., & Sweeney, J. (2013). Patient and family engagement: A framework for understanding the elements and developing interventions and policies. *Health Affairs, 32*(2), 223-231.

Center for Advancing Health. (2010). *A new definition of patient engagement: What is engagement and why is it important?* Retrieved from http://www.cfah.org/file/CFAH_Engagement_Behavior_Framework_current.pdf

Chambers, P., & Laughlin, C. (2013). Transcultural nursing care. In C.B. Laughlin (Ed.), *Core curriculum for ambulatory care nursing* (3rd ed., pp. 217-231). Pitman, NJ: American Academy of Ambulatory Care Nursing.

Chen, E.H., & Bodenheimer, T. (2011). Improving population health through team-based panel management. *Archives of Internal Medicine, 171*(17), 1558-1559.

Coulter, A., & Ellins, J. (2006). *Patient-focused interventions: A review of the evidence.* (2006). London, England: The Health Foundation.

Council on Linkages Between Academia and Public Health Practice. (2010). *About the core competencies for public health professionals.* Washington, DC: Public Health Foundation. Retrieved from http://www.phf.org/programs/corecompetencies

Cronenwett, L., Sherwood, G., Barnsteiner, J., Disch, J., Johnson, J., Mitchell, P., … Warren, J. (2007). Quality and safety education for nurses. *Nursing Outlook, 55*(3), 122-131.

Cronenwett, L., Sherwood, G., Pohl, J., Barnsteiner, J., Moore, S., Sullivan, D.T., … Warren, J. (2009). Quality and safety education for advanced nursing practice. *Nursing Outlook, 57*(6), 338-348.

Cusack, C.M., Knudsen, A.D., Kronstadt, J.L., Singer, R.F., & Brown, A.L. (2010). *Practice based population health: Information technology to support transformation to proactive primary care.* Rockville, MD: Agency for Healthcare Research and Quality.

Grundy, P., Davis, K., & Fisher, E. (2011). *Better to best value-driving elements of the patient centered medical home and accountable care organizations.* Retrieved from http://www.pcpcc.org/sites/default/files/media/better_best_guide_full_2011.pdf

Gulley, S.P., Rasch, E.K., & Chan, L. (2011). If we build it, who will come? Working-age adults with chronic health care needs and the medical home. *Medical Care, 49*(2), 149-155.

Gupta, R., & Bodenheimer, T. (2013). How primary care practices can improve continuity of care. *JAMA Internal Medicine, 173*(20), 1885-1886.

Halpern, R., & Boulter, P. (2000). *Population-based health care: Definitions and applications.* Boston, MA: Tufts Managed Care Institute.

Hibbard, J., & Lorig, K. (2012). The dos and don'ts of patient engagement in busy offices practices. *Journal of Ambulatory Care Management, 35*(2), 129-132.

Hibbard, J.H., Greene, J., & Overton, V. (2013). Patients with lower activation associated with higher costs: Delivery systems should know their patients' 'scores.' *Health Affairs, 32*(2), 216-222.

Hibbard, J.H., Stockard, J., Mahoney, E.R., & Tusler, M. (2004). Development of the patient activation measure (PAM): Conceptualizing and measuring activation in patients and consumers. *Health Services Research, 39*(4), 1005-1026.

Hodach, R. (2011). *The promise of population health management: New technologies are required to automate expanded physician workflow.* Retrieved from http://info.phytel.com/rs/phytel/images/population_health_final.pdf

Institute for Health Technology Transformation. (2012). *Population health management: A roadmap for provider-based automation in a new era of healthcare.* Retrieved from http://ihealthtran.com/pdf/PHMReport.pdf

Interprofessional Education Collaborative (IPEC). (2011). *Core competencies for interprofessional collaborative practice.* Retrieved from http://www.aacn.nche.edu/education-resources/ipecreport.pdf

Jessie, A.T., Johnson, S.A., & Trehearne, B.E. (2014). Population health management. In S.A Haas, B.A. Swan, & T.S. Haynes, *Care coordination and transition management core curriculum* (pp. 113-140). Pitman, NJ: American Academy of Ambulatory Care Nursing.

Katon, W.J., Lin, E.H., Von Korff, M., Ciechanowski, P., Ludman, E.J., … McCulloch, D. (2010). Collaborative care for patients with depression and chronic illnesses. *New England Journal of Medicine, 363*(27), 2611-2620.

Kim, C.S., & Flanders, S.A. (2013). In the clinic. Transitions of care. *Annals of Internal Medicine, 158*(5 Pt 1):ITC3-1. doi: 10.7326/0003-4819-158-5-20130305-01003

Laughlin, C.B. (Ed.). (2013). *Core curriculum for ambulatory care nursing* (3rd ed.). Pitman, NJ: American Academy of Ambulatory Care Nursing.

Lorig, K., Holman, H., Sobel, D., Laurent, D., Gonzalez, V., & Minor, M. (2012). *Living a healthy life with chronic conditions* (4th ed). Boulder, CO: Bull Publishing.

Moorehead, T., May, J., Ganda, K., & Jarm, L. (2012). *Population health management in physician practice: A call to action.* Retrieved from http://www.carecontinuumalliance.org/pdf/cca-report-10-23-12.pdf

National Wraparound Initiative. (2014). *Wraparound basics.* Retrieved from http://www.nwi.pdx.edu/wraparoundbasics.shtml

Philbin, E.F., & DiSalvo, T.G. (1999). Prediction of hospital readmission for heart failure: Development of a simple risk score based on administrative data. *Journal of the American College of Cardiology, 33*(6), 1560-1566.

QSEN Institute. (2014). *Pre-licensure KSAS.* Retrieved from http://qsen.org/competencies/pre-licensure-ksas

Rich, E., Lipson D., Libersky, J., & Parchman, M. (2012). *Coordinating care for adults with complex care needs in the patient-centered medical home: Challenges and solutions.* Rockville, MD: Agency for Healthcare Research and Quality.

Rutenberg, C., & Greenberg, M.E. (2012). *The art and science of telephone triage: How to practice nursing over the phone.* Hot Springs, AR: Telephone Triage Consulting, Inc.

U.S. Census Bureau. (2010). *2010 census data.* Retrieved from http://census.gov/2010census/data

Von Korff, M., Gruman, J., Schaefer, J., Curry, S.J., & Wagner, E.H. (1997). Collaborative management of chronic illness. *Annals of Internal Medicine, 127*(12), 1097-1102.

Wagner, E.H. (1998). Chronic disease management: What will it take to improve care for chronic conditions. *Effective Clinical Practice, 1*(1), 2-4.

# CHAPTER 11

# Care Coordination and Transition Management Between Acute Care and Ambulatory Care

*Janine Allbritton, MSN, RN*
*Mary Sue Dailey, APN-CNS*

## Learning Outcome Statement

The purpose of this chapter is to enable the reader to understand the outcomes a mutually developed, implemented, and continuously evaluated transition of care plan has on quality of care, patient satisfaction, and patient outcomes. In addition, recognizing the financial impact and understanding the importance of integrating evidence-based practice guidelines into a transition of care plan are essential components of the role of the registered nurse (RN) in Care Coordination and Transition Management (CCTM).

## Learning Objectives

After reading this chapter, the RN in the CCTM role will be able to:

- Identify opportunities for transition management within the continuum of care.
- Identify key elements of successful transition planning including identification of vulnerable populations.
- Review the most common factors influencing poor transition of care.
- Describe components of an evidence-based transition plan.
- List examples of transition of care models.
- Apply an evidence-based format to coordinate information transfer between sites of care.
- Demonstrate the knowledge, skills, and attitudes required for transitions in care (see Table 1).

## Competency Definition

*Transition of care* is the movement of a patient from one setting of care (hospital, ambulatory primary care practice, ambulatory specialty care practice, long-term care, home health, rehabilitation facility) to another (Centers for Medicare & Medicaid Services [CMS], 2013a). "It comprises a range of time-limited services that complement primary care and are designed to ensure health care continuity and avoid preventable poor outcomes among at-risk populations as they move from one level of care to another, among multiple providers and across settings" (Naylor, Aiken, Kurtzman, Olds, & Hirschman, 2011, p. 747). Transitional care is "a set of actions designed to ensure the coordination and continuity of health care as patients transfer between different locations or different levels of care within the same location" (Coleman & Boult, 2003, p. 555).

Until recently, much of the research conducted on transition of care events emphasized hospitals and the discharge planning process. It has become apparent there are numerous instances along the continuum of care during which the progress toward positive clinical outcomes has the potential to derail. It is also becoming apparent that responsibility for a person's care does not end when that person enters or exits another care setting. Through active involvement of the patient and caregiver and participation of providers of care from environments outside the hospital, in concert with discharge planning occurring during hospitalization, opportunities for preventing errors will be uncovered, preventable re-admissions will be decreased, and more conscientious use of the shrinking health care dollar will occur.

The coordination of patient care is an established standard of nursing practice, regardless of the practice environment. Engaging the patient and family to participate in determining the needs and preferences surrounding their care and providing education and securing essential equipment, supplies, and community resources to manage their care has long been part of the scope of the practicing registered nurse (RN). The American Nurses Association (ANA) released a position statement regarding the essential role of RNs in this endeavor. "Patient-centered care coordination is a core professional standard and competency for all registered nursing practice. Based on a partnership guided by the healthcare consumer's and family's needs and preferences, the registered nurse is integral to patient care quality, satisfaction, and the effective and efficient use of health care resources. Registered nurses are qualified and educated for the role of care coordination, especially with high risk and vulnerable populations" (ANA, 2012, para. 2). In October 2012, Medicare began linking hospital reimbursement to the quality of care. This increased focus on quality places more emphasis on better preparation of patients for managing their illness at home. The goal is to promote quality and cost savings through the reduction of after-hospital adverse events and prevent re-admissions. In particular, the ambulatory care RN plays a critical role in care coordination and transition management (CCTM) by focusing on prevention of illness, management of specific high-risk conditions, reduction or elimination of preventable complications, as well as promotion of healthy lifestyle changes and careful use of valuable health care resources. Management of a care transition generally begins when a patient is identified as having a status change (deterioration or improvement) that makes it appropriate to move to another setting or level of care (American Medical Directors Association [AMDA], 2010).

## I. Transition of Care Opportunities

A. Acute to ambulatory care which includes transition of care from hospital to primary care physician.
  1. This is one of the most common transitions of care to identify and one that has been researched the most.
  2. Provides an opportunity to have a major impact on quality of care with effective hand-off communication.
  3. Is the transition of care most likely to positively impact health care cost savings through implementation of strategies to reduce adverse events and hospital re-admission rates.
  4. Contains communication gaps between providers in the acute care and post-hospital care agencies which results in providers having an incomplete picture of the scope of the patient's needs.
  5. Requires collaboration between inpatient or acute care RN contact and the RN in CCTM in ambulatory care, Patient-Centered Medical Homes (PCMH), and outpatient settings, both having access to multidisciplinary health care teams.
  6. Provides opportunity for patients to further discuss and solidify goals discussed but not finalized in acute care settings.
  7. Home care agency must be made aware of pertinent care information and patient needs to maintain consistency in care and anticipate care needs.

B. Acute to sites within long-term care continuum requires RN points of contact to facilitate communication between health care team at different levels of care.
  1. Care transitions expose older adults to added risk for medical complications, decreased quality of life, and overuse of acute health care services (National Transitions of Care Coalition [NTOCC], 2011).
  2. Older adults now enter nursing homes with increasingly acute health conditions which means they are more vulnerable to poor health and quality-of-life outcomes.
  3. Nursing home residents are highly vulnerable to harm from poorly executed care transitions, including inadequate communication of critical information from the hospital, medication errors including omissions, delays in follow-up diagnostic tests, treatments, and repeated hospitalizations.
  4. The fundamental goal of those assisting older adults during transitions of care is to promote safe and person-centered transitions that are most likely to achieve patient and caregiver goals without complications (AMDA, 2010).

C. Ambulatory care and extended care to acute care.
  1. Acute care RNs are generally responsible for collecting data to establish a plan of care, but often have incomplete information regarding patient's prior health status, socioeconomic issues, support systems, and coping mechanisms. This is an opportunity for the RN in CCTM to facilitate the exchange of information.
  2. In current practice, information previously developed for a patient's ambulatory or extended care plan of care is seldom shared with the acute care medical team.
  3. The RN in CCTM can assist in facilitating the transfer of care to acute setting by ensuring and/or providing the following elements:
     a. The patient should have an accountable provider or a team of providers during all points of transition. This provider(s) should be clearly identified, will provide patient-centered care, and will serve as central coordinator across all settings and across other providers.
     b. The patient should have an up-to-date, proactive care plan that includes clearly defined goals, takes into consideration the patient's preferences, and is culturally appropriate.
     c. Whenever possible, the management and coordination of transitional care activities should be facilitated through the use of integrated electronic information systems that are interoperable and available to patients and providers.
     d. Information must be communicated to the acute care setting on current prescription and over-the-counter medications (including vitamins, herbs, laxatives, etc.) specifying name, dose, frequency, and duration.
     e. Strategies for appropriate communication with patients with limited English proficiency and health literacy must be defined.

f. Information on any known food/drug allergy or intolerance.
g. Recently completed lab and/or diagnostic procedure reports.
h. Information on any referrals currently being provided.
i. Current socioeconomic or psychosocial limitations.
j. Current use of outside agencies for durable medical supplies, home care, home-delivered meals, etc.
k. Name and contact information of caregiver at home.
l. Current advance directives.

D. Acute or ambulatory primary care providers to specialists.
1. Specialists often concentrate on single patient issue; not the whole person.
2. Communication between providers on plans/tests/results are often lacking due to deficiencies in integration of information between multiple types of electronic and paper medical records.
3. Many opportunities exist for improvement in collaboration between specialists to ensure plan of care congruent with patient goals.

E. Pediatric to young adult.
1. Transition from pediatric care to young adult is often overlooked.
2. This may be the first time the patient is autonomous as an adult.
3. Certain conditions such as pregnancy may suddenly change the patient's minority status, necessitating the RN's support in navigating the health care system.
4. Offers opportunity to empower patient during care decisions.

## II. Factors Influencing Poor Transition of Care

A. Deficiencies in communication between health care team members in current setting and the setting to which the patient is going (Basso, 2013).
1. No consistent tool or structured format utilized for hand-offs.
2. Perception that care responsibility ends with discharge from current setting.
3. Use of hospitalists for acute hospitalization adds an additional layer of providers needing information about the patient (Kim & Flanders, 2013).
a. Hospitalist often not familiar with patient's past history and may not have immediate access to outpatient medical records.
b. Hospitalist schedules may provide greater in-hospital coverage in terms of hours per day, but continuity of care may suffer due to lack of hand-off between hospitalists.
c. The majority of information exchanged is of a medical nature with little information pertaining to nursing, socioeconomic, psychosocial, and care issues.

B. Management of follow-up care left up to patient/family to navigate (Swan, 2012).
1. Health care systems have become more complex and difficult to navigate without direction.
2. Health literacy has a major impact on ability to manage care needs.

C. Lack of essential patient education on care at home (Manheim & Rifkin, 2010).
1. Multiple providers involved in care leads to confusion on who to call with problems or concerns.
2. Health care provider, rather than the patient, makes decisions on what is important for teaching.

D. Inability of patient/family to follow the plan of care (Jack, Paasche-Orlow, & Mitchell, 2013).
1. Resources available not thoroughly assessed.
2. Family/caregiver not involved in care; untapped resource.
3. Patient/family not actively involved in setting goals for care.
4. Patient encounters barriers that can include:
a. Cost of medications, care, and inadequacy of insurance coverage.
b. Lack of ease in making follow-up appointments.
c. Lack of transportation to appointments.

## III. Evidence-Based Transition Models

A. Community-based Care Transitions Program (CCTP) was developed by the CMS to test care transition interventions for currently enrolled Medicare persons who are at high-risk for re-admission following hospitalization (CMS, 2013a).

B. Nearly one in five Medicare patients discharged from a hospital – approximately 2.6 million seniors – are readmitted within 30 days, at a cost of over $26 billion every year (CMS, 2013a).

C. Various care models currently being used include (CMS, 2013b):
1. Better Outcomes by Optimizing Safe Transitions (BOOST) (Society of Hospital Medicine, 2014). Focus of Project BOOST is to:
a. Identify high-risk patients on admission and target risk-specific interventions through use of 8**P** screening tool which assesses:
(1) **P**roblems with medications: polypharmacy – i.e. ≥ 10 routine medications – or high-risk medication including anticoagulants, insulin, oral hypoglycemic agents, aspirin and clopidogrel dual therapy, digoxin, narcotics.
(2) **P**sychological: positive depression screen or history of depression diagnosis.

(3) **P**rincipal diagnosis: cancer, stroke, diabetes, heart failure, chronic obstructive pulmonary disease.
(4) **P**hysical limitations: deconditioning, frailty, or other physical limitations that impair ability to participate in self-care.
(5) **P**oor health literacy: inability to do "teach back."
(6) **P**atient support: social isolation, absence of support to assist with care, as well as insufficient or absent connection with primary care.
(7) **P**rior hospitalization: nonelective; in last 6 months.
(8) **P**alliative care: does the patient have an advanced or progressively worsening illness.

b. Reduce 30-day re-admission rates for general medicine patients.
c. Reduce length of stay.
d. Improve facility patient satisfaction and HCAHPS (Hospital Consumer Assessment of Healthcare Providers and Systems) scores.
e. Improve information flow between inpatient and outpatient providers.

2. Transitional Care Model (TCM) (Naylor et al., 1999; Naylor et al., 2004).
   a. Lead by a master's-prepared nurse to treat chronically ill, high-risk older patients before, during, and after hospitalization.
   b. One study that tested the TCM with Medicare beneficiaries hospitalized with common medical and surgical conditions resulted in total health care savings of $3,000 per patient for intervention versus control patients at 24 weeks ($3,630 vs. $6,661) (NTOCC, n.d.).
3. Care Transitions Intervention® (Coleman, Parry, Chalmers, & Min, 2006).
   a. Utilizes Transitions Coach® to coordinate the care of an assigned group of patients.
   b. The anticipated cost savings of one Transitions Coach (responsible for 350 chronically ill adults), after an initial hospitalization, over a period of 12 months, is $330,000 (NTOCC, n.d.).
4. Enhanced Discharge Planning Program (NTOCC, n.d.).
   a. Involves short-term post-discharge social work services to assess and intervene from biopsychosocial perspective.
   b. Cost analysis within Rush University Medical Center's (Chicago, IL) fee-for-service environment showed a $1,293 savings per patient.
5. Project Re-Engineered Discharge (RED) (Jack et al., 2013).
   a. Focus is on standardized discharge process to ensure patients are prepared when leaving the hospital.
   b. In 2008, researchers found patients discharged utilizing the RED program had a 30% lower rate of hospital utilization 30 days post discharge and re-admission or emergency department visit was prevented for every 7.3 subjects receiving the intervention (NTOCC, n.d.).
   c. Additionally, patients who received intervention had a 33.9% lower cost than those who did not receive intervention, which equated to a savings of $412 per patient (NTOCC, n.d.).
6. Transition Home for Patients with Heart Failure.
   a. Implemented at St. Luke's Hospital (Cedar Rapids, IA).
   b. Designed as part of the Institute for Healthcare Improvement's (IHI) Transforming Care at the Bedside [TCAB] program).
   c. Emphasized early and ongoing assessment of a patient's needs at discharge.
   d. Incorporated enhanced education and caregiver communication processes. Reduced the 30-day heart-failure-to-heart-failure re-admission rate for patients from 14% to 6%, and the all-cause heart failure re-admission rate to 15% to 17% (down from 23%).
7. State Action on Avoidable Rehospitalizations (STAAR) (Boutwell, Jencks, Nielsen, & Rutherford, 2009).
   a. IHI-partnered initiative to improve transitions in care and reduce rehospitalizations.
8. Geriatric Resources for Assessment and Care of Elders (GRACE) (Counsell, Callahan, Buttar, Clark, & Frank, 2006).
   a. Physician/practice-based care coordination model conducted over a long term.
   b. Requires nurse practitioner and social worker to offer in-home assessment and care management.
   c. In this randomized study the cost of this program was $315,040 ($1,432 per patient). The conclusion was the intervention was cost neutral for high-risk patients due to reductions in hospital care (NTOCC, n.d.).

D. Engagement of health care team (physician, RN, allied health providers, social work, care coordinator, etc.) to discuss and communicate patient goals and plan of care is essential. Elements identified as significant in the transition of care models include:
   1. Patient and caregiver education regarding self-management, assessing and acknowledging functional and cognitive status, and assessment of learning through "teach back."
   2. Identification of barriers to care, including psychosocial needs and resolutions.
   3. Completion of a General Assessment of Preparedness (GAP) checklist (Society of Hospital Medicine, 2008).

4. Completion of Patient Discharge Checklist such as identified as part of the BOOST program (Society of Hospital Medicine, 2008).
5. Evaluation of medication management including reconciliation of medication at discharge and post-discharge to identify adherence and resolve problems.
6. Coordination of follow-up appointments with primary physician and specialists; to include questions to ask and information to provide physicians.
7. Education of patients and caregivers regarding signs and symptoms that indicate worsening condition and steps to take (red flags).
8. Education of patient/significant other on communication skills to include how to speak with physicians to relay care needs.
9. Discussion regarding incomplete test results; when and how information will be communicated.
10. Communication and hand-off to all providers regarding patients' plans of care, which reflects patient and caregiver goals.
11. Arrangements for post-discharge home visit or follow-up via telephone within 72 hours for reinforcement of teaching, problem identification, and validation of receipt of medical/social services and equipment identified at discharge.
12. Incorporation of disease-specific care guideline into plan of care (coronary heart failure, myocardial infarction, hypertension, asthma, diabetes management) (Agency for Healthcare Research and Quality, n.d.). Due to overlap of guidelines for care of patients with multiple chronic conditions, the RN in CCTM needs to help guide the patient and caregiver through the health care maze to determine which guideline(s) are best suited based on the patient's goals.

## IV. Further Details of Selected Transition of Care Models

A. Better Outcomes by Optimizing Safe Transitions (BOOST) (Society of Hospital Medicine, 2014).
   1. Essential organizational steps for improving the discharge transition:
      a. Institutional support.
      b. Multidisciplinary team or steering committee.
      c. Engagement of patients and families.
      d. Data collection and reliable metrics.
      e. Specific aims or goals.
      f. Standardized discharge pathways to include:
         (1) Key medications.
         (2) Provision for medication changes.
         (3) Information on follow-up appointments.
         (4) Self-management instructions.
         (5) Pending test results and how these will be communicated.
      g. Institution-specific policies and procedures to guide the care team regarding:
         (1) Management of team communication.
         (2) Content of discharge summary.
         (3) Patient education.
         (4) Medication safety and polypharmacy.
         (5) Symptom management.
         (6) Discharge and follow-up care.
      h. Comprehensive education program for health care providers and patients.

B. Care Transitions Intervention (CTI) (Coleman, 2007).
   1. Model is composed of the following components.
      a. Personal health record (PHR).
      b. Discharge preparation checklist.
      c. Patient self-activation and management session with a Transitions Coach.
      d. Transitions Coach follow-up visits and phone calls.
   2. Intervention focuses on four conceptual areas (The Four Pillars®).
      a. Medication self-management.
      b. Patient understands and uses the PHR to communicate.
      c. Primary care and specialist follow-up.
      d. Knowledge of red flags.
         (1) Understanding of indications that condition is worsening.
         (2) Awareness of how to respond.

C. Geriatric Resources for Assessment and Care of Elders (GRACE) (Counsell et al., 2006).
   1. Foundational principles include:
      a. Specific targeting of older people at risk.
      b. Availability of collaborative expertise in geriatrics.
      c. Integration of program into primary care.
      d. Coordination of care across all sites of care.
      e. Use of electronic health record to support physician practices and facilitate monitoring of clinical parameters.
      f. Institutionally endorsed clinical practice guide.

## V. Application of Evidence-Based Tools

A. Case study: Shortness of breath/pneumonia (see Appendix 1).
B. Application of selected tools to case study.
   1. 8P tool RN-CCTM to Acute Care (see Appendix 2).
   2. 8P tool Acute Care to RN-CCTM in PCMH (see Appendix 3).
   3. Universal Patient Discharge Checklist with GAP (see Appendix 4).
   4. After hospital plan of care – medication schedule (see Appendix 5).
   5. Patient PASS: A Transition Record (see Appendix 6).

**Table 1.**
**CCTM Between Acute Care and Ambulatory Care: Knowledge, Skills, and Attitudes for Competency**

| Patient-Centered Care | | | |
|---|---|---|---|
| Recognize the patient or designee as the source of control and full partner in providing compassionate and coordinated care based on respect for patient's preferences, values, and needs (Cronenwett et al., 2007). | | | |
| **Knowledge** | **Skills** | **Attitudes** | **Sources** |
| Analyze multiple dimensions of patient-centered care including patient/family/community preferences and values, as well as social, cultural, psychological, and spiritual contexts.<br><br>*Types of transitions:*<br>• Acute to home<br>• Acute to subacute<br>• Home to acute<br>• Acute care to long-term acute care | Identify patient and caregiver main concerns regarding care after discharge, management of symptoms, attainable goals related to disease and prognosis.<br><br>Identify and create plans to address barriers in care settings that prevent fully integrating patient-centered care.<br><br>Engage patients or designated surrogates in active partnerships along the health-illness continuum. | Commit to the patient as the source of control and full partner in his/her care.<br><br>Commit to patient-centered, collaborative care planning.<br><br>Appreciate physical and other barriers to patient-centered care.<br><br>Value the involvement of patients and families in care decisions.<br><br>Respect preferences of patients related to their level of engagement in health care decision making. | Cronenwett et al., 2007 |
| Analyze patient-centered care in the context of care coordination, patient education, physical comfort, emotional support, and care transitions. | Work to address ethical and legal issues related to patients' rights to determine their care.<br><br>Work with patients to create plans of care that are defined by the patient. | Commit to respecting the rights of patients in determining their plan of care.<br><br>Recognize the need to work with family members to accept the patient's right for self-determination.<br><br>Value the decisions of patient and family in choosing best next level of care based on patient's goals. | Physician Orders for Life-Sustaining Treatment Paradigm (POLST), 2012 |
| Analyze strategies which empower patients and/or families involved in the health care process. | Engage patients and/or caregivers in developing active partnerships at all levels of care.<br><br>Eliminate barriers to family or other caregiver's presence during care discussions per patient's request. | Value the involvement of patients and families in care decisions.<br><br>Respect patient preferences for degree of active engagement in care process.<br><br>Honor active partnership with patients or their designated participants in planning, implementing, and evaluating care provided. | Cronenwett et al., 2007 |

*continued on next page*

**Source Note:** Cronenwett et al. (2007) reprinted form *Nursing Outlook, 55*(3), 122-131, with permission from Elsevier.

**Table 1. (continued)**
**CCTM Between Acute Care and Ambulatory Care: Knowledge, Skills, and Attitudes for Competency**

| Knowledge | Skills | Attitudes | Sources |
|---|---|---|---|
| **Safety** | | | |
| Minimize risk of harm to patients and providers through both system effectiveness and individual performance (Cronenwett et al., 2007). | | | |
| **Knowledge** | **Skills** | **Attitudes** | **Sources** |
| Identify best practices that promote patient, community, and provider safety in the practice setting. | Integrate strategies and safety practices to reduce risk of harm to patients, self, and others.<br>Essential elements of communication between providers during care hand-off to include:<br>• Re-admission risk.<br>• Overview of patient.<br>• Current problems.<br>• Outstanding tests.<br>• Patient preferences.<br>• Medication and allergies. | Commit to being a safety mentor and role model.<br>Value a systems approach to improving patient care instead of blaming individuals. | Cronenwett et al., 2007 |
| Describe evidence-based practices when responding to errors and good catches. | Use evidence-based best practices to create policies and processes to manage medical care such as National Clearinghouse Guidelines. | Commit to identifying errors and potential risks to improve quality and systems.<br>Value open and honest communication with patients and families about errors and hazards. | Cronennett et al., 2007 |
| **Teamwork and Collaboration** | | | |
| Function effectively within nursing and interprofessional teams, fostering open communication, mutual respect, and shared decision making to achieve quality patient care (Cronenwett et al., 2007). | | | |
| **Knowledge** | **Skills** | **Attitudes** | **Sources** |
| Understand the roles and scope of practice of each interprofessional team member including patients, in order to work effectively to provide the highest level of care possible. | Work with team members to identify goals for individual patients based on personal decisions for care.<br>Ensure inclusion of patients and family members as part of the team based on the patient and families preference to be included. | Respect the role of the patient within the family group.<br>Appreciate cultural differences and integration into care of the patient.<br>Value patients and families as the source of control for their health care. | Cronenwett et al., 2007 |
| | Demonstrate leadership in advancing interprofessional (IP) team function through a variety of strategies including, but not limited to:<br>• Reflection.<br>• Promotion of effective decision making. | Based on client/patient/family needs, consider that preferred practice is IP collaboration and willingly collaborate. | Interprofessional Education Collaborative (IPEC), 2011 |

*continued on next page*

Table 1. (continued)
CCTM Between Acute Care and Ambulatory Care: Knowledge, Skills, and Attitudes for Competency

| Teamwork and Collaboration (continued) | | | |
|---|---|---|---|
| **Knowledge** | **Skills** | **Attitudes** | **Sources** |
| | • Identification of factors that contribute to or hinder team collaboration, including power and hierarchy.<br>• Flexibility and adaptability.<br>• Able to assume diverse roles in the IP group and support others in their roles.<br>• Establish and maintain effective IP working relationship/ partnerships with clients/patients/ families and other team members, teams, and/or organizations to support achievement of common goals. | | |
| Describe appropriate hand-off communication practices. | Use communication practices that minimize risks associated with hand-offs among providers and across transitions of care<br>At a minimum, communication at hand-off should include:<br>• Medication management.<br>• Timely primary care/ specialist follow-up.<br>• Knowledge of red flags or warnings.<br>• Copy or access to patient-centered health record. | Appreciate the risks associated with missing information during hand-offs among providers and across transitions in care. | Cronenwett et al., 2007 |
| | Communicate effectively, including giving and receiving feedback.<br>Perform as an effective team member by:<br>• Sharing information.<br>• Listening attentively.<br>• Using understandable communications.<br>• Providing feedback to others.<br>• Responding to feedback of others. | Understand the potential barrier the use of medical jargon can have on patient/family understanding of communication. | IPEC, 2011 |

*continued on next page*

Table 1. (continued)
CCTM Between Acute Care and Ambulatory Care: Knowledge, Skills, and Attitudes for Competency

| Teamwork and Collaboration (continued) | | | |
|---|---|---|---|
| **Knowledge** | **Skills** | **Attitudes** | **Sources** |
| Analyze strategies that influence the ability to initiate and sustain effective partnerships with members of inpatient, office/clinic, and community interprofessional teams. | Integrate interprofessional competencies into practice. | Commit to collaborative practice with others involved in the patient's care.<br><br>Value the solutions obtained through systematic interprofessional collaborative efforts.<br><br>Value the team approach to providing high-quality care. | IPEC, 2011 |
| Analyze the impact of team-based practice. | Act with integrity, consistency, and respect for differing views. | Commit to being an effective team member. | Cronenwett et al., 2007 |
| | Continuously plan for improvement in self and others for effective transition management development and functioning.<br><br>Elicit input from other team members to improve individual and team performance. | Be open to continual assessment and improvement of skills as a team member.<br><br>Support the development of a safe team environment where issues can be addressed between team members and conflict can be resolved. | Mitchell et al., 2012 |
| **Evidence-Based Practice** | | | |
| Integrate best current evidence with clinical expertise and patient/family preferences and values for delivery of optimal health care (Cronenwett et al., 2007). | | | |
| **Knowledge** | **Skills** | **Attitudes** | **Sources** |
| Identify efficient and effective search strategies to locate reliable sources of evidence. | Employ efficient and effective search strategies to answer focused clinical or health system practices. | Value development of search skills for locating evidence for best practice. | Cronenwett et al., 2007 |
| Summarize current evidence regarding major diagnostic and treatment actions within the practice specialty and health care delivery system. | Exhibit contemporary knowledge of best evidence related to practice and health care systems. | Value cutting-edge knowledge of current practice. | Cronenwett et al., 2007 |
| | Promote research for evidence that is needed in practice specialty and health care system. | "Value working in an interactive manner with interdisciplinary team members" (p. 31). | IPEC, 2011 |

## References

Agency for Healthcare Research and Quality (AHRQ). (n.d.). *National guideline clearinghouse.* Retrieved from http://www.guideline.gov/

Agency for Healthcare Research and Quality (AHRQ). (2013). *Project RED (re-engineered discharge) training program.* Rockville, MD: Author. Retrieved from http://www.ahrq.gov/professionals/systems/hospital/red/index.html

American Medical Directors Association (AMDA). (2010). *Transitions of care in the long-term care continuum: Clinical practice guideline.* Columbia, MD: Author. Retrieved from http://www.amda.com/tools/clinical/toccpg.pdf

American Nurses Association (ANA). (2012). *Care coordination and registered nurses' essential role position statement.* Silver Spring, MD: Author.

Basso, C. (2013, November 11). Transitions of care – A path to quality outcomes. *Nurse.com,* 24-30.

Boutwell, A., Jencks, S., Nielsen, G.A., & Rutherford, P. (2009). *State Action on Avoidable Rehospitalizations (STAAR) initiative: Applying early evidence and experience in front-line process improvements to develop a state-based strategy.* Cambridge, MA: Institute for Healthcare Improvement.

Centers for Medicare & Medicaid Services (CMS). (2013a). *Community-based care transition programs.* Retrieved from http://innovation.cms.gov/initiatives/CCTP/?itemID=CMS1239313

Centers for Medicare & Medicaid Services (CMS). (2013b). *Partnership for patients: Readmissions and care transitions.* Retrieved from http://partnershipforpatients.cms.gov/p4p_resources/tsp-preventablereadmissions/toolpreventablereadmissions.html

Coleman, E.A. (2007). *The Care Transitions Program®.* Retrieved from http://www.caretransitions.org/structure.asp

Coleman, E.A., & Boult, C. (2003). Improving the quality of transitional care for persons with complex care needs. *Journal of the American Geriatrics Society, 51*(4), 556-557. doi:10.1046/j.1532-5415.2003.51186.x

Coleman, E., Parry, C., Chalmers, S., & Min, S. (2006). The care transitions intervention: Results of a randomized controlled trial. *Archives of Internal Medicine, 166,* 1822-1828.

Counsell, S.R., Callahan, C.M., Buttar, A.B., Clark, D.O., & Frank, K.I. (2006). Geriatric resources for assessment and care of elders (GRACE): A new model of primary care for low-income seniors. *Journal of the American Geriatric Society, 54*(7), 1136-1141.

Cronenwett, L., Sherwood, G., Barnsteiner, J., Disch, J., Johnson, J., Mitchell, P., ... Warren, J. (2007). Quality and safety education for nurses. *Nursing Outlook, 55*(3), 122-131. doi:10.1016/j.outlook.2007.02.006

Grimmer, K., Moss, J., Falco, J., & Kindness, H. (2006). Incorporating patient and carer concerns in discharge plans: The development of a practical patient-centered checklist. *Internet Journal of Allied Health Sciences and Practice, 4*(1).

Interprofessional Education Collaborative (IPEC). (2011). *Core competencies for interprofessional collaborative practice: Report of an expert panel.* Washington, DC: Author.

Jack, B.W., Paasche-Orlow, M.K., & Mitchell, S.M. (2013). *Re-engineered discharge (RED) toolkit.* AHRQ Publication No. 12(13)-0084. Rockville, MD: Agency for Healthcare Research and Quality. Retrieved from http://www.ahrq.gov/professionals/systems/hospital/toolkit/redtoolkit.pdf

Kim, C.S., & Flanders, S.A. (2013). Transitions of care. *Annals of Internal Medicine, 158*(5 Part 1), ITC3-1. doi:10.7326/0003-4819-158-5-201303050-01003

Manheim, J., & Rifkin, J. (2010). *Transitions of care: Physician to physician communication.* Denver, CO: The Colorado Health Foundation.

Mitchell, P., Wynia, M., Golden, B., McNellia, S., Okun, C.E., Webb, V., ... Kohorn, I.V. (2012). *Core principles & values of effective team-based health care.* Washington, DC: Institute of Medicine.

National Transitions of Care Coalition (NTOCC). (2011). *Care transition bundle: Seven essential intervention categories.* Retrieved from http://www.ntocc.org/Portals/0/PDF/Compendium/SevenEssentialElements.pdf

National Transitions of Care Coalition (NTOCC). (n.d.). *Improved transitions of patient care yield tangible savings.* Retrieved from http://www.ntocc.org/portals/0/pdf/resources/TangibleSavings.pdf

Naylor, M.D., Aiken, L.H., Kurtzman, E.T., Olds, D.M., & Hirschman, K.B. (2011). The care span: The importance of transitional care in achieving health reform. *Health Affairs, 30*(4), 746-754.

Naylor, M.D., Brooten, D., Campbell, R., Jacobsen, B.S., Mezey, M.D., Pauly, M.V., & Schwartz, J.S. (1999). Comprehensive discharge planning and home follow-up of hospitalized elders: A randomized clinical trial. *Journal of the American Medical Association, 281*(7), 613-620.

Naylor, M.D., Brooten, D.A., Campbell, R.L., Maislin, G., McCauley, K.M., & Schwartz, J.S. (2004). Transitional care of older adults hospitalized with heart failure: A randomized, controlled trial. *Journal of American Geriatric Society, 52*(5), 675-684.

Physician Orders for Life-Sustaining Treatment Paradigm (POLST). (2012). *What is POLST?* Retrieved from http://www.polst.org/advance-care-planning/

Society of Hospital Medicine. (2014). *The 8 Ps: Assessing your patient's risk for adverse events after discharge.* Philadelphia, PA: Author.

Swan, B.A. (2012). A nurse learns firsthand that you may fend for yourself after a hospital stay. *Health Affairs, 31*(11), 2579-2582. doi:10.1377/hlthaff.2012.0516

## Additional Readings

Coleman, E.A., & Boult, C. (2007). Improving the quality of transitional care for persons with complex care needs. *Assisted Living Consult, 3*(2), 30-32.

Hughes, R. (2008). *Patient safety and quality: An evidence-based handbook for nurses.* Rockville, MD: Agency for Healthcare Quality and Research.

Leff, B., Reider, L., Frick, K.D., Scharfstein, D.O., Boyd, C.M., Frey, K., ... & Boult, C. (2009). Guided care and the cost of complex healthcare: A preliminary report. *The American Journal of Managed Care, 15*(8), 555-559.

## Appendix 1.
## Application of Transition Tools to Sample Case Studies

The following case study illustrates how use of standardized tools such as those found in Project BOOST (Better Outcomes by Optimizing Safe Transitions) (Society of Hospital Medicine, 2014) and Project RED (AHRQ, 2013; Jack et al., 2013) can assist with communicating patient-specific needs at transitions of care. Components of Project BOOST include:

1. Risk stratification process (the 8P tool).
2. Risk-specific intervention plan linked to the 8P risk score summary.
3. Universal set of expectations for all patients being discharged from the hospital to home (the Universal Checklist).
4. General Assessment of Preparedness (GAP), a component list of issues important to providers and patients (and their caregivers) surrounding the readiness of patients for transition out of the hospital.

These assessment elements are often defined as TARGET (Tool for Addressing Risk: a Geriatric Evaluation for Transitions) but can be applied to multiple age groups. Aspects of the assessment may be completed by different members of the inpatient care team (e.g., nursing, case management, physicians, pharmacists, and social workers), and the tool can then act as a central repository of the information. Determining the individual (or preferably the *role* of the individual) who has ultimate ownership of the process is a critical step in improving the transition of care process. The "confirmed by" signature should be completed by whoever at the institution has final ownership of the transition process (e.g., the discharge planner or nurse).

*The 8Ps Risk Stratification Tool* is completed at admission, highlighting the need to identify patients at increased risk of adverse events post-hospitalization, and utilizing the duration of the hospitalization to mitigate these risks as much as possible. Risk-specific interventions correlate with problem areas identified on the 8P tool. This tool can be used as a hand-off between the RN in CCTM and nurses in the acute care setting, as well as from the acute care setting to the RN in CCTM who will follow the patient in the post-acute setting (home, skilled, or long-term care setting).

*Universal Patient Discharge Checklist* lists a universal set of expectations for all patients being discharged from the hospital to home.

*General Assessment of Preparedness (GAP)* is a list largely derived from a study of patient preferences of common logistical and psychological areas that, when not addressed, may act as barriers to a patient's ability to receive or obtain the care the patient needs (Grimmer et al., 2006). This practical patient-centered checklist is designed to be completed with the patient/caregiver prior to the patient leaving the acute or subacute care setting and proceeding to the next level of care. It incorporates patient and caregiver concerns into discharge plans. The following case study describes a patient situation and illustrates how the standardized tools can be applied to communicate patient-specific information between levels of care.

The Patient PASS: A Transition Record is also part of the Project BOOST toolkit. The content of this tool is designed to be written in terms the patient can understand and to prepare the patient to address health care situations after discharge successfully.

Project RED also has a number of tools to assist with safe transitions. The After Hospital Care Plan (AHCP) includes a medication schedule, appointment page, diagnosis information, and patient activation page to organize questions for the doctor.

In this case study, selected tools from both Project Boost and Project RED are utilized.

### Case Study: Shortness of Breath/Pneumonia
### Acute Care to RN in CCTM

Patricia P. is a 74-year-old African-American female hospitalized with shortness of breath. This is her second inpatient hospital admission in the last 2 weeks for shortness of breath and her fourth admission this year for similar symptoms. You are her case manager and when you meet her and ask what happened she replies, "I just couldn't breathe."

After review of previous admissions and the electronic medical record, you note her medical history includes congestive heart failure (CHF), chronic obstructive pulmonary disease (COPD), type 2 diabetes, hypertension, anxiety, and sleep apnea. Home medicines include enalapril, furosemide, potassium, inhalation aerosol (Advair®), bronchodilator (Spiriva®), metformin, Lantus® insulin, citalopram (Celexa®), and home oxygen. Her BMI is 45; she uses a continuous positive airway pressure machine at night and states she is compliant most of the time. She lives alone, but does have a grown son who visits her weekly and helps her with shopping. Socializing with friends has become increasingly difficult as her respiratory status has declined and she now requires oxygen and uses a walker for any ambulation.

As part of your care management assessment, you assess Patricia's risk for re-admission and realize her chronic conditions (COPD, diabetes), polypharmacy, recent hospital stay less than 30 days ago, as well as her age and ethnicity, put her at high risk for re-admission. The RN in CCTM called to give you report the morning after admission and utilized the BOOST tool as a framework to let you know compliance with medications and diet, as well as the availability of support and ownership of self-care, have been ongoing issues with this patient. When she was discharged last time, she went home on a prednisone taper and antibiotic for an exacerbation of COPD and bronchitis. The home health care nurse found her to be rather inconsistent in following the medication regime despite seeming to understand the importance of taking medications exactly as directed. Patricia said the antibiotics upset her stomach and the steroids made her "jittery." The home care nurse re-educated her, made sure she had a pill box, and helped her organize each day's medication. She called the primary care physician and got the antibiotic changed to one less likely to cause gastrointestinal upset. Patricia promised to take medications correctly but the home nurse found she was "forgetting" doses. Her son was supposed to take her to see her primary care provider 1 week after discharge but his work schedule changed and she missed the appointment due to lack of transportation. She is back in the hospital 10 days after her last discharge. The chest x-ray shows worsening infiltrates compared to previous reports, as well as mild CHF. Her weight has increased 5 kg over her discharge weight. Patricia is started on intravenous antibiotics and nebulizer treatments as well as additional diuretics.

*continued on next page*

 

## Appendix 1. (continued)
## Application of Transition Tools to Sample Case Studies

### Case Study: Shortness of Breath/Pneumonia
### Acute Care to RN in CCTM

As the inpatient case manager, you consult the multidisciplinary team to review and refine the plan of care developed at Patricia's last hospitalization. Her previous post-hospital care plan included information about her medications, diagnosis, follow-up physician appointments, home physical therapy, and a consult for visiting nurse. She was instructed to test her blood sugar and record it and weigh herself daily. She did this when reminded by the home care nurse but did not do consistently on the days the nurse did not come.

When you sit down with Patricia and utilize "teach back" to explore possible reasons for her difficulty in following her home plan of care, you uncover some gaps. She appears to not understand the connection between infection, antibiotics, and steroids for her COPD exacerbation or the multiple causes for her shortness of breath. Even though she states the importance of "not eating salt" in terms of her CHF, she keeps TV dinners and soup for the times she needs quick easy foods because she does not want to spend a lot of time in the kitchen.

Despite being on insulin for many years, she does not understand sick day management and/or realize the need to call her physician if she is experiencing distressing side effects from her medications. Since she hadn't been feeling well, she was eating mostly processed foods and few fresh fruits and vegetables. Even though the hospital does discharge call backs, Patricia states she never got a follow-up phone call.

Determined to do your best with Patricia, you realize there are many problems to tackle and lifestyle change is an important aspect of her compliance. With the multidisciplinary team, you brainstorm what to do better with this patient and strategies to motivate and assist her to comply with her prescribed therapy. With Patricia's permission, you call her son and see if he is willing to come to the hospital to discuss in person the after-hospital plan of care. Due to his work and family commitments, he is not able to do this, but is willing to discuss the plan with you over the phone. You send him an electronic version and review it over the phone, especially noting the importance of assisting and encouraging his Mom to comply with medications and diet and making sure she monitors her blood sugar and weight. You ask if he can take her for a 1-week post-hospital follow-up appointment and arrange the appointment at a time convenient for the son. After verifying the cost of new medications, you fax her new prescriptions to an outpatient pharmacy and they deliver them to the hospital room before she leaves. The visiting nurse and home therapy are reinstated.

In reviewing Patricia's After Hospital Plan of Care (AHPC) with her, you review the information sheets you gave her on pneumonia, CHF, and COPD. You go over all medications and help her develop a medication schedule. Patricia fills in the time and reason for each of her medications as well as common side effects. It specifically states she should not skip or stop any medications without talking to her physician. The Patient PASS lists her upcoming primary care appointment and doctor's phone number, reminds her to weigh herself daily and write it down on the calendar provided, and includes a spot to write down questions. It includes specifics on what to do if she gains more than 3 pounds in a day, experiences increasing shortness of breath, or develops chest pain or a worsening cough. You remind her a nurse will call her in the next few days to check on her condition and review the after-hospital care plan. You also make sure she has the name and phone number of the home care agency who will be coming out to see her. You remind her to bring the AHCP to her primary care appointment next week.

The final step you take as her inpatient case manager is to transition her back to the RN in CCTM in the primary care provider's office. You complete the hand-off tool and send it electronically. You then call to note specific areas the RN in CCTM should focus on: medication compliance, weight monitoring, diet compliance, and keeping medical appointments. You make the appointment for her to see the primary care physician as well as get a follow-up chest x-ray and see the pulmonologist. You ask the RN in CCTM to assist the patient in developing a long-term dietary compliance plan for both her diabetes and CHF.

 

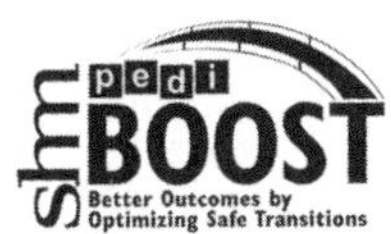

## Appendix 2.
## The 8Ps: Assessing Your Patient's Risk for Adverse Events After Discharge
## RN in CCTM Transitioning Patient to Acute Care
## SOB/Pneumonia

*Note: Bold/italic areas apply to sample case study.*

| Risk Assessment: 8P Screening Tool (Check all that apply) | | Risk-Specific Intervention | Signature of Individual Responsible for Ensuring Intervention Administered |
|---|---|---|---|
| **Problems with medications** (polypharmacy – i.e. ≥ 10 routine meds – or high risk medication including: anticoagulants, insulin, oral hypoglycemic agents, aspirin and clopidogrel dual therapy, digoxin, narcotics) ☒ | ☒ | Medication specific education using "teach back" provided to patient and caregiver. ***Have reinforced correct use of medications, but patient stopped taking steroids and antibiotics due to feeling nauseated and jittery and felt the steroids made her blood sugar increase. Home care nurse noticed that patient sometimes forgot to take medications, especially when there was more than one dose/day.*** | |
| | ☐ | Elimination of unnecessary medications. | |
| | ☒ | Simplification of medication scheduling to improve adherence. ***Recently worked with Dr. Primary to adjust insulin so patient was not doing a sliding scale type coverage at meal times because she was inconsistent. Lantus insulin is new to her in last few months; she is able to afford it.*** ***Home care nurse has made sure she has medication box with compartments but she still forgets to take medications at times.*** | |
| | ☒ | Monitoring plan developed and communicated to patient and after-care providers, where relevant (e.g., warfarin, digoxin, and insulin). ***Patient has a blood glucose meter but is not consistent in blood sugar testing BID.*** | |
| | ☐ | Specific strategies for managing adverse drug events reviewed with patient/caregiver. | |
| | ☐ | Follow-up phone call at 72 hours to assess adherence and complications. | |
| **Psychological** (depression screen positive or history of depression diagnosis) ☒ | ☐ | Assessment of need for psychiatric after-care if not in place. | |
| | ☐ | Communication with primary care provider, highlighting this issue if new. | |
| | ☒ | Involvement/awareness of support network ensured. ***This patient is very anxious and has minimal family support. Her breathing tends to worsen when she gets the least bit anxious. Son is not that available due to work schedule and due to $O_2$ dependancy, patient is not as able to get out to see her church friends like she did previously. Does have a counselor Mary and is on Celexa, which was started about 3 months ago. States she feels safe in the hospital.*** | |
| **Principal diagnosis** (cancer, stroke, diabetes mellitus, COPD, heart failure) ☒ | ☐ | Review of National Discharge Guidelines, where available. | |
| | ☒ | Disease-specific education using "teach back" with patient/caregiver. ***Appears overwhelmed by trying to balance diabetic as well as heart failure diet, blood sugar, and weight monitoring.*** | |
| | ☒ | Action plan reviewed with patient/caregivers regarding what to do and who to contact in the event of worsening or new symptoms. ***Patient has been instructed to call the RN in CCTM or home care RN for SOB, elevated blood sugar, but she panics and calls ambulance before reaching out for help before her symptoms worsen.*** | |
| | ☒ | Discussed goals of care and chronic illness model with patient/caregiver. ***Patient's goal is to be social with her friends from church, she is limited by need for $O_2$ and easy fatigability, and recent nausea from antibiotics.*** | |

*continued on next page*

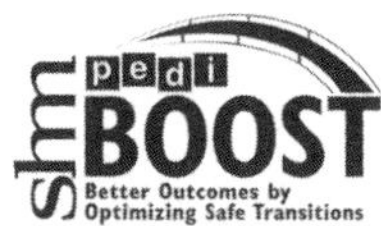


Appendix 2. (continued)
The 8Ps: Assessing Your Patient's Risk for Adverse Events After Discharge
RN in CCTM Transitioning Patient to Acute Care
SOB/Pneumonia
*Note: Bold/italic areas apply to sample case study.*

| Risk Assessment: 8P Screening Tool (Check all that apply) | | Risk-Specific Intervention | Signature of Individual Responsible for Ensuring Intervention Administered |
|---|---|---|---|
| **Physical limitations** (patients with deconditioning, frailty, or other physical limitations that impair their ability to participate in their own care) ☒ | ☒ | Engage family/caregivers to ensure ability to assist with post-discharge care assistance. ***Patient has limited mobility due to shortness of breath. Son can take her to medical appointments on his day off.*** | |
| | ☒ | Assessment of home services to address limitations and care needs. ***Visiting nurse and home therapy were in place prior to admission. Patient not consistent in testing blood sugar, weighing self, and taking medications.*** | |
| | ☐ | Follow-up phone call at 72 hours to assess ability to adhere to the care plan with services and support in place. | |
| **Poor health literacy** (inability to do "teach back") ☒ | ☐ | Committed caregiver involved in planning/administration of all general and risk-specific interventions. | |
| | ☐ | Post-hospital care plan education using "teach back" provided to patient and caregiver. | |
| | ☒ | Link to community resources for additional patient/caregiver support. ***Has home care nurse through Superior Home Care and also home therapy to work on activity spacing.*** ***Would pulmonary rehab be beneficial to this patient, both from an educational and support standpoint? She is able to take the subsidized city taxi when feeling well.*** | |
| | ☒ | **Follow-up phone call at 72 hours to assess adherence and complications.** | |
| **Patient support** (social isolation, absence of support to assist with care, as well as insufficient or absent connection with primary care) ☒ | ☐ | Follow-up phone call at 72 hours to assess condition, adherence, and complications. | |
| | ☒ | Follow-up appointment with appropriate medical provider within 7 days after hospitalization. ***She missed her hospital follow-up appointment last hospitalization because her son had to work and she did not feel well enough to take the taxi. Please make sure any appointments are made on son's day off or try to see if she has another person she can ask to give her a ride (maybe a church friend?).*** | |
| | ☒ | Involvement of home care providers of services with clear communications of discharge plan to those providers. ***Has had home care RN for 3x week visits as well as home therapy, has home oxygen which she has had for about a year.*** | |
| | ☐ | Engage a transition coach. | |

*continued on next page*

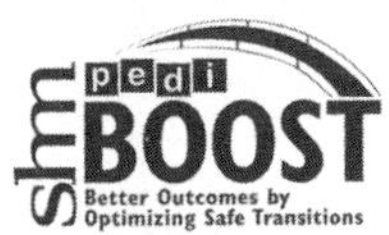


**Appendix 2. (continued)**
**The 8Ps: Assessing Your Patient's Risk for Adverse Events After Discharge**
**RN in CCTM Transitioning Patient to Acute Care**
**SOB/Pneumonia**
*Note: Bold/italic areas apply to sample case study.*

| Risk Assessment: 8P Screening Tool (Check all that apply) | Risk-Specific Intervention | Signature of Individual Responsible for Ensuring Intervention Administered |
|---|---|---|
| **Prior hospitalization** (nonelective; in last 6 months) ☒ | ☒ Review reasons for rehospitalization in context of prior hospitalization. ***Patient does not really feel it is a problem to be back in the hospital because she feels safe. Need to reinforce that frequent re-admissions are not in her best interests and need to explore ways to keep her safe and healthy at home.*** <br> ***Not really sure what can motivate this patient to adhere to medical plan to optimize condition (maybe a pulmonary support group?).*** <br> ☐ Follow-up phone call at 72 hours to assess condition, adherence, and complications. <br> ☒ Follow-up appointment with medical provider within 7 days of hospital discharge. ***Please make sure any appointments are made on son's day off.*** <br> ☐ Engage a transition coach. | |
| **Palliative care** (Would you be surprised if this patient died in the next year? **Does this patient have an advanced or progressive serious illness?**) "No" to 1st or "Yes" to 2nd = positive screen ☐ | ☐ Assess need for palliative care services. <br> ☒ **Identify goals of care and therapeutic options.** <br> ☒ **Communicate prognosis with patient/family/caregiver.** <br> ☒ **Assess and address bothersome symptoms (i.e., shortness of breath).** <br> ☐ Identify services or benefits available to patient based on advanced disease status. <br> ☐ Discuss with patient/family/caregiver role of palliative care services and benefits and services available to the patient. | N/A |

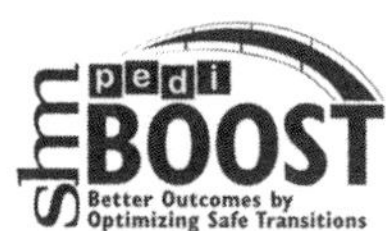


## Appendix 3.
## Tool for Addressing Risk: A Geriatric Evaluation for Transitions Hand-Off Tool – Acute Care to RN in CCTM in PCMH SOB/Pneumonia

*Note: Bold/italic areas apply to sample case study.*

| Risk Assessment: 8P Screening Tool (Check all that apply) | | Risk-Specific Intervention | Signature of Individual Responsible for Ensuring Intervention Administered |
|---|---|---|---|
| **Problems with medications** (polypharmacy – i.e. ≥ 10 routine meds – or high risk medication including: anticoagulants, ***insulin,*** oral hypoglycemic agents, aspirin and clopidogrel dual therapy, digoxin, narcotics) ☒ | ☒ | Medication specific education using "teach back" provided to patient and caregiver. ***After last discharge 3 weeks ago, patient stopped taking antibiotics and steroids before completing. Stressed need to finish as prescribed. Has another course of prednisone taper and Cipro.*** | N/A |
| | ☒ | Monitoring plan developed and communicated to patient and after-care providers, where relevant (e.g., warfarin, digoxin, and ***insulin***). ***Test blood sugar BID at home and call primary MD if greater than 300 for more than 1 day.*** | |
| | ☒ | Specific strategies for managing adverse drug events reviewed with patient/caregiver. If patients gets nauseated or jittery, call RN in CCTM. Don't stop taking medications. | |
| | ☒ | Follow-up phone call at 72 hours to assess adherence and complications. ***Outpatient pharmacy delivered new medications and a pill box to her room in hospital. Please verify med compliance.*** | |
| **Psychological** (depression screen positive or history of depression diagnosis) ☒ | ☒ | Assessment of need for psychiatric after-care if not in place. ***Has history of anxiety and sees counselor, on Celexa. Please ensure she makes a follow-up appointment with her counselor.*** | |
| | ☐ | Communication with after-care providers, highlighting this issue if new. | |
| | ☐ | Involvement/awareness of support network ensured. | |
| **Principal diagnosis** (cancer, stroke, ***diabetes mellitus, COPD, heart failure***) ☒ | ☒ | Review of National Discharge Guidelines, where available CHF. | |
| | ☒ | Disease-specific education using "teach back" with patient/caregiver. ***CHF discharge instructions, has a scale, needs reinforcement of diet and practical suggestions for when she doesn't feel well. Patient has appointment with dietician in Dr. Primary office on 11/25 right before she sees the MD.*** | |
| | ☒ | Action plan reviewed with patient/caregivers regarding what to do and who to contact in the event of worsening or new symptoms. | |
| | ☒ | Discuss goals of care and chronic illness model discussed with patient/caregiver. Discussed options to deal with symptoms and what to do if she gets SOB or gains weight. | |
| **Physical limitations** (patients with deconditioning, frailty, or other physical limitations that impair their ability to participate in their own care) ☒ | ☒ | Engage family/caregivers to ensure ability to assist with post-discharge care assistance. ***Patient has limited mobility due to shortness of breath. Son will take to 1 week follow-up; made appointment on his day off.*** | |
| | ☒ | Assessment of home services to address limitations and care needs. ***Visiting nurse and home therapy re-ordered. Please make sure visiting nurse monitors medication compliance, blood sugar monitoring, and reviews patient weight record.*** | |
| | ☒ | Follow-up phone call at 72 hours to assess ability to adhere to the care plan with services and support in place. | |

*continued on next page*

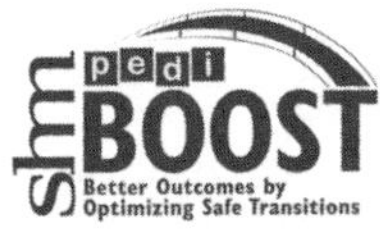

## Appendix 3. (continued)
## Tool for Addressing Risk: A Geriatric Evaluation for Transitions
## Hand-Off Tool – Acute Care to RN in CCTM in PCMH
## SOB/Pneumonia

*Note: Bold/italic areas apply to sample case study.*

| Risk Assessment: 8P Screening Tool (Check all that apply) | Risk-Specific Intervention | Signature of Individual Responsible for Ensuring Intervention Administered |
|---|---|---|
| **Poor health literacy** (inability to do "teach back") ☒ | ☒ Committed caregiver involved in planning/administration of all general and risk-specific interventions. ***Son helps with shopping but not available for day-to-day help.***<br>☒ After-care plan education using "teach back" provided to patient and caregiver. ***Patient has Patient Pass Transition Record. Please reinforce.***<br>☐ Link to community resources for additional patient/caregiver support.<br>☒ Follow-up phone call at 72 hours to assess adherence and complications. | |
| **Patient support** (social isolation, absence of support to assist with care, as well as insufficient or absent connection with primary care) ☒ | ☒ Follow-up phone call at 72 hours to assess condition, adherence, and complications.<br>☒ Follow-up appointment with after-care medical provider within 7 days. ***Has appointment with Dr. Primary 11/25 and Dr. Lung 11/30 (needs chest x-ray before Dr. Lung appointment). Has prescription. Please remind to have it done.***<br>☒ Involvement of home care providers of services with clear communications of discharge plan to those providers. ***Visiting RN set up through Superior Home Care, already has home $O_2$. Son can take to appointments if made on his day off from work, otherwise she uses a subsidized taxi program (already registered). Reviewed all DC instructions with son by phone as he was not available at hospital. Patient does not appear to understand link between steroids, blood sugar, weight gain, and shortness of breath.*** | |
| **Prior hospitalization** (nonelective; in last 6 months) ☒ | ☒ **Review reasons for rehospitalization in context of prior hospitalization.**<br>☒ **Follow-up phone call at 72 hours to assess condition, adherence, and complications.**<br>☒ **Follow-up appointment with after-care medical provider within 7 days.** | |
| **Palliative care** (Would you be surprised if this patient died in the next year? **Does this patient have an advanced or progressive serious illness?**) "No" to 1st or "Yes" to 2nd = positive screen ☒ | ☐ Assess need for palliative care services.<br>☐ Identify goals of care and therapeutic options.<br>☐ Communicate prognosis with patient/family/caregiver.<br>☒ **Assess and address bothersome symptoms.**<br>☐ Identify services or benefits available to patients based on advanced disease status.<br>☐ Discuss with patient/family/caregiver role of palliative care services and benefits and services available. ***Currently a full code. Would not discuss in hospital.*** | |

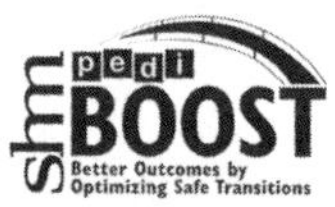


## Appendix 4.
## Universal Discharge Checklist and GAP

*Note: Bold/italic areas apply to sample case study.*

| Universal Patient Discharge Checklist – *COMPLETED BY ACUTE CARE RN* | | | Initials |
|---|---|---|---|
| 1. GAP assessment (see below) completed with issues addressed. | ☒ ***YES*** | ☐ NO | |
| 2. Medications reconciled with pre-admission list. | ☒ ***YES*** | ☐ NO | |
| 3. Medication use/side effects reviewed using "teach back" with patient/caregiver(s). | ☒ ***YES*** | ☐ NO | |
| 4. "Teach back" used to confirm patient/caregiver understanding of disease, prognosis, and self-care requirements. | ☒ ***YES*** | ☐ NO | |
| 5. Action plan for management of symptoms/side effects/complications requiring medical attention established and shared with patient/caregiver using "teach back." | ☒ ***YES*** | ☐ NO | |
| 6. Discharge plan (including educational materials; medication list with reason for use and highlighted new/changed/discontinued drugs; follow-up plans) taught with written copy provided to patient/caregiver at discharge. | ☒ ***YES*** | ☐ NO | |
| 7. Discharge communication provided to principal care provider(s). | ☒ ***YES*** | ☐ NO | |
| 8. Documented receipt of discharge information from principal care provider(s). | ☒ ***YES*** | ☐ NO | |
| 9. Arrangements made for outpatient follow-up with principal care provider(s). | ☒ ***YES*** | ☐ NO | |
| **For increased-risk patients, consider:** | | | |
| 1. Interdisciplinary rounds with patient/caregiver prior to discharge to review after-care plan. | ☒ ***YES*** | ☐ NO | |
| 2. Direct communication with principal care provider before discharge. | ☒ ***YES*** | ☐ NO | |
| 3. Phone contact with patient/caregiver arranged within 72 hours post-discharge to assess condition, discharge plan comprehension and adherence, and to reinforce follow-up. | ☒ ***YES*** | ☐ NO | |
| 4. Follow-up appointment with principal care provider within 7 days of discharge. | ☒ ***YES*** | ☐ NO | |
| 5. Direct contact information for hospital personnel familiar with patient's course provided to patient/caregiver to address questions/concerns *if unable to reach principal care provider* prior to first follow-up. | ☒ ***YES*** | ☐ NO | |

Confirmed by: ______________________ ______________________ ___/___/___

Signature — Print Name — Date

**General Assessment of Preparedness (GAP)**
Prior to discharge, evaluate the following areas with the patient/caregiver(s). Communicate concerns identified as appropriate to principal care providers.
**A** = beginning upon Admission; **P** = Prior to discharge; **D** = at Discharge

| Logistical Issues | | | |
|---|---|---|---|
| 1. Functional status assessment completed (P). | ☒ ***YES*** | ☐ NO | ☐ N/A |
| 2. Access (e.g., keys) to home ensured (P). | ☒ ***YES*** | ☐ NO | ☐ N/A |
| 3. Home prepared for patient's arrival (P) (e.g., medical equipment, safety evaluation, food). | ☒ ***YES*** | ☐ NO | ☐ N/A |
| 4. Financial resources for care needs assessed (P). | ☒ ***YES*** | ☐ NO | ☐ N/A |
| 5. Ability to obtain medications confirmed (P). | ☒ ***YES*** | ☐ NO | ☐ N/A |
| 6. Responsible party for ensuring medication adherence. Identified/prepared; if not patient (P). | ☒ YES | ☐ NO | ☐ N/A |
| 7. Transportation to initial follow-up arranged (D). | ☒ ***YES*** | ☐ NO | ☐ N/A |
| 8. Transportation home arranged (D). | ☒ ***YES*** | ☐ NO | ☐ N/A |

*continued on next page*

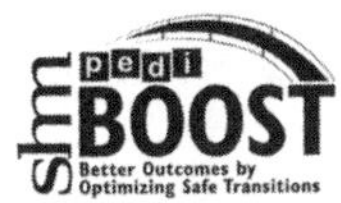

## Appendix 4. (continued)
## Universal Discharge Checklist and GAP

*Note: Bold/italic areas apply to sample case study.*

**General Assessment of Preparedness (GAP)**
Prior to discharge, evaluate the following areas with the patient/caregiver(s). Communicate concerns identified as appropriate to principal care providers.
**A** = beginning upon Admission; **P** = Prior to discharge; **D** = at Discharge

| Psychosocial Issues | | | |
|---|---|---|---|
| 1. Substance abuse/dependence evaluated (A). | ☒ ***YES*** | ☐ NO | ☐ N/A |
| 2. Abuse/neglect presence assessed (A). | ☒ ***YES*** | ☐ NO | ☐ N/A |
| 3. Cognitive status assessed (A); makes own decisions. | ☒ ***YES*** | ☐ NO | ☐ N/A |
| 4. Advanced care planning documented (A). | ☒ ***YES*** | ☐ NO | ☐ N/A |
| 5. Support circle for patient identified (P). | ☒ ***YES*** | ☐ NO | ☐ N/A |
| 6. Contact information for home care services. Obtained and provided to patient (D). | ☒ ***YES*** | ☐ NO | ☐ N/A |

Confirmed by: ______________________ ______________________ ___/___/___
Signature Print Name Date

# Appendix 5.
# Medication Schedule
## After Hospital Care Plan for: Patricia P.
## Discharge Date: 11/20/2013

**Your Doctors:**
Primary Care Physician (PCP) – Dr. Primary
Lung – Dr. Lung

**Your Nurse:**
Jackie Green, RN, CCTM

**EACH DAY, follow this schedule:**

| MEDICINES | | | | |
|---|---|---|---|---|
| What Time of Day Do I Take This Medicine? | Why Am I Taking This Medicine? | Medicine Name & Amount | How Many Do I Take? | How Do I Take This Medicine? |
| Morning | Breathing – steroid | Prednisone 10 mg | 4 pills<br>Nov. 21, 22, 23,<br>3 pills<br>Nov. 24, 25, 26,<br>2 pills<br>Nov. 27, 28, 29,<br>1 pill<br>Nov. 29, 30, Dec. 1<br>then stop | By mouth |
| | Infection | Ciprofloxacin (Cipro®) 500 mg | 1 pill<br>Nov. 21, 22, 23, 24, 25<br>then stop | By mouth |
| | Blood pressure | Enalapril (Vasotec®) 20 mg | 1 | By mouth |
| | Water pill (diuretic) | Furosemide (Lasix®) 40 mg | 1 | By mouth |
| | Breathing | Advair® 250/50 mcg/puff | 1 puff | Inhaler |
| | Breathing | Spiriva® 18 mcg | 1 pill into special inhaler | Inhaler |
| | Blood sugar | Lantus® insulin 25 units | Shot | Injection |
| | Blood sugar | Metformin 500 mg | 1 pill | By mouth |
| | Anxiety | Celexa® 40 mg | 1 pill | By mouth |
| | Potassium supplement | K-Dur 20 mEq | 1 pill | By mouth |
| Noon | Water pill (diuretic) | Lasix® 40 mg | 1 pill | By mouth |
| Evening | Breathing | Prednisone 10 mg | 4 pills<br>Nov. 21, 22, then stop<br>nighttime dose | By mouth |
| | Breathing | Singulair® 10 mg | 1 pill | By mouth |
| | Blood sugar | Metformin® 500 mg | 1 pill | By mouth |
| Bedtime | Infection | Cipro® 500 mg | 1 pill<br>Nov. 21, 22, 23, 24, 25<br>then stop | By mouth |
| | Breathing | Advair® 250/50 mcg/puff | 1 puff | Inhaler |
| Only when needed | Anxiety | Xanax® 1 mg<br>You can take up to twice a day | 1 pill | By mouth |
| Only when needed | Breathing | Albuterol (ProAir HFA®)<br>You can take this every 6 hours | 2 puffs | Inhaler |

## Appendix 6.
## Medication Schedule from Patient PASS: A Transition Record

### Patient Preparation to Address Situations (after discharge) Successfully
### Patricia P. – Shortness of Breath and Pneumonia

<table>
<tr><th colspan="3">I was in the hospital because of shortness of breath and pneumonia.</th></tr>
<tr><th>If I have the following problems…</th><th>I should…</th><th>Important Contact Information</th></tr>
<tr><td>1. Hard time breathing, chest pain, worsening cough, more phlegm, fever</td><td>1. Stop and rest, take 2 puffs of Advair, put on oxygen, and make sure tank is not empty; call RN Jackie 555-991-0000.</td><td>My primary doctor:<br>Dr. Primary 555-333-4444</td></tr>
<tr><td>2. Gain more than 3 pounds in 1 day</td><td>2. Make sure to take all medications and call Dr. Primary office for possible medication adjustment.</td><td>My hospital doctor:<br>Dr. Jones 555-444-5555</td></tr>
<tr><td>3. Nauseated or jittery</td><td>3. Call RN Jackie; don't just skip medicine.</td><td>My lung doctor:<br>Dr. Lung 555-444-5555</td></tr>
<tr><td>4. Blood sugar over 300 for more than 1 day</td><td>4. Call Dr. Primary office.</td><td>My visiting nurse:<br>Superior Home Care 555-555-6666</td></tr>
<tr><td>My appointments:<br>Debbie: dietician – 11/25 10:00 a.m.<br>Dr. Primary: 11/25 11:00 a.m. for hospital follow-up<br>Dr. Lung: 11/30 1:00 p.m. to check if pneumonia better<br>Mary: counselor – call for appointment</td><td>Tests and issues I need to talk with my doctor(s) about at my clinic visit:<br>1. Results of chest x-ray: make sure to get it done before appointment on 11/30.<br>2. Review weight and blood pressure charts.</td><td>My pharmacy:<br>Walgreens 555-543-5555</td></tr>
<tr><td colspan="2">Other Instructions<br>1. Get chest x-ray before Dr. Lung appointment on 11/03. X-ray is in same building as his office. Bring order that hospital gave you.<br>2. Check blood sugar before eating breakfast and dinner (evening meal) and write it on the chart.<br>3. Weigh yourself daily. Call Dr. Primary if weight is up more than 3 pounds in a day.<br>4. Wear CPAP at night and when napping.<br>5. Low fat, low salt diet. No sweets. Do not add salt to your food.</td><td>I understand my treatment plan. I feel willing and able to participate actively in my care.<br><br>______________________<br>Patient/Caregiver Signature<br><br>______________________<br>Provider Signature<br>Date 11/20/13</td></tr>
</table>

**Source:** Agency for Healthcare Research and Quality, 2013.

# CHAPTER 12

# Informatics Nursing Practice

*Rosemary Kennedy, PhD, MBA, RN, FAAN*
*Ida M. Androwich, PhD, RN, BC-NI, FAAN*
*Carol Mannone, MSN, RN, CH-GC*
*Naomi Mercier, MSN, RN-BC*

## Learning Outcome Statement

The purpose of this chapter is to enable the reader to demonstrate the elements of competency in informatics nursing practice that are required for the registered nurse (RN) in the Care Coordination and Transition Management (CCTM) role. Specific learning outcomes and objectives have been identified for each competency.

The competencies that will be addressed in this chapter include:

- *Competency 1:* The use of health information technology that is aligned with the RN-CCTM Model.
- *Competency 2:* Explain why information and technology skills are essential for safe patient care (Cronenwett et al., 2007).
- *Competency 3:* Integration of National Quality Strategy requirements within use of health information technology to improve care coordination and transition management.

*Note:* Additional resources related to nursing informatics are found in Androwich and Kraft (2013).

## Competency Definitions

*Nursing informatics* (NI) is defined by the American Nurses Association (2010) as a "specialty that integrates nursing science, computer science, and information science to manage and communicate data, information, knowledge, and wisdom in nursing practice. NI supports consumers, patients, nurses, and other providers in decision-making in all roles and settings. This support is accomplished through the use of information structures, information processes, and information technology" (p. 65). *Health information technology* (HIT), as an important component in care coordination, is the application of computers and technology to the provision of health care in all settings, including all stakeholders involved in health (Hersch, 2009). Because HIT plays a critical role in communication, frequently the terms *information* and *communications technology* are used along with HIT.

There are different technologies that are included under the umbrella term of HIT. One of national importance is the *electronic health record* (EHR), which includes comprehensive and longitudinal information about the patient, supporting care across all settings (acute, home, ambulatory, clinic, etc.). The Healthcare Information and Management Systems Society (HIMSS) defines an EHR as a secure, real-time, point-of-care, patient-centric information resource for clinicians (HIMSS, 2003). *Personal health records* (PHRs) store health care information that is entered and managed by the patient and/or consumer of health care (Healthit.gov, n.d.a). PHRs typically contain patient-reported care compliance and clinical status, and outcome information that is critical data for effective care coordination. Patient access to the information in their EHRs is enabled with the use of patient portals, that provide secure online 24-hour access to personal health information, such as medications, laboratory results, and care plans, from any location through the Internet (HealthIT.gov, n.d.b).

*Mobile technology* and *cloud computing* play a major role in care coordination and transition management. The major advantage of cloud computing for care coordination is "on demand" access to information without requiring human interaction with individual service providers. The advent of cloud computing allows for ubiquitous, convenient, on-demand network access to a pool of applications, servers, and services that can be accessed with minimal effort (Mell & Grance, 2011). With the appropriate security and patient privacy software, cloud computing can be a tool to facilitate information exchange across geographic settings, providers, and patients. As nurses advise and educate patients, it is important to assess the Internet sources of education using criteria ensuring the entity posting the information is a valid and reliable source of evidence-based content, that original sources of publication are provided, and that the information is reviewed by someone with the appropriate credentials before it is posted.

 

# I. Competency 1: The Use of Health Information Technology that Is Aligned with the RN-CCTM Model

## Learning Outcome Statement

- Integrate the application of information science within the RN-CCTM Model to manage data, information, and knowledge during CCTM.
- Recognize the importance of using nationally recognized standardized terminologies to support cross-setting communication and transition across all domains of the patient-centered medical home.
- Describe the application of standardized terminologies to support all aspects of the nursing process including documentation of assessments, diagnoses, interventions, goals, and outcomes as described in the RN-CCTM Model.
- Understand the importance of using standardized data structures and messaging standards to communicate information during CCTM across providers and geographical settings.
- Describe the integration of the knowledge, skills, and attitudes between the RN-CCTM Model and nursing informatics (see Table 1).

## Learning Objectives

- Explain why valid, reliable, and structured data/information is essential for safe and effective CCTM.
- Identify essential information that must be available in a database to support coordination of care across providers and geographical settings.
- Describe the data, information, and knowledge required for use within health information technology to support CCTM.
- Describe the role of standardized terminologies in supporting communication of information between disparate electronic systems across providers and geographical settings.
- Show how the RN-CCTM Model can be used to identify the requirements for HIT to support CCTM.
- Evaluate requirements for the electronic care plan that support the RN-CCTM Model to support self-care management, cross-setting communication, and identification of high-risk and population management.
- Recognize the importance of the entire clinical team, including the patient/family/caregiver, in defining requirements for HIT to support care coordination.

Although nursing informatics is a highly specialized area of practice, there are fundamental competencies that all practicing nurses need to achieve for safe, quality, and competent Care Coordination and Transition Management in the current technological environment. A nursing informatics competency is defined as "adequate knowledge, skills, and the ability to perform specific informatics tasks" (McGonigle, Hunter, & Hebda, 2013, p. 239). Information systems that support nursing practice require the incorporation of clinical knowledge/clinical content within HIT.

The Technology Informatics Guiding Education Reform (TIGER) was formed to develop informatics recommendations for all practicing nurses and graduating nursing students. The TIGER Informatics Competency Collaborative performed an extensive review of literature for informatics, which resulted in over 1,000 individual competency statements. This body of work was then synthesized to create the TIGER Informatics Competency Model.

The 2012 Quality and Safety Education for Nurses (QSEN) competencies for informatics focus on the use of information and technology to communicate, manage knowledge, mitigate error, and support decision making. These competencies are closely aligned with the competencies in the RN-CCTM Model, which evolved from an effort to standardize work that ambulatory care nurses do using evidence from the interdisciplinary literature on Care Coordination and Transition Management.

Health information technology can support the activities related to care coordination, facilitate transfer of information, enable communication between parties in different locations, and provide real-time decision support. Care coordination, combined with the use of HIT, has the potential to reduce cost and improve outcomes for all populations in all health care settings. The most impressive outcomes occur in high-risk populations whose complex health issues involve costly treatments and repeated hospitalizations (National Quality Forum, 2010). HIT, as a modality of delivery of services by RNs in CCTM, requires knowledge of data standards, EHRs, health information exchanges (HIEs), and communication technologies as they apply to care coordination and transition management.

A. Role of HIT and communication technologies.
   1. Health information technology.
      a. Serves as an important component in care coordination.
      b. Facilitates person-centered care.
      c. Leverages important information and communications technologies. Provides ubiquitous access to information, evidence-based alerts and reminders across people, function, and sites over time.

   d. Closes the gap in care and facilitates evidence-based decision making.
   e. Supports the care "triple aim:" to improve health outcomes, lower costs, and enhance the patient experience (Hersch, 2009).
2. Knowledge of HIT in relation to care coordination.
   a. Supports the use of HIT in all domains of care coordination.
      (1) Health care home.
      (2) Proactive and longitudinal care plan.
      (3) Communication and hand-offs within and between settings of care.
      (4) Transition management.
   b. Allows recognition of the role of HIEs in sharing information.
      (1) Uses HIEs to sharing information between and among facilities.
      (2) Integrates HIEs into practice, education, and research.
      (3) Recognizes the importance of HIEs to exchange information spanning different organizations across diverse regions of care delivery.
3. The nurse's knowledge of HIT in relation to the patient/person/caregiver allows:
   a. Understanding of the role of PHRs in consumer engagement, safety, and quality.
   b. Recognition of the importance of mobile technology platforms, such as iPads and smartphones.
   c. Practice using mobile technology for on-demand access to information, serving multiple users at once (nurse, physician, patient, caregiver, consumer).
4. Nursing use of the Internet.
   a. Supports practice using the Internet as a source for access to evidence-based content.
   b. Allows articulation of criteria used to assess sources of information found on the Internet.
   c. Leads to practices using a structure and process for evaluating sources of content on the Internet prior to integration with CCTM functions.
   d. Recognizes the role of the Internet in supporting coordination of care from one setting to another.

## II. Competency 2: Explain Why Information and Technology Skills Are Essential for Safe Patient Care (Cronenwett et al., 2007)

### Learning Outcome Statement

- Demonstrate understanding of the different health IT solutions and their value in enhancing CCTM.
- Understand the role of clinical decision-support tools in Care Coordination and Transition Management, recognizing that they are to be utilized to support decision making in concert with critical thinking and clinical judgment rather than dictate practice.
- Identify functions related to CCTM that can be supported with HIT (e.g., problem list communication, clinical decision support, and care plan management).
- Integrate quality reporting and performance improvement within health IT use to support quality measurement.
- Understand the importance of standardized terminology in clinical practice and care coordination.
- Demonstrate ability to translate the information needs of caregivers to those designing the actual systems to capture and communicate patient care data.
- Integrate various health IT solutions, such as EHRs, PHRs, the Internet, smart phones, and HIEs into CCTM using the RN-CCTM Model as the foundation.
- Identify safety functions related to CCTM that can be supported with HIT (e.g., alerts for out-of-range findings, suggestion of potential problems based on documentation, and access to evidence-based guidelines in real time during CCTM).

### Learning Objectives

- Describe ways in which various forms of HIT support CCTM in accordance with the RN-CCTM Model.
- Demonstrate effective use of technology and standardized practices that support safety and quality using the RN-CCTM Model.
- Demonstrate the role various HIT solutions, such as EHRs, PHRs, the Internet, smart phones, and HIEs, have in enhancing CCTM.
- Describe the application of professional practice standards to the use of HIT within the RN in CCTM role in ambulatory care.
- Demonstrate the skills needed to use HIT to support CCTM within the scope of the RN in CCTM role in ambulatory care.
- Contrast benefits and limitations of different communication technologies and their impact on safety and quality.
- Describe the benefits and limitations of selected safety-enhancing technologies (e.g., barcodes, computer provider order entry, medication pumps, and automatic alerts/alarms), when coordinating care and transitioning patients from one level of care to another (Cronenwett et al., 2007; 2009).

Electronic health records are essential to improving patient safety (Sittig & Singh, 2012). The information contained within EHRs and other forms of HIT provide information to caregivers necessary to diagnose health problems, reduce errors in care delivery, and provide better quality at lower costs. For instance, HIT solutions can be designed to provide alerts that a medication is missing from the patient medication list when the patient transitions from one setting of care to another.

HIT can support clinical decision support at a patient level through alerts, reminders, and evidence-based guidelines to enhance CCTM. In addition, HIT supports decision making at an aggregate level through analysis of patient outcomes using data mining techniques. Essentially, HIT-enabled clinical decision support helps prevent adverse events, improve the quality of care, and increase satisfaction with care (HealthIT.gov, n.d.c).

The use of multiple sources of HIT solutions (e.g., use of EHR systems, remote care management and monitoring, linkages to web-based services and information, computer-driven algorithms, tracking clinical and nonclinical metrics, dynamic and remote health assessments, and provider communication and coordination of care), when well integrated, enhance the value of population health management and care coordination. Integration is key to achieving this goal. HIEs currently under development with support from the Health Information Technology for Economic and Clinical Health (HITECH) Act (2010) will increasingly become information sources for data collection and analysis.

A. Role of HIT in safety.
   1. Support multiple uses of data contained within HIT systems during CCTM to monitor safety events.
   2. Allow the identification of data necessary to track outcomes over time.
   3. Allow capture of the data elements related to safety events using the Agency for Healthcare Research and Quality (AHRQ, 2010) common format structure.
   4. Allow capture of data to help nurses in monitoring safety while also providing the necessary information to move towards quality management across populations of patients.
   5. Support the evaluation of population health outcomes to ensure patients receive appropriate and timely preventive and chronic care.
   6. Support team collaboration in the use of HIT to stratify patient health status indices.

B. Identification of data and data types in HIT important for health prevention and top chronic conditions, including:
   1. Preventive health markers.
      a. Immunizations.
      b. Lab test examples:
         (1) Cholesterol, LDL, HDL.
         (2) HbA1c.
      c. Mammography.
      d. Colonoscopy.
      e. Tuberculin testing.
      f. Body mass index (weight & height).
   2. Chronic condition screening.
      a. Diabetes.
      b. Heart disease.
      c. Renal disease.
   3. Can also be used to notify patients of test results.

C. Decision-support systems.

Nurse leaders are constantly challenged to keep up with the rapidly growing and constantly changing information relevant to practice. HIT can assist in this process by bringing necessary information to the nurse in forms that will leverage the information-seeking and decision-making processes. HIT systems provide decision support by bringing evidence, expertise, and scarce resources to the provider at the point of care. Nurse leaders must use all available evidence to increase the probability of "doing the right thing." In the future, institutions will be successful in delivering quality care to the extent they have comparable, reliable, and relevant data for cost, utilization, and outcome studies; for guideline development; for quality management; and for identification of best practices (Androwich & Kraft, 2013).

   1. An automated decision-support system provides the nurse with a tool that enhances the nurse's ability to make effective and timely decisions in semi-structured and uncertain situations.
   2. Structure of any decision-support system.
      a. Some type of user interface that facilitates or triggers inquiries.
      b. A knowledge base (database) containing expert information organized to promote decision making.
      c. An inference engine with analytic models that can generate alternative solutions.
      d. A terminology infrastructure that enables syntactic and semantic representation of rules and guidelines.
   3. An example of how a decision-support system might operate in a clinical setting is the scheduling of immunizations.
      a. The terminology infrastructure would enable both syntactic and semantic representation of rules and guidelines.
      b. The system would ask for input of the child's date of birth, weight, immunization history, and other pertinent facts.
      c. The database would use the information provided to compare with accepted practice standards contained in the knowledge base.
      d. The algorithm in the inference engine would then be used to provide a recommendation for the next immunization to be scheduled.

D. Characteristics of a decision-support system.
   1. Ability to organize and interpret large amounts of data.

2. Standardized decision-making criteria.
3. Provision of expert-level assistance to novice.
4. Allow for capturing (extracting and documenting) knowledge of experts.

E. The goal is to develop an "intelligent health care system;" a learning organization that promotes a culture of knowledge and empowerment among its members.

F. The trend in ambulatory patient care is to organize care around targeted patient populations (e.g., high cost or high volume).

G. Accountable Care Organizations and the implementation of "meaningful use" will require collection and reporting of data and will progressively attach rewards/incentives and penalties to clinicians and organizations for meeting these data requirements.

H. Population-based decision support is one type of decision-support system. Data from a number of patients are aggregated and used to provide information to support patient care for individual patients.
1. These systems are essential for disaster preparedness to enable the early detection of trends via syndromic surveillance, as well as providing resource management and decision support in actual disasters (O'Carroll, Yasnoff, Ward, Ripp, & Martin, 2003).
2. The term "syndromic surveillance" applies to surveillance using health-related data (typically symptom clusters) that precede a given diagnosis and signal a sufficient probability of a number of cases or a potential population outbreak that would warrant further response.
3. Though historically the syndromic surveillance has been used to target the investigation of potential cases, public health officials are increasingly exploring the usefulness of syndromic surveillance methods in detecting outbreaks associated with bioterrorism (Haas & Androwich, 2011).

I. Evidence-based practice is the integration of the best research evidence with clinical experience to facilitate clinical decision making (Sackett, Strauss, Richardson, Rosenberg, & Haynes, 2000). This same principle can be used in planning care for patient populations. Evidence-based nursing sources of evidence include:
1. Computerized literature databases, such as the Cumulative Index of Nursing and Allied Health Literature (CINAHL) and the National Library of Medicine's Medline.
2. On-line, published, systematic evidence reviews, such as The Cochrane Collaboration, the Agency for Healthcare Research and Quality, Zynx Health for interdisciplinary plans of care, and CINAHL's Clinical Innovations Database.

J. The goal of evidence-based practice for nurses is to:
1. Determine the best care options.
2. Answer clinical questions.
3. Identify areas for care improvement. Care planning and care coordination rely upon identifying best practice models from the literature that derive recommendations from large population studies.

K. An example of an evidence-based decision support in care coordination is the Project BOOST (Society for Hospital Medicine, n.d.), designed to provide safe transitions in care and prevent unnecessary rehospitalization. One component of the tool is the "Essential Elements for Improving the Discharge Transition" which includes:
1. Institutional support for and prioritization of this initiative, expressed as a meaningful investment in time, equipment, informatics, and personnel in the effort.
2. A multidisciplinary team or steering committee that is focused on improving the quality of care transitions in the institution.
3. Engagement of patients and families and recognition of the central role they play in executing the post-hospital care plan.
4. Data collection and reliable metrics that, at a minimum, reflect any relevant Centers for Medicare & Medicaid Services (2014) core measures and the relevant Physician Quality Reporting Initiative measures. These data should be transformed into reports that inform the team and front-line workers of progress and problem areas to address.
5. Specific aims, or goals, that are time defined, measurable, and achievable.
6. Standardized discharge pathways that highlight key medications and any medication changes, important follow-up and self-management instructions, and any pending tests.
7. Policies and procedures that are institution specific and that support the order sets and promote their safest and most effective use. These documents must be widely disseminated and used and when possible embedded in the order set. A high-reliability design should be used to enhance effective implementation. These policies and procedures should outline and guide the care team in:
    a. Team communication.
    b. Content of the discharge summary.
    c. Patient education.
    d. Medication safety and polypharmacy.
    e. Symptom management.
    f. Discharge and follow-up care.
    g. Comprehensive education programs for health care providers and patients, reinforcing both general and institution-specific information about the discharge process and use of specific tool (Society of Hospital Medicine, 2008).

# III. Competency 3: Integration of National Quality Strategy Requirements within Use of HIT to Improve CCTM

## Learning Outcome Statement

- Use of the National Quality Strategy to guide care coordination, such as clinical decision support to identify populations at risk and measure impact of nursing care on quality, with a focus on improving performance.
- Demonstrate understanding of the different health IT solutions and their value in enhancing health across populations.
- Describe models for population health management and care coordination and associated data elements needed for assessment, planning, intervention, and evaluation of care outcomes.

## Learning Objectives

- Describe how health IT can help nurses improve health at a national level through CCTM.
- Identify data elements that are needed to measure individual and population health process and outcomes.
- Describe the key elements of an evidence-based methodology for improving the discharge transition.

In 2011, the National Quality Strategy (NQS) Relationship to Care Coordination focused national attention on care coordination, aligning efforts on the use of HIT to focus on effective communication to coordinate care. Integral to these efforts is the use of HIT to capture, aggregate, and report data to enable more standardized and efficient care delivery at both the patient and population level (AHRQ, 2012).

The use of HIT is important to meet the goals of the NQS and to this extent, the Health Information Technology for Economic and Clinical Health (HITEC) Act of 2009 fosters adoption of "meaningful use" of certified EHRs to improve quality and reduce health care costs through financial incentives (Harle, Huerta, Ford, Diana, & Menachemi, 2013). This has significant implications for care coordination, as "meaningful use" requires the exchange of electronic health information with other systems and to also integrate the information into care delivery (American Recovery and Reinvestment Act, 2009). The exchange of information within and between sources of care, whether HIT or providers of care, is an integral function of care coordination, therefore the "meaningful use" requirements are aligned to support care coordination activities.

A. Coordination of care and population health management are systems designed to meet the "triple aim" health care goals. Both systems are dependent on the EMR to facilitate communication and the transfer of information.
   1. Coordination of care is the integration of care across the continuum of the patient's health care conditions, needs, and experiences which incorporates transfer of information to:
      a. Patients.
      b. Families.
      c. Caregivers.
      d. Health care teams.
   2. Primary care and family practice providers are the pivotal members of the health care team.
      a. Sharing information within and outside of the practice.
      b. Integrating specialty care.
      c. Transferring information across and up and down all the settings of care.

B. Changes in primary care: there are six principle tasks for effective communication in care coordination.
   1. Maintaining patient continuity with a primary care clinician team.
   2. Documenting and compiling patient information generated within and outside the primary care office.
   3. Using information to manage and coordinate care delivered in primary care practice.
      a. Access and assess patient data.
      b. Manage and coordinate care.
      c. Population-based tracking for patient panel.
   4. Referring and consulting (initiation, communication, and ongoing tracking).
   5. Sharing care with clinicians across practices and settings.
   6. Providing care and/or exchanging information for transitions and emergency care.

C. Data elements required for primary care and population health management.
   1. Assessment.
   2. Planning.
   3. Intervention.
   4. Evaluation of care outcomes.

D. Assessment, process, and outcome indicators need to be developed and embedded in nursing documentation screens, coded in standardized terminology (ICN or SnoMed-CT) so RN CCTM interventions can be tracked and contributions can be understood.

**Table 1.**
**Professional Informatics Practice: Knowledge, Skills, and Attitudes for Competency**

| COMPETENCY 1: Use of Health Information Technology that Is Aligned with the RN-CCTM Model | | | |
|---|---|---|---|
| **Knowledge** | **Skills** | **Attitudes** | **Sources** |
| Describe ways in which various forms of health information technology (HIT) support care coordination and transition management (CCTM) in accordance with the RN-CCTM Model. | Demonstrate accountability by practicing using HIT within CCTM.<br>Describe methods for using HIT including electronic health records (EHRs), health information exchanges (HIEs), personal health rocords (PHRs), mobile technology, and the Internet in professional practice.<br>Communicate the role of HIT to other professionals, patients, consumers, and stakeholders in health care. | Value systems thinking and use of HIT to improve coordination of care.<br>Value the professional role of the RN in HIT; use to improve coordination of care.<br>Recognize the potential for improvement in HIT using the RN-CCTM Model as input. | Androwich & Kraft, 2013<br>Sheer, 2007 |
| Demonstrate the role that various health IT solutions, such as EHRs, PHRs, the Internet, smart phones, and HIEs have in enhancing care coordination and transition management. | Identify ways in which HIT can enhance CCTM.<br>Evaluate use of HIT and impact on care coordination.<br>Demonstrate ability to translate the information needs of caregivers to those designing the actual systems to capture and communicate patient care data. | Appreciate ways in which HIT can support professional practices.<br>Respect the intersection of nursing practice and HIT in care coordination.<br>Appreciate the ways HIT can be designed to improve care coordination. | Hersch, 2009<br>National Quality Forum, 2006 |
| Describe the application of professional practice standards to use of health IT within the RN in CCTM role in ambulatory care. | Demonstrate accountability by practicing within own scope of competence and training.<br>Recognize and implement nursing best practices in use of HIT to support CCTM. | Value legal, ethical, and professional standards of practice.<br>Value the professional role of the RN and recognize differences in scope of practice of RNs, licensed practical nurses/ licensed vocational nurses, and the role of unlicensed assistive personnel.<br>Recognize the potential for improved practices through continuing education. | Cronenwett et al., 2007 |

*continued on next page*

**Source Note:** Cronenwett et al. (2007) reprinted form *Nursing Outlook, 55*(3), 122-131, with permission from Elsevier.

**Table 1. (continued)**
**Professional Informatics Practice: Knowledge, Skills, and Attitudes for Competency**

| COMPETENCY 1: Use of Health Information Technology That Is Aligned with the RN-CCTM Model | | | |
|---|---|---|---|
| **Knowledge** | **Skills** | **Attitudes** | **Sources** |
| Recognize the importance of HIT skills in enhancing practice. | Demonstrate skills in using HIT to support CCTM within the scope of the RN in CCTM role. | Value functionality contained within all forms of HIT to enhance nursing practice. | Harle et al., 2004 |
| Analyze systems theory and design as applied to health informatics. | Use performance-improvement tools (e.g., Lean, Six Sigma, Plan-Do-Study-Act) in system analysis and design to assess use of technology to improve care.<br>Use project management methods in relation to implementation of new technologies.<br>Model behaviors that support theories and methods of change management. | Value systems thinking and use of technology to improve patient safety and quality.<br>Appreciate the Systems Development Lifecycle in the design of information systems. | Cronenwett et al., 2007 |
| "Evaluate the strengths and weaknesses of information systems in practice." | "Participate in the selection, design, implementation, and evaluation of information systems."<br>Consistently "communicate the integral role of information technology in nurses' work."<br>"Model behaviors that support implementation and an appropriate use of EHRs."<br>"Assist team members in adopting IT by piloting and evaluating proposed information technologies." | "Recognize nursing's important role in selecting, designing, implementing, and evaluating health information systems for practice environments."<br>"Appreciate the need for an interprofessional team to make final decisions related to selection and use of new information systems."<br>"Value the use of information technologies in practice." | American Association of Colleges of Nursing (AACN), 2012, p. 15 |

*continued on next page*

**Table 1. (continued)**
**Professional Informatics Practice: Knowledge, Skills, and Attitudes for Competency**

| COMPETENCY 2: Explain Why Information and Technology Skills Are Essential for Safe Patient Care | | | |
|---|---|---|---|
| **Knowledge** | **Skills** | **Attitudes** | **Sources** |
| Demonstrate understanding of the different HIT solutions and value in enhancing CCTM. | Contrast benefits and limitations of common IT strategies used in the delivery of patient care.<br>Evaluate the strengths and weaknesses of information systems used in patient care.<br>Participate in the selection, design, implementation, and appropriate use of EHRs.<br>Assist team members to adopt IT by piloting and evaluating proposed technologies. | Communicate the value and integral role of information technology in nurses' work. | Cronenwett et al., 2007 |
| Understand the role of clinical decision-support tools in CCTM, recognizing they are to be utilized to support decision making rather than to dictate practice. | Work to develop and maintain an extensive knowledge base to support design and use of HIT to enhance clinical decision making.<br>Use decision-support tools but apply clinical judgment and critical thinking.<br>Avoid over-reliance on decision-support tools.<br>Demonstrate skills in searching, retrieving, and managing data to make decisions at the point of care and an aggregate level across populations to make decisions. | Respect the patient's right to participate in care planning and make his or her own decision about course of action.<br>Recognize the final decision maker is usually the patient/caregiver while remaining sensitive to situations in which the nurse needs to act on the patient's behalf to assure his or her safety.<br>Appreciate the value of decision-support tools to enhance the nurse's knowledge base and as a check list to avoid clinical oversights. | Cronenwett et al., 2007 |
| Understand the major components of automated decision-support tools. | Recognize requirements for decision support including the use of knowledge bases, analytical tools, and user interfaces.<br>Articulate system requirements using nursing practice as the foundation. | Appreciate how HIT could work to support practice, such as reminders related to immunizations, access to evidence-based protocols, and suggestions related to treatment. | Androwich & Kraft, 2013 |

*continued on next page*

Table 1. (continued)
Professional Informatics Practice: Knowledge, Skills, and Attitudes for Competency

| COMPETENCY 2: Explain Why Information and Technology Skills Are Essential for Safe Patient Care | | | |
|---|---|---|---|
| **Knowledge** | **Skills** | **Attitudes** | **Sources** |
| Understand the benefits and limitations of selected safety-enhancing technologies. | Describe the role of HIT in promoting safety.<br>Recognize HIT limitations in safety while articulating the role of nursing judgment when using HIT.<br>Identify metrics to measure HIT impact on safety. | Appreciate the role of pre/post measurement in using HIT to improve safety.<br>Appreciate the role of nursing practice and workflow as a critical lever in improving safety. | Cronenwett et al., 2007 |
| Evaluate benefits and limitations of common information systems strategies to improve safety and quality. | Participate in the design of clinical decision-support systems (e.g., alerts and reminders in EHRs).<br>Anticipate unintended consequences of new technology. | | AACN, 2012 |
| "Know the current regulatory requirements for information systems use." | "Use federal and other regulations related to information systems in selecting and implementing information systems in practice." | "Appreciate the role that federal regulation plays in developing and implementing information systems that will improve patient care and create more effective delivery systems." | AACN, 2012, p. 15 |
| "Evaluate benefits and limitations of different health information technologies and their impact on safety and quality" (p. 16). | "Promote access to patient care information for all who provide care" (p. 16).<br>"Serve as a resource for documentation of nursing care at basic and advanced levels" (p. 16).<br>"Develop safeguards for protected health information" (p. 16).<br>"Comply with HIPAA (Health Insurance Portability and Accountability Act) regulations in the use of EHRs and other sources of patient information" (p. 16).<br>"Champion communication technologies that support clinical decision making, error prevention, care coordination, interprofessional collaboration, and protection of patient privacy" (p. 16). | "Appreciate the need for consensus and collaboration in developing systems to manage information in practice" (p. 16).<br>"Value the confidentiality and security of all electronic information" (p. 15). | AACN, 2012 |

*continued on next page*

**Table 1. (continued)**
**Professional Informatics Practice: Knowledge, Skills, and Attitudes for Competency**

| COMPETENCY 3: Integration of National Quality Strategy Requirements within Use of HIT to Improve Care Coordination and Transition Management | | | |
|---|---|---|---|
| **Knowledge** | **Skills** | **Attitudes** | **Sources** |
| Identify components of the National Quality Strategy six aims. | Articulate the six aims of the National Quality Strategy and use of HIT.<br>Identify methods for HIT design to support the National Quality Strategy related to care coordination and person-centered care.<br>Engage in public policy decision making to enhance the National Quality Strategy. | Value the importance of improving health for populations of patients.<br>Value the important role of public policy in nursing practice. | Agency for Healthcare Research & Quality, 2012<br>American Recovery and Reinvestment Act of 2009<br>Centers for Medicare & Medicaid Services, 2014<br>Hersch, 2009<br>National Quality Forum, 2006<br>Samal et al., 2012 |
| Analyze data sets to identify nursing care impact on outcomes. | Demonstrate efficient use of standardized terminologies and HIT applications to technology to perform role.<br>Use standards as defined in the "meaningful use" rule as a guide for top-priority conditions for analysis of quality.<br>"Use the existing coding and billing system to appropriately reflect the level and type of service delivered in practice" (p. 16).<br>"Model behaviors that support implementation and appropriate use of data accessed through databases, EHRs, dashboards, remote monitoring devices, telemedicine, and other technologies" (p. 15). | "Appreciate the importance of valid, reliable, and significant data to improve quality and provide efficient care" (p. 15). | AACN, 2012 |

## References

Agency for Healthcare Research and Quality. (2010). *PSO privacy protection center.* Retrieved from https://www.psoppc.org/web/patientsafety

Agency for Healthcare Research and Quality (AHRQ). (2012). *National quality strategy (NQS).* Retrieved from http://www.ahrq.gov/working forquality/

America Association at Colleges of Nursing (AACN), QSEN Education Consortium. (2012). *Graduate-level QSEN competencies, knowledge, skills and attitudes.* Retrieved from http://www.aacn.nche.edu/faculty/qsen/competencies.pdf

American Nurses Association (ANA). (2010). *Nursing: Scope and standards of practice* (2nd ed.). Silver Spring, MD: Author.

American Recovery and Reinvestment Act of 2009. (P.L. 111-5). 111th Congress of the United States of America.

Androwich, I., & Kraft, M.R. (2013). Informatics. In C.B. Laughlin (Ed.), *Core curriculum for ambulatory care nursing* (3rd ed., pp. 63-75). Pitman, NJ: American Academy of Ambulatory Care Nursing.

Centers for Medicare & Medicaid Services. (2014). *Clinical quality measures (CQMs).* Retrieved from http://www.cms.gov/Regulations-and-Guidance/Legislation/EHRIncentivePrograms/ClinicalQuality Measures.html

Cronenwett, L., Sherwood, G., Barnsteiner, J., Disch, J., Johnson, J., Mitchell, P., ... Warren, J. (2007). Quality and safety education for nurses. *Nursing Outlook, 55*(3), 122-131.

Cronenwett, L., Sherwood, G., Pohl, J., Barnsteiner, J., Moore, S., Sullivan, D.T., ... Warren, J. (2009). Quality and safety education for advanced nursing practice. *Nursing Outlook, 57*(6), 338-348.

Haas, S., & Androwich, I. (2011). Ambulatory care nursing: Concerns and challenges. In P.S. Cowen & S. Moorhead, *Current issues in nursing* (8th ed., Chapter 19). St. Louis, MO: Elsevier.

Harle, C., Huerta, T., Ford, E., Diana, M., & Menachemi, N. (2013). Overcoming challenges to achieving meaningful use: Insights from hospitals that successfully received Centers for Medicare & Medicaid Services payments in 2011. *Journal of the American Medical Informatics Association, 20*(2), 233-237.

Health Information Technology for Economic and Clinical Health (HITECH) Act. (2010). Washington, DC: U.S. Department of Health & Human Services.

Healthcare Information and Management Systems Society (HIMSS). (2003). *HIMSS electronic health record definitional model: Version 1.0, 1-8.* Chicago, IL: Author.

HealthIT.gov. (n.d.a). *Basics of health IT.* Retrieved from http://www.healthit.gov/patients-families/basics-health-it

HealthIT.gov. (n.d.b). *Learn ERT basics.* Retrieved from http://healthit.gov/providers-professionals/learn-ehr-basics

HealthIT.gov. (n.d.c). *Clinical decision support (CDS).* Retrieved from http://www.healthit.gov/policy-researchers-implementers/clinical-decision-support-cds

Hersch, W. (2009). A stimulus to define informatics and health information technology. *BMC Medical Informatics and Decision Making, 9,* 24.

McGonigle, D., Hunter, K. & Hebda, T. (2013). How can we promote nursing informatics? *Online Journal of Nursing Informatics (OJNI), 17*(1). Retrieved from http://ojni.org/issues/?p=2391

Mell, P., & Grance, T. (2011). *The NIST definition of cloud computing, recommendations of the National Institute of Standards and Technology.* Washington, DC: U.S. Department of Commerce.

National Quality Forum. (2006). *National Quality Forum-endorsed definition and framework for measuring care coordination.* Washington, DC: Author.

O'Carroll, P.W., Yasnoff, W.A., Ward, M.E., Ripp, L.H., & Martin, E.L. (Eds.) (2003). *Public health informatics and information systems.* New York, NY: Springer.

Sackett, D.L., Strauss, S.E., Richardson, W.S., Rosenberg, W., & Haynes, R.B. (2000). *Evidence-based medicine: How to practice and teach EBM* (2nd ed.). Edinburgh, Scotland: Churchill Livingstone.

Samal, L., Dykes, P.C., Greenberg, J., Hasan, O., Venkatesh, A.K., Volk, A., & Bates, D.W. (2012). *Environmental analysis of health information technology to support care coordination and care transitions.* Washington, DC: National Quality Forum.

Sheer, B. (2007). *Highlights of the International Council of Nurses 2007 Annual Conference, Yokohama, Japan.* Retrieved from http://www.medscape.com/viewarticle/559912

Sittig, D., & Singh, N. (2012). Electronic health records and national patient-safety goals. *New England Journal of Medicine, 367,* 1854-1860.

Society for Hospital Medicine. (n.d.). *Improving the care of patients as they transition from hospital to home.* Retrieved from http://www.hospitalmedicine.org/ResourceRoomRedesign/RR_Care Transitions/PDFs/Project_BOOST_Fact_SheetFinal.pdf

Society of Hospital Medicine. (2008). *Essential first steps in quality improvement.* Retrieved from http://www.hospitalmedicine.org/Resource RoomRedesign/RR_CareTransitions/html_CC/02FirstSteps/00_First Steps.cfm

## Additional Reading

Agency for Healthcare Research and Quality (AHRQ). (2013). *Findings and lessons from the AHRQ: Ambulatory and safety quality program.* Rockville, MD: Author.

# CHAPTER 13

# Telehealth Nursing Practice

*M. Elizabeth Greenberg, PhD, RN-BC, C-TNP*
*Carol Rutenberg, MNSc, RN-BC, C-TNP*
*Kathryn B. Scheidt, MSN, MS, BSN, RN*

## Learning Outcome Statement

The purpose of this chapter is to enable the reader to demonstrate the elements of competency in professional telehealth nursing practice that are required for the registered nurse (RN) in the Care Coordination and Transition Management (CCTM) role.

## Learning Objectives

After reading this chapter, the RN working in the CCTM role will be able to:

- Integrate knowledge, skills, and attitudes requisite to competency in telehealth nursing with knowledge, skills, and attitudes requisite to CCTM competencies.
- Recognize the importance of and understand the specialized telehealth triage skills necessary for safe and effective CCTM practice for the RN.
- Describe principles of successful communication and collaboration unique to telehealth nursing and provision of care in the non-face-to-face setting.
- Practice safe, timely, and effective care coordination and transition management in ambulatory care setting using telehealth principles, practices, and appropriate telecommunication technologies.
- Describe the existing legal, ethical, and professional standards associated with telehealth nursing practice in the RN in CCTM role.
- Verbalize the importance of continuing education to maintain/enhance knowledge base in telehealth nursing for CCTM.
- List the principles of telehealth triage in the RN in CCTM role.
- Collaborate with patient/family/caregiver to facilitate CCTM when using telecommunications technology to collaborate.
- Practice interdisciplinary collaboration when using telecommunication technology.
- Employ appropriate teamwork and delegation within the domain of telehealth nursing.
- Demonstrate the knowledge, skills, and attitudes required for telehealth nursing practice for the RN in the CCTM role (see Tables 1-5).

## Competency Definition

"Telehealth is the inclusive term used to describe the wide range of health services delivered, managed, and coordinated by all health related disciplines via electronic information and telecommunications technologies" (Greenberg, Espensen, Becker, & Cartwright, 2003, p. 8). "Telehealth Nursing is a subset of telehealth that focuses on the delivery, management, and coordination of care and services provided via telecommunications technology within the domain of nursing" (Greenberg et al., 2003, p. 9).

Telehealth nursing practices utilize a vast array of telecommunications technologies, including telephone, fax, electronic mail, internet, video monitoring, and interactive video. Telehealth nursing interventions are continually evolving to support and coordinate patient care through virtual information exchange (Greenberg et al., 2003). "This exchange of information can include symptom triage, consumer education, disease or condition management, appointment scheduling and confirmation, specialist referrals...and more" (American Academy of Ambulatory Care Nursing [AAACN], 2011, p. 14). Care coordination and transition management in ambulatory care settings requires both interaction with the patient and family and communication with and transfer of information across providers, agencies, and venues.

When engaged in Care Coordination and Transition Management (CCTM), the use of telecommunications technology will be ubiquitous, and thus competence in telehealth nursing practice is a foundational element for effective practice in each of the specific CCTM dimension(s). The role of the RN in CCTM requires competency in each of five essential elements of telehealth practice. These essential elements are: professional practice, triage principles and practice, effective communication, teamwork and collaboration, and technology know-how. For safe and effective practice, it is particularly important the RN in CCTM accepts the fact that when interacting with a patient via telecommunication technology, there is always the potential for triage and therefore a specialized telehealth triage skill set is required for nurses engaged in CCTM. In this chapter, the five essential elements will be described, along with the requisite knowledge, skills, and attitudes that are needed to attain competence. Although some of these elements are common to nursing in the face-to-face setting, the information addressed herein incorporates nuances and distinct practice differences necessary for the provision of care using telecommunications technology.

## I. Professional Telehealth Practice

Telehealth nursing practice must comply with basic standards put forth by the nursing profession (Rutenberg & Greenberg, 2012). Telehealth as a modality of delivery of CCTM services requires knowledge of specific legal, ethical, and professional standards as they apply to care delivery.

A. Application of standards to telehealth practices.
   1. Legal standards.
      a. Complies with licensure requirements.
      b. Practices consistent with Nurse Practice Act(s) in applicable jurisdiction(s).
      c. Has knowledge of issues related to interstate practice and Nurse Licensure Compact (National Council of State Boards of Nursing, 2014).
      d. Practices within the guidelines set forth by Health Insurance Portability and Accountability Act (HIPAA).
      e. Maintains workstation standards according to Occupational Safety and Health Administration (OSHA).
   2. Professional standards.
      a. Practices consistent with *Scope and Standards of Practice for Professional Telehealth Nursing* (AAACN, 2011).
      b. Utilizes the nursing process in all telehealth encounters.
      c. Recognizes telehealth nursing as a highly collaborative practice; however, functions autonomously and maintains accountability for own actions and associated patient outcomes.
      d. Documents all telehealth encounters thoroughly, accurately, and promptly.
   3. Ethical standards.
      a. Complies with American Nurses Association Code of Ethics (2001).
      b. Recognizes patient right to self-determination, but in all cases acts in the best interest of the patient to ensure safety.
   4. Need for ongoing professional development in telehealth.
      a. Recognizes the rapidly evolving state of the art in telehealth nursing.
      b. Remains current in the use of relevant telecommunication technology.
      c. Engages in continuing education to maintain comprehensive clinical knowledge base.
      d. Actively seeks to supplement existing knowledge deficits.

## II. Telehealth Triage Principles and Practice

RNs in CCTM who provide care using telecommunications technology must be poised and ready to perform triage. Because triage in the telehealth setting involves identifying and managing patients with unknown medical diagnoses, the nurse must possess a significant depth and breadth of knowledge to determine the nature and urgency of the patient's problem(s) and to refer them to the appropriate level of care, providing counseling and support as necessary (see Table 2).

The ability to triage a patient using telehealth technology may be required even when the focus of the nurse-patient interaction is on care coordination and transition management. Therefore, in each nurse-patient interaction, the nurse must actively look for existing symptoms and be prepared to triage the patient as necessary.

A. Application of the nursing process in telehealth triage.
   1. Performs an adequate assessment including relevant subjective and objective data.
   2. Formulates diagnostic statement to include the nature and urgency of the problem and any potential confounding factors.
   3. Identifies desired outcomes as a basis for development of plan of care to ensure patient safety.
   4. Collaboratively develops an individualized plan of care to assure achievement of desired outcomes.
   5. Implements plan/intervention with attention to continuity of care.
   6. Evaluates effectiveness of triage intervention.
B. Principles of telehealth triage in the RN in CCTM role (Rutenberg & Greenberg, 2012).
   1. Considers the possibility of, and actively looks for, unexpected problems and rules out the worst possible clinical presentation.
   2. Consistently errs on side of caution to ensure patient safety.
   3. Interacts directly with patient when possible in order to perform accurate assessment.
   4. Is not misled by patient's self-diagnosis.
   5. Avoids jumping to a conclusion about the nature of the patient's problem.
   6. Exercises critical thinking and judgment in use of support tools.
   7. Provides support and collaboration as needed by the individual.
   8. Recognizes that interpretation of health care language is required throughout each telehealth encounter (Greenberg, 2009).

## III. Effective Communication Using Telehealth Technology

The RN in CCTM must use telehealth technology "to communicate effectively using a variety of formats, tools, and technologies to build professional relationships and to deliver care…" (AAACN, 2011, p. 31). When using telecommunication technology, the RN in CCTM must identify and implement communication strategies that accurately and effectively elicit and provide information to patients, nurses, and other team members. For example, depending on the telecommunication technology used, the nurse will be communicating via visual, auditory, or written means, or a combination of these. Furthermore the communication may be synchronous or asynchronous. The RN in CCTM must therefore recognize that the skills necessary for effective communication must be adapted when the nurse is not in the physical presence of the patient, his or her family/caregiver, or other members of the health care team (Rutenberg & Greenberg, 2012) (see Table 3).

A. Limitations/challenges with non-face-to-face communication.
   1. Utilizes visualization as a technique to gain a clear picture of the patient's problem and confirms understanding by verifying impression with patient.
   2. Employs effective verbal and nonverbal communication techniques when interacting with patient/family/caregiver using telecommunications technology.
   3. Confirms patient comfort with the information/direction given and the plan of care.
   4. Clearly and promptly documents telehealth interactions so they are accessible to members of the health care team.
B. Endeavors to establish rapport with patient and family/caregiver by creating an interpersonal connection in non-face-to-face encounters.
   1. Introduces self and role in RN in CCTM.
   2. Expresses empathy, is attentive to patient input, and acknowledges patient perspective.
   3. Interprets (e.g., rephrases) information when necessary to increase understanding.
   4. Utilizes verbal and nonverbal strategies to connect with the patient.
C. Enlists the services of an interpreter when necessary.
   1. Effectively interacts with Relay Operator for the Hearing Impaired.
   2. When using TTY or TDD technology, understands patient phraseology.
   3. Effectively utilizes an approved language line or interpreter when necessary for language interpretation.

## IV. Teamwork and Collaboration

While utilizing telehealth technology, the RN in CCTM must actively foster open communication, facilitate mutual respect, engage in shared decision making, participate in team learning, delegate as appropriate, and work to achieve optimal care coordination and transition management (Cronenwett et al., 2007). Effective teamwork and collaboration requires knowledge of interdisciplinary roles and practices (see Table 4).

A. Collaborates with patient/family/caregiver to facilitate CCTM when using telecommunications technology.
   1. Recognizes and respects patient/family/caregiver role in decision making.
   2. Identifies, acknowledges, and addresses patient agenda (e.g., request or desired outcome) in the telehealth encounter.
B. Facilitates interdisciplinary collaboration when using telecommunication technology.
   1. Possesses knowledge of interdisciplinary roles and practices.
   2. Recognizes and avoids risks associated with transferring patient care responsibilities to another professional ("hand-off") during transitions in care, especially in the telehealth setting.
   3. Applies principles of successful communication and collaboration unique to telehealth nursing during interdisciplinary interactions.
C. Facilitates appropriate teamwork and delegation within the domain of telehealth nursing.
   1. Delegate as appropriate and necessary to enhance efficiency within telehealth encounters.
   2. Delegates to licensed practical nurses (LPNs) and unlicensed assistive personnel (UAPs) as appropriate to their level of education, scope of practice, and licensure.
   3. Adheres to the five rights of delegation when providing care utilizing telecommunication technology.

## V. Technology Know-How

The RN in CCTM must be able to appropriately, safely, and efficiently use telecommunications technology to meet the needs of the patient or population. The telecommunications technology used by the RN in CCTM will differ across settings. The RN in CCTM is responsible to attain and maintain competence in daily use (see Table 5).

A. Proficient in the use of telecommunication technology used in their setting.
   1. Possesses a basic understanding of how technology works.
   2. Is able to troubleshoot connectivity issues.
   3. Understands documentation and storage of data.
   4. Is familiar with contingency plan in the event of technology breakdown.
B. Maintains patient safety and confidentiality when using telehealth technology.
   1. Confirms with whom they are interacting when using telecommunication technology.
   2. Maintains patient privacy while using telecommunication technology.
   3. Uses certified practices and systems for secure management of data.

 

**Table 1.**
**Professional Telehealth Practice: Knowledge, Skills, and Attitudes for Competency**

| Knowledge | Skills | Attitudes | Sources |
|---|---|---|---|
| Understand the existing legal, ethical, and professional standards associated with telehealth nursing.<br>Recognize the importance of continuing education to maintain/enhance knowledge base in telehealth nursing. | Demonstrate accountability by practicing within own scope of competence and training.<br>Assure patient safety in compliance with professional standards and scope of practice laws and regulations.<br>Recognize and implements telehealth best practices in care coordination and transition management. | Value legal, ethical, and professional standards of practice.<br>Value the professional role of the RN and recognizes differences in scope of practice of RNs, licensed practical nurses/licensed vocational nurses (LPN/LVNs), and the role of unlicensed assistive personnel (UAP).<br>Recognize the potential for improved practices through continuing education. | Cronenwett et al., 2007 |
| Understand the concept of accountability and responsibility for telehealth nursing practice and for the outcome of that practice. | Uphold and practice within legal, ethical, and professional standards of telehealth nursing practice.<br>Adhere to existing patient privacy, confidentiality, and security laws related to patient information especially as it pertains to practice using telecommunications technology.<br>Appropriately delegate functions to LPNs, LVNs, and UAP.<br>Adhere to patient privacy, confidentiality, and security principles related to sharing/display/storage of patient records and information. | Accept responsibility for own behavior.<br>Value legal and ethical principles and patient right to privacy.<br>Appreciate the importance of remaining current in a rapidly changing practice. | AAACN, 2011<br>International Council of Nurses (ICN), 2007 |
| Articulate the elements of the nursing process as they apply to telehealth encounters. | Adhere to the *Scope and Standards of Practice for Professional Telehealth Nursing.*<br>Participate in lifelong learning specific to telehealth nursing, seeking new education and training opportunities as new practice opportunities become available. | Is committed to lifelong learning. | AAACN, 2011 |

*continued on next page*

**Table 1. (continued)**
**Professional Telehealth Practice: Knowledge, Skills, and Attitudes for Competency**

| Knowledge | Skills | Attitudes | Sources |
|---|---|---|---|
| Understand legal and ethical principles related to sharing patient information. | Apply the nursing process in all telehealth patient encounters.<br>When care is provided across state lines:<br>• Maintain licensure in states in which he/she is practicing.<br>• Practice within the RN scope of practice in the state in which care is regarded as being provided by the rolovant board of nursing. | Value patient's rights.<br>Value the nursing process as the basic standard of nursing practice and recognizes the importance of utilizing all elements of nursing process in telehealth interactions.<br>Recognize and values the importance of licensure in the practice of nursing across state lines.<br>Appreciate that regulations and standards exist to protect the public, which is a sovereign responsibility of each board of nursing.<br>Is committed to providing high-quality, safe, and effective patient care coordination and transition management. | AAACN, 2011<br>Rutenberg & Greenberg, 2012 |

Table 2.
Telehealth Triage Principles and Practice: Knowledge, Skills, and Attitudes for Competency

| Knowledge | Skills | Attitudes | Sources |
|---|---|---|---|
| Acknowledge the necessity of collaboration in development of a plan of care to achieve desired outcomes. | Elicit care expectations of patient and family.<br>Collaborate with the patient/caregiver to develop a plan of care to attain desired outcomes that are realistic and achievable. | Value patient safety.<br>Respect the patient and caregiver as reliable sources of information.<br>Respect the patient's right to participate in care planning and making his or her own decision about the course of action.<br>Recognize that patient expectations influence outcomes in management of symptoms.<br>Respect the patient's perspective, valuing patient self-determination. | Cronenwett et al., 2007 |
| Identify strategies for implementing the plan of care as appropriate for the individual patient and within the clinical context. | Collaborate with the patient/caregiver to identify desired outcomes for the triage encounter.<br>Implement the plan of care in collaboration with the patient/caregiver and other members of the health care team as appropriate. | Recognize the key role of the patient/caregiver in implementation of the plan of care in any telehealth encounter. | Cronenwett et al., 2009 |
| Identify assessment techniques to collect both subjective and objective data using telecommunication technologies.<br>Understand the role of outcomes identification in individualizing care using telecommunications technology.<br>Is knowledgeable about the process of evaluation of a telehealth encounter to achieve desired outcomes. | Establish a therapeutic relationship with the patient when using technology.<br>Conduct assessments including both subjective and objective data using an array of available resources.<br>Prioritize plan and intervention based on assessment data.<br>Involve other members of the health care team in development of a plan of care as appropriate and necessary.<br>Implement an interdisciplinary plan of care directly or via geographically remote site person(s) to achieve desired outcomes.<br>Evaluate the patient's progress toward attainment of expected outcomes. | Recognize the duty of nurse to provide safe and effective care.<br>Realize desired outcomes must be individualized and that the patient/caregiver has an important role in their development.<br>Recognize the telehealth encounter doesn't end with implementation of the plan of care, but that the nurse has a responsibility to follow-up, when indicated, to measure attainment of desired outcomes and assure patient safety. | ICN, 2007 |

*continued on next page*

**Source Note:** Cronenwett et al. (2007) reprinted form *Nursing Outlook, 55*(3), 122-131, with permission from Elsevier.

**Table 2. (continued)**
**Telehealth Triage Principles and Practice: Knowledge, Skills, and Attitudes for Competency**

| Knowledge | Skills | Attitudes | Sources |
|---|---|---|---|
| Understand the need to function within a professional code of ethics that ensures individual rights.<br>Understand that implementation in the telehealth setting by necessity must include other individuals since the telehealth nurse is unable to provide physical care or services directly to the patient. | Work toward identifying and honoring the patient's wishes.<br>Employ creative strategies when patient desires conflict with patient health and safety. | Recognize the highly collaborative nature of telehealth nursing.<br>Understand that a plan of care must be individualized to each patient and might be impacted by patient motivation and available resources.<br>Understand the need to balance patient self-determination with assuring patient safety. Is sensitive to the fact telehealth nursing is highly collaborative.<br>Recognize the final decision maker in a telehealth encounter is usually the patient/caregiver while remaining sensitive to situations in which the nurse needs to act on the patient's behalf to assure his or her safety.<br>Employ strategies to reduce risk in the performance of triage using telecommunications technology. | AAACN, 2011 |
| Demonstrate comprehensive knowledge of the interpersonal, clinical, and technical skills needed to perform triage in non-face-to-face settings.<br>Comprehend the complexity of patient assessment utilizing telecommunications technology.<br>Develop nursing diagnostic statements based on assessment.<br>Possess a wide and diverse clinical knowledge base.<br>Has knowledge of patient and community resources as well as organizational policies relevant to development of an individualized plan of care.<br>Understand the role of clinical decision support tools in triage, recognizing they are to be utilized to support decision making rather than to dictate decision making.<br>Recognize clinical pitfalls in the practice of telehealth triage.<br>Explain the minimum skill set for provision of triage services in the non-face-to-face setting. | Assess presence and extent of symptoms.<br>Develop assessment techniques that compensate for the nurse's inability to see or touch the patient.<br>Formulate diagnostic statements that address patient's presenting problems and include the nature and urgency of the patient's problem and related needs.<br>Address the patient's ability to carry out the plan of care and other factors that might impact continuity of care.<br>Assure continuity of care in implementation of the plan of care.<br>Facilitate actions to assure patient safety.<br>Document a complete, accurate, and prompt account of the interaction.<br>Follow-up when appropriate and necessary, based on assessment of the likelihood the patient will be able to carry out the plan of care and the risk associated with failure to do so. | Recognize the ability of the patient and caregiver to provide health data utilizing their visual, tactile, auditory, and olfactory senses with individualized coaching.<br>Recognize the duty of nurse to provide safe and effective care.<br>Is sensitive to the complexity of the health care system and the patient's likely need for support and coaching in navigating the system.<br>Value the role of the team in providing care to a patient and recognizes the important contributions of the patient, family, telehealth nurse, and other members of the health care team as well as appropriate community resources.<br>Value lifelong learning and understands that patients may present with a wide variety of clinical and social problems which the nurse must recognize and address.<br>Value the role of critical thinking and clinical judgment in the provision of care during a triage encounter.<br>Appreciate the value of decision support tools to enhance the nurse's knowledge base and as a checklist to avoid clinical oversights.<br>Value the unique nature of triage outside of the face-to-face setting and understands that in the absence of face-to-face assessment and a known medical diagnosis, it requires a somewhat different, often more conservative approach to patient management. | Rutenberg & Greenberg, 2012 |

*continued on next page*

**Table 2. (continued)**
**Telehealth Triage Principles and Practice: Knowledge, Skills, and Attitudes for Competency**

| Knowledge | Skills | Attitudes | Sources |
|---|---|---|---|
| *(continued from previous page)* | Work to develop and maintain an extensive knowledge base to support clinical decision making in triage encounters.<br>Consistently utilize decision support tools during triage, but applies clinical judgment and critical thinking.<br>Avoid overreliance on decision support tools.<br>Practice in a manner that assures patient safety.<br>Perform an adequate assessment with all symptom-based encounters, regardless of the nature of the patient or complaint, or the technology used.<br>Consistently err on the side of caution.<br>Avoid accepting patient self-diagnosis without adequate investigation.<br>Avoid stereotyping the patient.<br>Interact directly with the patient whenever possible.<br>Recognize the perils associated with fatigue and haste.<br>Use critical thinking to recognize and address all concerns, remaining on the alert for unexpected problems.<br>Anticipate problems to be worst possible until proven otherwise.<br>Advocate for the patient, even when it is difficult to do so.<br>Follow-up when indicated by the nursing care plan.<br>Facilitate continuity of care, recognizing the telehealth encounter is often not the endpoint of care, but rather the beginning. | Understand all patients are potentially in crisis and their concerns must be identified and addressed in a professional and empathetic manner.<br>Recognize the importance of the role of the RN in telehealth encounters.<br>Approach each encounter with caution and recognizes the inherent risk in the provision of care using telecommunications technology.<br>Value patient health and safety. | Rutenberg & Greenberg, 2012 |

**Table 3.**
**Effective Communication: Knowledge, Skills, and Attitudes for Competency**

| Knowledge | Skills | Attitudes | Sources |
|---|---|---|---|
| Examine how the safety, quality, and cost effectiveness of health care can be improved through the active involvement of patients and families. | Elicit and validate patient values, preferences, and expressed needs. | Respect patient preferences, values, and needs.<br>Value various forms of communication and accepts that others may have differing ways of communicating. | Cronenwett et al., 2007 |
| Analyze differences in communication styles, preferences among patients, nurses, and other members of the health care team. | | Value inter-professional collaboration and communication. | Cronenwett et al., 2009 |
| Recognize subtle changes in interpersonal communications patterns of patients and providers that may indicate potential problems or important changes in status that require attention.<br>Recognize need to create therapeutic relationship with patient. | Adapt communication style to the goals of the patient and the technology used.<br>Create therapeutic environment using telehealth technologies.<br>Use a variety of formats, tools, and technologies to build professional relationships and to coordinate care.<br>Communicate patient values, preferences, and expressed needs as appropriate to other members of the health care team. | Recognize own responsibility for contributing to effective communication.<br>Acknowledge role of continuous quality improvement. | ICN, 2007 |
| Identify a variety of communication strategies using technology including the effective use of both verbal and nonverbal communication.<br>Coordinate care within and across settings via telecommunication technology. | Evaluate personal skills and styles of communication via technology to identify areas needing improvement or education.<br>Share communication experiences with peers and asks for feedback and evaluation of effectiveness.<br>Facilitate identification and delivery of services via communication technology. | Understand that effective communication is essential to a telehealth encounter.<br>Value medical record as a communication tool and endeavors to document the encounter in such a way as to be relevant to other members of the team. | AAACN, 2011 |

*continued on next page*

**Table 3.**
**Effective Communication: Knowledge, Skills, and Attitudes for Competency**

| Knowledge | Skills | Attitudes | Sources |
|---|---|---|---|
| Recognize the limitations inherent in non-face-to-face communication.<br>Discuss strategies used to "connect" with others when using communicating via technology. | Identify self with name and licensure.<br>Engage in active listening.<br>Clarify statements when necessary.<br>Allow patients to tell their story in their own way, communicating their concerns in a manner most comfortable to and effective for them.<br>Use self-disclosure when appropriate and necessary to connect with the patient/family/ caregiver.<br>Encourage the patient to take notes during telehealth encounter.<br>Document as appropriate and maintains clear records of communi-cations. | Recognize self-disclosure as a strategy which can either enhance or interrupt connection with the patient/family caregiver and realizes it must be used judiciously when it is believed that it will enhance the nurse's ability to meet the patient's needs without instead shifting the focus from the patient/family/caregiver to the RN.<br>Understand effective communication is essential to a telehealth encounter. | Rutenberg & Greenberg, 2012 |
| Recognize information needs of patients, providers, and other members of the health care team.<br>Recognize which elements of communication tools improve telehealth interactions and promote positive results. | Verify caller/contact identity and relationship to patient and identifies need or desired outcome of the communication.<br>Adapt communication style as needed to fit the technology used (e.g., tone of voice, facial expression, clear written word, appropriate literacy level).<br>Participate in evaluation of communication tools and encounter forms. | Recognize own responsibility for contributing to effective communication. | Rutenberg & Greenberg, 2012 |

**Table 4.**
**Teamwork and Collaboration: Knowledge, Skills, and Attitudes for Competency**

| Knowledge | Skills | Attitudes | Sources |
|---|---|---|---|
| Discuss how authority and hierarchy in non-face-to-face settings influence teamwork and patient safety.<br>Identify barriers and facilitators that the use of telecommunication technologies bring to effective team functioning.<br>Understand the impact of effective team functioning on safety and quality of care.<br>Describe scope of practice and roles of interdisciplinary and nursing telehealth care team members. | Assert own position/ perspective in coordination of patient care.<br>Initiate a plan for self-development as a team member.<br>Participate in designing systems that support effective teamwork.<br>Follow(s) communication practices that minimize risks associated with hand-offs among providers and across transitions in care, especially in the telehealth environment.<br>Function(s) competently within own scope of practice as a member of the telehealth care team.<br>Assume(s) the role of team member or leader based on the situation.<br>Initiate requests for assistance when situation warrants.<br>Integrate the contributions of others in assisting patient/family to achieve health goals.<br>Demonstrate self-awareness of strengths and limitations as a team member.<br>Recognize strengths and limitations of telecommunication technology in functioning as a member of a CCTM team.<br>Identify contributions of other individuals in meeting CCTM needs of patients and families. | Value the perspectives and expertise of all health team members.<br>Recognize a shared responsibility for effective team functioning in non-face-to-face settings.<br>Value own role in preventing errors.<br>Appreciate the importance of teamwork and collaboration in the telehealth setting.<br>Appreciate the value of what individuals and teams can do to meet client needs in the telehealth setting.<br>Value(s) the influence of system solutions in achieving team functioning in the telehealth setting.<br>Respect(s) the centrality of the patient and family as core members of any health care team, especially in the telehealth environment. | Cronenwett et al., 2007 |

*continued on next page*

**Table 4. (continued)**
**Teamwork and Collaboration: Knowledge, Skills, and Attitudes for Competency**

| Knowledge | Skills | Attitudes | Sources |
|---|---|---|---|
| Analyze strategies associated with technology that influence the ability to initiate and sustain effective partnerships with members of nursing and inter-professional teams.<br>Analyze strategies for identifying and managing overlaps in team member roles and accountabilities.<br>Recognize the risks associated with transferring patient care responsibilities to another professional ("hand-off") during transitions in care, especially in the telehealth setting. | Lead or participate in the design and implementation of telehealth systems that support effective teamwork.<br>Manage, within the scope of practice, areas of overlap in role and/or accountability in team member functioning.<br>Act with integrity, consistency, and respect for differing views when coordinating care using telecommunications technology. | Value(s) the influence of system solutions in achieving team functioning in the telehealth setting (p. 342).<br>Respect(s) the centrality of the patient and family as core members of any health care team, especially in the telehealth environment (p. 341).<br>Appreciate the risks associated with hand-offs among providers and across transitions in care, especially in the telehealth setting. | Cronenwett et al., 2009 |
| | Assure that the patient and the team members understand safety issues.<br>Identify and advocates for patient goals in each encounter.<br>Document the process and results of care within electronic record or approved organizational method whereby approved multidisciplinary providers at authorized locations have access to the data. | | ICN, 2007 |
| Recognize the need for teamwork and collaboration to coordinate care within the telehealth domain. | Utilize telecommunications technology effectively when functioning in the RN in CCTM role.<br>Demonstrate principles of delegation of duties to team members.<br>Ensure authentic identities of practitioners and clients when coordinating care using telecommunications technology.<br>Implement and communicate via technology an interdisciplinary plan of care to achieve and improve patient outcomes. | Appreciate the importance of teamwork and collaboration in the telehealth setting. | AAACN, 2011 |

**Table 5.**
**Technology Know-How: Knowledge, Skills, and Attitudes for Competency**

| Knowledge | Skills | Attitudes | Sources |
|---|---|---|---|
| Explain knowledge and skills required to provide care and to communicate via specific telecommunications technologies.<br>Analyze features of technology that support or pose barriers to coordinating care and managing transitions. | Demonstrate efficient use of technology devices to perform role.<br>Apply appropriate telecommunication technology to support CCTM.<br>Champion(s) communication technologies that support care coordination.<br>Assure safety of self and others when using telehealth technology. | Value technologies that support care coordination.<br>Appreciate the need for continuing education.<br>Value patient safety, privacy, and confidentiality.<br>Value confidentiality and security of all electronic information. | Cronenwett et al., 2007 |
| Has knowledge and familiarity (technical competence) with the technology used.<br>Identify safety principles associated with the use of telecommunications technology.<br>Identify the rapid changes associated with technology.<br>Is knowledgeable about organizational policies related to utilization of telecommunications technology. | Use technology appropriately and safely to coordinate care for patients.<br>Provide direction and support for other users.<br>Establish a positive working relationship with key technical support person(s) to ensure that technical problems/ questions can be addressed in expedient fashion.<br>Examine strategies for improving systems to support team functioning.<br>Follow safety precautions.<br>Acquire training on telehealth technology used in their organization.<br>Anticipate potential technical problems by having back-up plan or alternative action ready.<br>Acquire knowledge and experience as technology changes.<br>Utilize technology according to organizational or agency policy.<br>Participate in the selection, design, implementation, and evaluation of technology.<br>Maintain competence in technology use. | Value safety and efficiency.<br>Value patient preferences.<br>Accept personal responsibility for performance. | ICN, 2007 |

*continued on next page*

 

**Table 5. (continued)**
**Technology Know-How: Knowledge, Skills, and Attitudes for Competency**

| Knowledge | Skills | Attitudes | Sources |
|---|---|---|---|
| Is aware of geographic and time constraints that may accompany use of telecommunications technology. | Follow ergonomic guidelines to prevent harm.<br>Engage others in active partnerships using technology.<br>Plan ahead, meets time commitments. | Honor active partnerships with others in planning, implementation, and evaluation of care.<br>Respect patient and provider preferences for degree of active engagement in use of technology. | AAACN, 2011 |

## References

American Academy of Ambulatory Care Nursing (AAACN). (2011). *Scope and standards of practice for professional telehealth nursing* (5th ed.). Pitman, NJ: Author.

American Nurses Association. (2001). *Code of ethics for nurses.* Washington, DC: Author.

Cronenwett, L., Sherwood, G., Barnsteiner, J., Disch J., Johnson, J., Mitchell, P., … Warren, J. (2007). Quality and safety education for nurses. *Nursing Outlook, 55*(3), 122-131.

Cronenwett, L., Sherwood, G., Pohl, J., Barnsteiner, J., Moore, S., Sullivan, D., … Warren, J. (2009). Quality and safety education for advanced nursing practice. *Nursing Outlook, 57*(6), 338-348.

Greenberg, M.E. (2009). A comprehensive model of the process of telephone nursing. *Journal of Advanced Nursing, 65*(12), 2621-2629.

Greenberg, M.E., Espensen, M., Becker, C., & Cartwright, J. (2003). Telehealth nursing practice special interest group adopts teleterms. *ViewPoint, 25*(1), 8-10.

International Council of Nurses (ICN). (2007). *International competencies for telenursing.* Geneva, Switzerland: Author.

National Council of State Boards of Nursing. (2014). *Nurse licensure compact.* Retrieved from https://www.ncsbn.org/nlc.htm

Rutenberg, C., & Greenberg, M.E. (2012). *The art and science of telephone triage: How to practice nursing over the phone.* Hot Springs, AR: Telephone Triage Consulting, Inc.

## Additional Readings

American Nurses Association. (1998). *Core principles on telehealth.* Washington, DC: Author.

Espensen, M. (Ed.). (2009). *Telehealth nursing practice essentials.* Pitman, NJ: American Academy of Ambulatory Care Nursing.

Laughlin, C.B. (Ed.). (2013). *Core curriculum for ambulatory care nursing* (3rd ed.). Pitman, NJ: American Academy of Ambulatory Care Nursing.

Massachusetts Department of Higher Education Nurse of the Future Competency Committee. (2010). *Nurse of the future nursing core competencies.* Boston, MA: Massachusetts Department of Higher Education.

# Glossary*

**5 A's Behavior Change Model Adapted for Self-Management Support Improvement** – An interactive closed-loop model for implementing self-management strategies.

**Abandonment** – Relationship between patient and health care provider is terminated abruptly; provider disregards legal and ethical obligations to facilitate continuity of care and to avoid harm caused by terminating the relationship prematurely.

**Accessibility of Care** – Refers to the ease with which consumers can initiate interaction with a clinician about health problems; includes activities to eliminate barriers raised by geography, financing, culture, race, language, etc.

**Accreditation Association for Ambulatory Health Care (AAAHC)** – A private, nonprofit agency that offers voluntary, peer-based review of the quality of health care services of ambulatory health organizations, including ambulatory and office-based surgery centers, managed care organizations, as well as Indian and student health centers, among others.

**Active Listening** – A way of listening and responding to another person that improves mutual understanding. Active listening skills are conversational techniques that enable better understanding and more productive communication.

**Acute Care Nursing** – Nursing care of patients typically in a hospital setting who are receiving treatment for illness, accident, trauma, or surgical procedure with the goal of promoting, restoring, or maintaining optimal health.

**Advance Directives** – Allow competent adults to make certain kinds of health care decisions in advance of an acute (such as a car accident) or chronic (such as Alzheimer's or cancer) incapacity, thus ensuring their wishes are respected even if they are unable to communicate them directly. Three types are living wills, durable power of attorney for health care, and DNR ("Do Not Resuscitate") order.

**Advocacy** – Act or process of advocating or supporting (a cause or proposal) on behalf of another.

**Algorithm** – A step-by-step procedure that is explicit and in a logical order to achieve a specific result.

**Ambulatory Care** – Outpatient care in which patients stay less than 24 hours and are discharged to their normal residential situation after care.

**Ambulatory Care Nursing** – A specialty practice area that is characterized by nurses responding rapidly to high volumes of patients in a short span of time while dealing with issues that are not always predictable.

**Ambulatory Patient Classifications (APCs)** – Used by the Centers for Medicare & Medicaid Services for prospective payment in hospital outpatient departments and ambulatory surgery centers; based on procedures and adjusted for severity.

**Ambulatory Patient Groups (APGs)** – Patient classification system designed to explain amount and type of resource used in ambulatory care visit.

**Americans with Disabilities Act (ADA)** – Prohibits discrimination on the basis of disability in employment, state and local government, public accommodations, commercial facilities, transportation, and telecommunications.

**Autonomy** – The right to self-determine a course of action; support of independent decision making.

**Balanced Scorecard** – Graphic or pictorial display of the organization's indicators chosen to support the strategic plan and vision of the organization; allows for examination of relationships among the separate indicators (care, quality, financial, operational, etc.).

**Benchmarking** – A continuous measurement of a process, product, or service in comparison to those of the toughest competitor, to those considered industry leaders, or to similar activities in the organization and using the information to change/improve practices, resulting in superior performance as determined by measured outcomes.

**Beneficence** – Doing good; requires defining what is meant by "good" in the situation.

**Better Outcomes by Optimizing Safe Transitions (BOOST)** – A national initiative led by the Society of Hospital Medicine to improve the care of patients as they transition from hospital to home. Project BOOST has developed tools to assist in transitions.

**CAGE-AID** – A questionnaire that focuses on both drug and alcohol abuse.

**Capitation** – Method for funding expenses of enrollees in prepaid health plans; pays providers a fixed fee per member regardless of whether or not the service is provided. For example, a plan pays a per member per month (PMPM) amount to a physician group to provide primary care services for each enrollee in the plan.

**Care Coordination** – (1) A process that seeks to achieve the optimal cost-effective use of scarce resources by helping individuals obtain health and appropriate social and life-support services that meet their unique needs at a given point in time or across the lifespan.

(2) The deliberate organization of patient care activities between two or more participants (including the patient) involved in a patient's care to facilitate the appropriate delivery of health care services. Organizing care involves the marshalling of personnel and other resources needed to carry out all required patient care activities and is often managed by the exchange of information among participants responsible for different aspects of care.

(3) An information-rich, patient-centric endeavor that seeks to deliver the right care (and only the right care) to the right patient at the right time. A function that helps ensure the patient's needs and preferences for health services and information sharing across people, functions, and sites are met over time. Care coordination maximizes the value of services delivered to patients by facilitating beneficial, efficient, safe, and high-quality patient experiences and improved health care outcomes.

**Care Transitions** – A change in the level of service or location of providers of care as patients move within the health system.

**Case Management** – A collaborative process of assessment, planning, facilitation, and advocacy for options and services to meet an individual's health needs through communication and available resources to promote quality cost-effective outcomes; a method for managing the provision of health care to members/patients with catastrophic or high-cost medical conditions.

**Centers for Medicare & Medicaid Services (CMS)** – Formerly Health Care Financing Administration (HCFA); division within the U.S. Department of Health and Human Services that determines the standard rules and reporting mechanisms for health care services.

**Certification** – Process that uses predetermined standards to validate and recognize an individual's knowledge, skills, and abilities in a defined functional and clinical area of specialty practice approved by the American Nurses Association as an area of specialty practice.

**Clinical Care Classification (CCC)** – Formerly Home Health Care Classification (HHCC); Saba's Georgetown System for Patient Problems, Interventions, and Outcomes.

**Clinical Practice Guidelines** – Statements that have been systematically developed based on evidence to assist practitioners and patients in making decisions about appropriate health care for specific clinical circumstances.

**Cognitive Impairment** – Failing of short and long-term recall and general thinking logic skills.

**Collaboration** – Working together toward a common goal; to pursue a common purpose and a sharing of knowledge to resolve problems, decide issues, and set goals within a structure of collegiality.

**Commercial Indemnity Plans** – A type of insurance contract in which the insurer pays for care received up to a fixed amount per encounter or episode of illness.

**Competence** – Having the ability to demonstrate the knowledge, technical, critical thinking, and interpersonal skills necessary to perform one's job responsibilities.

**Competency** – An expected level of performance that integrates knowledge, skills, abilities, and judgement.

**Complementary, Alternative, and Integrative Therapies (CAM)** – Care that includes nontraditional therapies either in place of or together with conventional medicine.

**Confidentiality** – To protect the patient's and family's right to privacy regarding information the nurse or institution holds about the patient.

**Confusion** – Disorientation, inappropriate behavior or communication, and/or hallucinations.

**Co-Payment** – Out-of-pocket expense paid by an individual for a specific service defined in the insurance plan.

**Core Competencies for Nursing** – A standard set of performance "domains" in which it is necessary to demonstrate proficiency to enter into professional practice.

**Cost Benefit Analysis** – A formal financial analysis completed by organizations to determine the cost of a program, projected revenues, and to identify and quantify program benefits; includes assumptions about specific expenses and potential revenue based on projected volumes.

**CPT** – The Physicians' Current Procedural Terminology, published by the American Medical Association; the internationally recognized coding system for reporting medical services and procedures.

**Credentialing** – Review and verification of credentials (education, training, licensure, certification, experience). In some cases (such as in most nursing homes and an increasing number of other health care facilities), this includes performing criminal background checks.

**Critical Thinking** – A deliberate nonlinear process of collecting, interpreting, analyzing, drawing conclusions about, presenting, and evaluating information that is both factually and belief based. This is demonstrated in nursing by clinical judgment, which includes ethical, diagnostic, and therapeutic dimensions and research.

**Cultural Competence** – Requires developing cultural awareness (conscious learning process through which one becomes appreciative and sensitive to the cultures of other people), cultural knowledge (process of understanding the key aspects of a group's culture), cultural skills (ability to collect relevant data regarding health histories and perform culturally specific assessments), and cultural encounters (process that encourages one to engage directly in cross-cultural interactions with people from culturally diverse backgrounds).

**Cultural Safety** – Providing culturally safe care requires the nurse to be respectful of nationality, culture, age, sex, and political and religious beliefs.

**Decision Support System –** Automated tool that enhances the nurse's ability to make decisions in semi-structured, uncertain situations by bringing necessary information, evidence, expertise, and resources to the point of care.

**Deductible –** Amount an insured individual is responsible to pay before insurance pays. For example, an individual may have to pay a $200 deductible for hospitalization before the remainder of the hospital stay is covered by insurance.

**Delegation –** The transfer of responsibility for the performance of a task from one person to another.

**Deontology –** Also known as duty-based ethics; based on the belief there are duties to which one must be faithful and which one is obligated to carry out because these duties are owed to all human beings and because of the expectations implied by one's professional role.

**Depression (Major) –** Possessing five or more symptoms of depression (e.g., insomnia, fatigue, weight loss or gain, low self-esteem, sudden bursts of anger, excessive sleeping).

**Diagnosis-Related Groups (DRGs) –** A system for classifying hospital inpatients into groups requiring similar quantities of resources according to characteristics such as diagnosis, age, procedure, complications, and co-morbidities.

**Distance Learning –** Provides access to learning modalities initially designed to reach/include persons in rural/isolated areas, providing educational opportunities/resources.

**Domain of Ambulatory Nursing Practice –** The overall scope of nursing practice in the ambulatory arena; it includes attributes of the environment in which practice occurs, patient requirements for care, and specific nursing role dimensions.

**Drug Abuse Screening Test (DAST) –** 20 or 28-item self-report scale for abuse of drugs other than alcohol.

**Education Process –** Systematic planned course of action consisting of two major interdependent operations: teaching and learning.

**Electronic Health Record –** A secure, real-time, point-of-care, patient-centric information resource for clinicians.

**Emergency Medical Treatment and Active Labor Act (EMTALA) –** Federal law passed in 1986 to ensure patient access to emergency services regardless of ability to pay.

**Emotional Intelligence –** Ability to accurately perceive one's own and others' emotions, to understand the signals that emotions send about the relationship, and to manage one's own and others' emotions.

**Engagement in Health Care –** Actions individuals must take to obtain the greatest benefit from the health care services available to them.

**Environmental Management –** The assurance of appropriate management plans to provide a safe, accessible, effective, and functional environment of care.

**Equal Employment Opportunity Commission (EEOC) –** A federal agency that enforces regulations concerning equal opportunity.

**Ethics –** A philosophical framework for examining values as they relate to human behaviors; how behaviors are viewed as right or wrong, good or bad, concerned with both the motives and the outcomes of actions.

**Evidence-Based Practice –** The conscientious, explicit, and judicious use of current best evidence in making decisions about the care of individual patients; combines research and clinical expertise.

**Existential Distress –** Occurs at a time when a person is questioning the meaning of his or her life. This response encompasses the physical, psychosocial, and spiritual angst that may occur at the end of life.

**Fee for Service –** Reimbursement method in which payment is made for each service or item.

**Fidelity –** Faithfulness; involves duty owed to patients, families, and colleagues to do what one says.

**Fixed Costs –** Costs do not change with volume of service units or activity, such as patient visits.

**Generalized Anxiety Scale (GAD-7) –** A self-reported questionnaire for screening and severity measuring of generalized anxiety disorder (GAD).

**Geriatric Resources for Assessment and Care of Elders (GRACE) –** A team-developed care plan to improve the quality of geriatric care and optimize health and functional status, decrease excess health care use, and prevent long-term nursing home placement.

**Get Up and Go Test –** A timed test for measurement of mobility. It includes a number of tasks such as standing from a seated position, walking, turning, stopping, and sitting down.

**Grief –** The individualized feelings and responses that a person makes to real, perceived, or anticipated loss.

**Health Care Financing Administration (HCFA) –** See Centers for Medicare & Medicaid Services (CMS).

**Health Care Financing Administration (HCFA) Common Procedure Coding System (HCPCS) –** A uniform method for health care providers and medical suppliers to report professional services, procedures, and supplies to health care plans.

**Health Care Reform –** As described by the Patient Protection and Affordable Care Act (PPACA) of 2010, introduces changes related to health insurance coverage, access to services, quality of care, costs of health care, and overall population health.

**Health Care Team –** Includes the patient, family, and other members of the health care system who are involved in the development and implementation of the care plan.

**Health Coaching –** A practice that educates patients while promoting self-management of individualized health goals.

**Health Education –** Any combination of planned learning experiences based on sound theories that provide individuals, groups, and communities the opportunity to acquire the information and skills needed to make quality health decisions.

**Health Information Exchange (HIE) –** The transmission of health care related data among facilities, health information organizations (HIO), and government agencies according to national standards. HIE is an integral component of the health information technology (HIT) infrastructure under development in the United States and the associated National Health Information Network (NHIN).

**Health Information Technology (HIT) –** The application of computers and technology to the provision of health care in all settings, including all stakeholders involved in health.

**Health Insurance Portability and Accountability Act (HIPAA) –** Federal law that establishes a "floor" for privacy protection and implementing privacy and security regulations; applies to all health plans, health care clearinghouses, and those health care providers (including nurses) who bill electronically for their services; provides that patients have a right to control their information and must "authorize" use or disclosure of their health information.

**Health Literacy –** Cognitive and social skills that determine the motivation and ability of individuals to gain access to and understand and use information in ways that promote and maintain good health.

**Health Maintenance Organization (HMO) –** A health plan that uses physicians as gatekeepers. In this model, the patient chooses a primary care provider (PCP) who is responsible for all aspects of care management and who must authorize (gatekeeper) or give permission for referral to other providers; another model of HMO places risk on the providers for medical expenses. In this instance, providers are encouraged to provide appropriate medical services, but not medically unnecessary services.

**Healthy People 2020 –** Federal government's health care improvement priorities managed by federal agencies; provides measurable objectives applicable at national, state, and local levels; increases public awareness and understanding of determinants of health.

**HEDIS® –** A set of standardized performance measures designed to assure purchasers and consumers have the information they need to reliably compare the performance of health plans; sponsored and maintained by NCQA.

**Hospice –** Comprehensive, noncurative services are provided to a terminally ill patient and his or her family by an interdisciplinary team (including physicians, nurses, social workers, chaplains, counselors, certified nursing assistants, therapists, and volunteers) wherever the patient is.

**ICD-9-CM (International Classification of Diseases, 9th revision, Clinical Modification) –** Published by the U.S. National Center for Health Statistics; the internationally recognized system for the purpose of international morbidity and mortality reporting; in the United States, used for coding and billing purposes.

**ICD-10-CM (International Classification of Diseases, 10th edition, Clinical Modification Procedure Coding System) –** New classification system that captures more detailed clinical information to reflect advances in clinical medicine; uses 3-7 alpha or numeric digits.

**Independent Practice Association (IPA) –** A legal entity whose members are independent physicians who contract with the IPA for the purpose of having the IPA contract with one or more HMOs.

**Index of Independence in Activities of Daily Living (IADL) –** An instrument used in assessing functional status when measuring a patient's ability to perform activities of daily living independently.

**Informatics –** Use and support the use of information and technology to communicate, manage knowledge, mitigate error, and support decision making.

**Informed Consent –** Process by which a patient is provided relevant information about a proposed procedure, test, or course of treatment; given an opportunity to ask questions; and asked to voluntarily agree.

**Institute of Medicine (IOM) –** An independent, nonprofit organization that works to provide unbiased and authoritative advice to decision-makers and the public to improve health.

**Interprofessional Team –** A group of individuals from different disciplines working and communicating with each other, providing his/her knowledge, skills, and attitudes to augment and support the contributions of others.

**Interstate Compacts** – Allow that nurses may practice across state lines, physically or electronically, unless under discipline or a monitoring agreement that restricts interstate practice. Nurses are licensed where they live (the "home state").

**The Joint Commission (Formerly The Joint Commission on Accreditation of Healthcare Organizations [JCAHO])** – An independent, nonprofit organization that evaluates and accredits more than 15,000 health care programs in the United States.

**Justice** – Fair, equitable distribution of resources.

**Logic Model** – A tool used to clarify and graphically display; most often used by managers and evaluators of programs to evaluate the effectiveness of a program.

**Magnet Recognition Program®** – American Nurses Credentialing Center's program to recognize health care organizations that provide the very best in nursing care and uphold the tradition within professional nursing practice.

**Managed Care** – A system that combines financing and care delivery through comprehensive benefits delivered by selected providers and financial incentives for enrolled members to use these providers; goals of managed care are quality, cost effectiveness, and accessible health care. It is a coordinated system of health care, which achieves outcomes (reduced utilization and improved population health) through preventive care, case management, and the provision of medically necessary and appropriate care.

**Meaningful Use (MU)** – In a health information technology (HIT) context, it is the use of electronic health records (EHR) and related technology within a health care organization.

**Medicaid** – A plan jointly funded by federal and state governments, introduced in 1966 to cover low-income individuals; it is managed by each state.

**Mini Cog** – An assessment tool to determine the mental status of older adults and identify patients in need of further evaluation by a neurologist.

**Mini-Mental State Examination (MMSE)** – A brief 30-point questionnaire used to screen for cognitive impairment.

**Modified Caregiver Strain Index** – 13-question tool that measures strain related to care provision.

**Modified LACE** – An assessment tool that incorporates Length of stay, Acuity of admission, Co-morbidity, and Emergency department visits to identify patients with a high-predicted risk for re-admission or death.

**Montreal Cognitive Assessment (MoCA)** – A cognitive screening test designed to assist health professionals detect mild cognitive impairment.

**Motivational Interviewing (MI)** – A skillful clinical communication style for eliciting from patients their own motivations for making behavior changes in the interest of their health.

**Mourning** – The outward, social expression of loss; often dictated by cultural norms, customs, and practices, including rituals and traditions; is also influenced by the individual's personality and life experiences.

**National Committee for Quality Assurance (NCQA)** – An independent, nonprofit organization that assesses, evaluates, and publicly reports on the quality of health plans, health care provider groups, and individual physicians.

**National Database of Nursing Quality Indicators (NDNQI)** – A repository for nursing-sensitive indicators; contains data collected at the nursing unit level to make informed staffing decisions and improve patient care and outcomes.

**National Patient Safety Goals (NPSGs)** – The Joint Commission's series of specific actions that accredited organizations are required to meet with the purpose of preventing medical errors and improving processes for patient safety.

**Negligence** – A duty of care owed to the patient is breached, with a reasonable direct relationship to the patient suffering damages.

**Nonmaleficence** – Acting in such a way that avoids harm, either intentional harm or harm as an unintended outcome.

**North American Nursing Diagnosis Association (NANDA) Nomenclature** – Terminology used by nurses to document diagnoses in all settings where nursing care is delivered.

**Nursing** – The protection, promotion, and optimization of health and abilities; prevention of illness and injury; alleviation of suffering through the diagnosis and treatment of human response; and advocacy in the care of individuals, families, communities, and populations.

**Nursing Code of Ethics** – A guide for carrying out nursing responsibilities in a manner consistent with quality in nursing care; an expression of nursing's own understanding of its commitment to society; the ethical obligations and duties of every individual who enters the nursing profession.

**Nursing Informatics** – A specialty that integrates nursing science, computer science, and information science to manage and communicate data, information, and knowledge in nursing practice.

**Nursing Informatics Competency** – Adequate knowledge, skills, and abilities to perform specific informatics tasks.

**Nursing Interventions Classification (NIC)** – Taxonomy for classifying nursing interventions; used in all settings where care is delivered to document nursing interventions; developed by a team at University of Iowa, led by McCloskey and Bulechek.

**Nursing Minimum Data Set (NMDS)** – A concept developed to ensure all data important to nursing was collected in a standardized manner in every encounter, across all settings; includes 16 data elements; not widely implemented in practice.

**Nursing Plan of Care** – A nursing care plan outlines the nursing care to be provided to an individual/family/community. It is a set of actions the nurse will implement to resolve/support nursing diagnoses identified by nursing assessment; and guides in the ongoing provision of nursing care and assists in the evaluation of that care.

**Nursing Process** – The essential core of practice for the registered nurse to deliver holistic, patient-focused care.

**Nursing-Sensitive Outcomes** – Changes in the actual or potential health status, behavior, or perceptions of individuals, families, or populations that can be attributed to nursing interventions provided.

**Nursing Services** – Organized services delivered to groups of patients by nursing staff; includes nursing care as well as services to support or facilitate direct care, such as referral and coordination of care.

**Occupational Safety and Health Administration (OSHA)** – Branch of the U.S. Department of Labor responsible for enforcing laws and regulations on workplace safety.

**Orientation** – A structured plan created by the organization to "on-board" new staff to provide smooth assimilation into a new position; key components include a general organizational overview, department specifics, and individualized job duties.

**Out-of-Pocket Expense** – Refers to the portion of health care cost for which the individual is responsible.

**Ozbolt's Patient Care Data Set (PCDS)** – Taxonomy used by nurses to document care in all settings, but primarily developed for the acute care setting; comprises nursing diagnoses, patient care actions, and nursing outcomes.

**Pain** – An unpleasant sensory and emotional experience associated with actual or potential tissue damage, or described in terms of such damage.

**Palliative Care** – Both a philosophy of care and an organized, highly structured system for delivery of care; its goal is to prevent and relieve suffering and to support the best possible quality of life for patients and their families, regardless of the stage of the disease or the need for other therapies.

**Patient Activation Measure® (PAM®)** – An assessment that gauges the knowledge, skills, and confidence essential to managing one's own health and health care.

**Patient Advocacy** – The support and empowerment of patients to make informed decisions, navigate the health care system to access appropriate care, and build strong partnerships with providers, while working towards system improvement to support patient-centered care.

**Patient- and Family-Centered Care** – An approach to the planning, delivery, and evaluation of health care that is grounded in mutually beneficial partnerships among health care providers, patients, and families.

**Patient-Centered Care** – Recognizing the patient or designee as the source of control and full partner in providing compassionate and coordinated care based on respect for patient's preferences, values, and needs.

**Patient-Centered Medical Home (PCMH)** – A care delivery model that facilitates partnerships between individual patients, their health care team, and, when appropriate, the patient's family; attributes include patient centeredness, continuous improvement, and care that is comprehensive, coordinated, and accessible.

**Patient Education** – (1) The process of influencing patient behavior and producing the changes in knowledge, skills, and attitudes necessary to maintain or improve health.

(2) A process of assisting people to learn health-related behaviors that they can incorporate into everyday life with the goal of optimal health and independence in self-care.

**Patient Health Questionnaire (PHQ-2 or 9)** – A multipurpose instrument used to assess signs and symptoms of depression.

**Patient Protection and Affordable Care Act (PPACA)** – U.S. law passed in 2010 to reform health care, focused on health promotion, disease prevention, and increased access through insurance reform.

**Pay for Performance** – Government and other third-party payer programs to incentivize adherence to suggested evidence-based guidelines that lead to improved patient outcomes.

**Peer Review** – Process of reviewing and assessing the clinical competence and conduct of health professionals on an ongoing basis; an integral part of quality assessment and improvement processes.

**Performance Improvement** – Systematic analysis of the structure, processes, and outcomes within systems for the purpose of improving the delivery of care.

**Personal Health Records (PHRs)** – Store health care information that is entered and managed by the patient and/or consumer of health care.

**Physician Hospital Organization (PHO)** – Legal organization often developed for purposes of contracting with managed care plans; links physicians to specific hospitals for hospitalization care.

**Point of Service (POS)** – A plan that defines service providers in the service area outside of the usual preferred provider network.

**Polypharmacy** – Involves clients with one or more conditions who are using multiple medications, some of which are not clinically indicated.

**Population Health** – Encompasses the ability to assess the health needs of a specific population; implement and evaluate interventions to improve the health of that population; and provide care for individual patients in the context of the culture, health status, and health needs of the populations of which that patient is a member.

**Practice-Based Population Health (PBPH)** – An approach to care that uses information on a group of patients within a primary care practice or group of practices to improve the care and clinical outcomes of patients within that practice.

**Pre-Visit Chart Review** – Collaborate review of patients chart 24-48 hours before patient visit.

**Precertification** – Process of obtaining authorization or certification from a health plan for hospital admissions, referrals, procedures, or tests.

**Preferred Provider Organization (PPO)** – Program in which contracts exist between the health plan and care providers at a discount for services; typically, the plan provides incentives for patients to use in-network providers as opposed to nonparticipating providers (independent/noncontracted) through decreased co-payments.

**Presence** – Effective listening; occurs at five different levels: hearing, understanding, retaining information, analyzing and evaluating information, and helping/active empathizing.

**Primary Care** – The provision of integrated, accessible health care services by clinicians who are accountable for addressing a large majority of personal health care needs, developing a sustained partnership with patients, and practicing in the context of family and community.

**Primary Prevention** – Includes health promotion (HP) interventions and specific protections (SP); may be directed at individuals, groups, or populations; targeted at well populations or those already ill (e.g., HP = nutrition education; SP = use of seatbelts, avoidance of allergens, or importance of inoculations).

**Productivity** – Measure of the efficiency with which labor and materials are converted into service or care; volume of output related to amount of resources consumed/used to produce a specified output/service.

**Quality Improvement** – A systematic and continuous action leading to measurable improvement in health care services and the health status of targeted patient groups.

**Quality Improvement Using Evidence-Based Practice** – Evaluation of practice evidence and research using data to monitor the outcomes of care processes and improvement methods to design and test changes to continuously improve the quality and safety of health care systems.

**Re-Engineered Discharge (Project RED)** – A training program that is a patient-centered, standardized approach to discharge planning designed to help hospitals re-engineer their discharge process.

**The Registered Nurse Care Coordination Transition Management Model (RN-CCTM)** – Standardizes the work of ambulatory care health care providers as well as providers in other settings across the continuum using evidence from interdisciplinary literature on care coordination and transition management.

**Report Cards** – Identify performance measures that include quality indicators (immunization, Pap smear, and mammogram rates), utilization indicators (membership, access, finances, hospital, and emergency department admission), and satisfaction levels; consumers use report card data to compare the performance of different organizations against a predetermined standard/best practice.

**Research Utilization** – A process of using research findings as a basis for practice; typically based on a single study.

**Resource-Based Relative Value Scale (RBRVS)** – A classification system that attempts to assign the resource requirements within a defined setting based on weights, according to relative cost of each service.

**Revenue** – Total amount of income received or that is entitled to be received based on services rendered or goods provided.

**Risk Management** – An organization-wide program to identify risks, control occurrences, prevent damage, and control legal liability; a process whereby risks to an institution are evaluated and controlled.

**Risk Stratification** – Proactively identify and outreach to at-risk patients to develop patient-centered care planning.

**Root Cause Analysis** – A method to determine the fundamental reason that causes variation in performance.

**Secondary Prevention** – Involves early diagnosis and prompt treatment to avoid disability (e.g., screening, biopsies, medication, surgery).

**Self-Care** – Patients learn to care for themselves and participate in collaborative goal setting and decision making.

**Self-Efficacy** – A person's confidence in his/her ability to carry out behaviors necessary to achieve the desired goal.

**Self-Management Support** – The systematic provision of education and supportive interventions by health care staff to increase patients' skills and confidence in managing their health problems, including regular assessment of progress and problems, goal setting, and problem-solving support.

**SMART Goals** – SMART is a mnemonic, giving criteria to guide in the setting of objectives: Specific, Measurable, Attainable, Realistic, and Timely.

**SNOMED-CT®** – Systematic Nomenclature for Medicine-Reference Terminology (College of American Pathologists); comprehensive, multi-axial nomenclature classification system created for the indexing of the entire medical and health care vocabulary.

**Standard** – An authoritative statement developed and disseminated by a professional organization or governmental or regulatory agency by which the quality of practice, services, research, or education can be judged.

**State Practice Acts** – A combination of laws and regulations that define and regulate the practice of medicine, nursing, and other health professions.

**Strategic Planning** – The continuous process of systematically evaluating the nature of the organization, defining its long-term objectives, identifying quantifiable goals, developing strategies to reach these objectives and goals, and allocating resources to carry out these strategies.

**Supervision** – The direction and oversight of the performance of others.

**"Teach Back"** – A method of teaching patients; providing clear information for patients and families and confirming understanding.

**Team Building and Collaboration** – To build, support, and participate effectively within nursing and interprofessional teams, fostering open communication, mutual respect, and shared decision making to achieve quality patient care during care transitions.

**Teamwork and Collaboration** – Effectively functioning within nursing and interdisciplinary teams, fostering open communication, mutual respect, and shared decision making to achieve quality patient care.

**Teamwork in Health Care** – A dynamic process involving two or more health professionals with complementary backgrounds and skills, sharing common health goals and exercising concerted physical and mental effort in assessing, planning, or evaluating patient care.

**Telehealth** – A wide range of health services delivered, managed, and coordinated by all health-related disciplines via electronic information and telecommunications technologies.

**Telehealth Nursing** – Delivery, management, and coordination of care and services provided via telecommunications technology within the domain of nursing; encompassing practices that incorporate a vast array of telecommunications technologies (telephone, fax, electronic mail, Internet, video monitoring, and interactive video) to remove time and distance barriers for the delivery of nursing care.

**Telephone Nursing** – All care and services within the scope of nursing practice that are delivered over the telephone; component of telehealth nursing practice restricted to the telephone.

**Telephone Triage** – An interactive process between the nurse and patient that occurs over the telephone; involves identifying the nature and urgency of client health care needs and determining the appropriate disposition; a component of telephone nursing practice that focuses on assessment and prioritization and referral to the appropriate level of care.

**Tertiary Prevention** – Involves rehabilitation to return to maximum use of remaining capacities (such as maximizing functional status of the patient with COPD pulmonary toilet and oxygen administration).

**Transition Management in the Context of Ambulatory Care RNs** – The ongoing support of patients and their families over time as they navigate care and relationships among more than one provider and/or more than one health care setting and/or more than one health care service. The need for transition management is not determined by age, time, place, or health care condition, but rather by patients' and/or families' needs for support for ongoing, longitudinal individualized plans of care and followup plans of care within the context of health care delivery.

**Transitional Care** – (1) A set of actions designed to ensure the coordination and continuity of health care as patients transfer between different locations or different levels of care within the same location. Representative locations include (but are not limited to) hospitals, sub-acute and post-acute nursing facilities, the patient's home, primary and specialty care offices, and long-term care.

(2) A broad range of time-limited services designed to ensure health care continuity, avoid preventable poor outcomes among at-risk populations, and promote the safe and timely transfer of patients from one level of care to another or from one type of setting to another.

**Translational Research** – Involves use of theory to guide development, implementation, diffusion, and evaluation of effectiveness and sustainability of evidence-based practice.

**Transtheoretical Model** – Describes behavioral change which takes into account the patient's desire to change. Created and tested by DiClemente and Prochaska.

**TriCare** – A federal program providing coverage to families of active duty military personnel, military retirees, spouses, and dependents (replaced CHAMPUS (Civilian Health and Medical Program of the United States)].

**U.S. Preventive Services Task Force (USPSTF)** – Non-governmental expert panel of primary care, evidence-based medicine experts who review current preventive services and make practice recommendations.

**Usual, Customary, and Reasonable (UCR)** – A method used to determine if a fee is usual, customary, and reasonable; customary is based on a percentile of aggregated fees charged in the geographic area for the same service; usually refers to fees normally charged by a doctor or health care provider for a service.

**Utilitarianism** – Also known as consequence-based ethics; the theory that seeks to choose the thing that will offer the most good to the greatest number of people, increase pleasure, and avoid pain.

**Utilization Management** – The second process of care coordination across the continuum of care; the management and evaluation of the medical necessity, appropriateness, and efficiency of the use of health care services, procedures, and facilities under the auspices of the applicable health benefit plan.

**Variable Costs** – Costs that vary with changes in volumes of service units, such as patient visits.

**Veracity** – Truth telling.

**Zarit Burden Interview** – A 22-item caregiver self-reported questionnaire that identifies the stresses experienced by caregivers.

* Definitions compiled from cited definitions/work located in each chapter of this text.

# Resources

| Resources (discussed in text) | Description | Resource/Website |
|---|---|---|
| Better Outcomes by Optimizing Safe Transitions (BOOST) | A national initiative led by the Society of Hospital Medicine to improve the care of patients as they transition from hospital to home. Project BOOST has developed tools to assist in transitions. | **Society of Hospital Medicine**<br>http://www.hospitalmedicine.org |
| CAGE-AID | A questionnaire that focuses on both drug and alcohol abuse. | **PartnersAgainstPain.com**<br>http://www.partnersagainstpain.com/printouts/A7012DA4.pdf<br>**Washington State Agency Medical Directors' Group**<br>http://www.agencymeddirectors.wa.gov/Files/cageover.pdf |
| Drug Abuse Screening Test (DAST) | 20 or 28 item self-report scale for abuse of drugs other than alcohol. | **Counselling Resources.com**<br>http://counsellingresource.com/lib/quizzes/drug-testing/drug-abuse/<br>**The Drug Abuse Screening Test (DAST)**<br>http://www.drtepp.com/pdf/substance_abuse.pdf |
| Generalized Anxiety Scale (GAD-7) | A self-reported questionnaire for screening and severity measuring of generalized anxiety disorder (GAD). | **Anxiety and Depression Association of America**<br>http://www.adaa.org/sites/default/files/GAD-7_Anxiety-updated.pdf |
| Geriatric Resources for Assessment and Care of Elders (GRACE) | A team-developed care plan to improve the quality of geriatric care and optimize health and functional status, decrease excess health care use, and prevent long-term nursing home placement. | ***Journal of the American Geriatrics Society***<br>http://onlinelibrary.wiley.com/doi/10.1111/j.1532-5415.2006.00791.x/abstract |
| Get Up and Go Test | A timed test for measurement of mobility. It includes a number of tasks such as standing from a seating position, walking, turning, stopping, and sitting down. | **Centers for Disease Control and Prevention**<br>http://www.cdc.gov/homeandrecreationalsafety/pdf/steadi/timed_up_and_go_test.pdf |
| Index of Independence in Activities of Daily Living (IADL) | An instrument used in assessing functional status when measuring a patient's ability to perform activities of daily living independently. | **Abramson Center for Jewish Life**<br>http://www.abramsoncenter.org/PRI/documents/IADL.pdf |
| Mini Cog | An assessment tool to determine the mental status of older adults and identify patients in need of further evaluation by a neurologist. | ***International Journal of Geriatric Psychiatry***<br>http://www.ncbi.nlm.nih.gov/pubmed/11113982<br>**Society of Hospital Medicine**<br>http://www.hospitalmedicine.org/geriresource/toolbox/pdfs/clock_drawing_test.pdf |
| Mini-Mental State Examination (MMSE) | A brief 30-point questionnaire used to screen for cognitive impairment. | **PAR®**<br>http://www.minimental.com/ |
| Modified Caregiver Strain Index | 13-question tool that measures strain related to care provision. | **ConsultGeriRN.org**<br>http://consultgerirn.org/uploads/File/trythis/try_this_14.pdf |

*continued on next page*

| Resources (discussed in text) | Description | Resource/Website |
|---|---|---|
| Modified LACE | An assessment tool that incorporates **L**ength of stay, **A**cuity of admission, **C**o-morbidity, **E**mergency department visits to identify patients with a high predicted risk for re-admission or death. | **RAADPlan**<br>http://readmissionalertdischargeplan.com/yahoo_site_admin/assets/docs/Modified_LACE_Tool.157211759.pdf |
| Montreal Cognitive Assessment (MoCA) | A cognitive screening test designed to assist health professionals for detection of mild cognitive impairment. | **Dr. Z. Nasreddine**<br>http://www.mocatest.org/ |
| Patient Activation Measure® (PAM®) | An assessment that gauges the knowledge, skills, and confidence essential to managing one's own health and health care. | **Insignia Health**<br>http://www.insigniahealth.com/solutions/patient-activation-measure<br>***Health Services Research***<br>http://www.ncbi.nlm.nih.gov/pmc/articles/PMC1361231/ |
| Patient Health Questionnaire (PHQ-2 or 9) | A multi-purpose instrument used to assess signs and symptoms of depression. | **American Psychological Association**<br>http://www.apa.org/pi/about/publications/caregivers/practice-settings/assessment/tools/patient-health.aspx<br>**Pfizer**<br>http://phqscreeners.com/ |
| Re-Engineered Discharge (Project RED) | A training program that is a patient-centered, standardized approach to discharge planning designed to help hospitals re-engineer their discharge process. | **Project RED (Re-Engineered Discharge)**<br>http://www.bu.edu/fammed/projectred/ |
| Resource-Based Relative Value Scale (RBRVS) | A classification system that attempts to assign the resource requirements within a defined setting based on weights, according to relative cost of each service. | **American Medical Association**<br>http://www.ama-assn.org |
| Zarit Burden Interview | A 22-item caregiver self-reported questionnaire that identifies the stresses experienced by caregivers. | **American Psychological Association**<br>http://www.apa.org/pi/about/publications/caregivers/practice-settings/assessment/tools/zarit.aspx<br>**University of Iowa Health Care**<br>http://www.healthcare.uiowa.edu/igec/tools/caregivers/burdenInterview.pdf |

American Academy of Ambulatory Care Nursing

*Many settings. Multiple roles. One unifying specialty.*

## Mission

Advance the art and science of ambulatory care nursing.

## Vision

Professional registered nurses are the recognized leaders in ambulatory care environments. They are valued and rewarded as essential to quality health care.

## Strategic Message

AAACN is a welcoming, unifying community for registered nurses in all ambulatory care settings. This professional organization offers:

- connections with others in similar roles,
- help in advancing practice and leadership skills, and
- advocacy that promotes greater appreciation for the specialty of ambulatory care nursing.

## Core Values

Individually and collectively, our members are guided by our deep belief in:

- Responsible health care delivery for individuals, families, and communities
- Visionary and accountable leadership
- Productive partnerships, alliances, and collaborations
- Appreciation of diversity
- Continual advancement of professional ambulatory care nursing practice

## Strategic Goals

1. *Serve Our Members* – Enhance the professional growth and career advancement of our members.
2. *Expand Our Influence* – Expand the influence of AAACN and ambulatory care nurses to achieve a greater positive impact on the quality of ambulatory care.
3. *Strengthen Our Core* – Ensure a healthy organization committed to serving our members and expanding our influence.

## Membership

Over 3,000 registered nurses who practice in varying ambulatory care settings such as hospital-based outpatient clinics/centers, solo/group medical practices, telehealth call centers, university hospitals, community hospitals, military and VA settings, managed care/HMOs/PPOs, colleges/educational institutions, patient homes, and free-standing facilities. Members are managers and supervisors, administrators and directors, staff nurses, care coordinators, educators, consultants, advanced practice nurses, and researchers.

## Membership Benefits

Academy membership benefits include discounted rates to the AAACN National Preconference and Conference offering multiple practice innovations, industry exhibits, and numerous networking opportunities. Other benefits include distance learning programs, special member rates on publications and the fee to take the ANCC ambulatory care nursing certification exam; the bimonthly newsletter, *ViewPoint;* subscription to one of three journals – *Nursing Economic$, MEDSURG Nursing, or Pediatric Nursing;* opportunity to join a special interest group in the area of: Leadership, Patient/Staff Education, Pediatrics, Telehealth Nursing Practice, Veterans Affairs, or Tri-Service Military; awards and scholarship programs; access to national experts and colleagues through the AAACN online membership directory, monthly E-newsletter, email discussion lists, Online Library, an Expert Panel, website **aaacn.org**, and online Career Center; Position Statement and Paper on the Role of the Registered Nurse in Ambulatory Care.

## AAACN Courses

Ambulatory Care Nursing Certification Review Course*
Care Coordination and Transition Management (CCTM) Course

*This course can be presented at your location – call the National Office for details. Site Licenses for multiple users are available. Course also available on DVD and in the Online Library at www.aaacn.org/library

## AAACN Publications/Education Resources

*Ambulatory Care Nursing Certification Review Course Syllabus*

*Ambulatory Care Nursing Certification Review Course* (DVD)

*Ambulatory Care Nursing Orientation and Competency Assessment Guide*

*Ambulatory Care Nursing Review Questions*

*Care Coordination and Transition Management Core Curriculum*

*Core Curriculum for Ambulatory Care Nursing*

*Scope and Standards of Practice for Professional Ambulatory Care Nursing*

*Scope and Standards of Practice for Professional Telehealth Nursing*

*Telehealth Nursing Practice Essentials*

## Annual Conference

AAACN provides cutting-edge information and education at its annual conference, usually held in the month of March or April. Nurses from across the country as well as international colleagues come together to network, learn from each other, and share knowledge and skills. Renowned speakers in the field of ambulatory care present topics of current interest offering over 24 contact hours. An Exhibit Hall featuring the products and services of vendors serving the ambulatory care and telehealth community provides information and resources to attendees.

## Certification

AAACN values the importance of certification and promotes achieving this level of competency through its educational products to prepare nurses to take the ambulatory care nursing certification examination. AAACN strongly encourages all telehealth nurses to become certified in ambulatory care nursing. Because telehealth nurses provide nursing care to patients who are in ambulatory settings, they must possess the knowledge and competencies to appropriately provide ambulatory care. Ambulatory certification is and will continue to be the gold standard credential for any nursing position within ambulatory care.

## Corporate Collaborations

Together, working with corporate colleagues, AAACN continues to advance the delivery of ambulatory care to patients. AAACN is open to alliances or collaborations with corporate industry to achieve mutual goals. Corporations are encouraged to contact the National Office to suggest ways AAACN can work with them to advance the practice of ambulatory care nursing.

***American Academy of Ambulatory Care Nursing***
**P.O. Box 56, Pitman, NJ 08071-0056**
**Phone: 800-262-6877 Fax: 856-589-7463**
**Email: aaacn@ajj.com**
**Website: www.aaacn.org**

# INDEX

Note: **Bold** page numbers indicate location of glossary definitions. Page numbers followed by *t* and *f* indicate tables and figures, respectively.

## A

## B



## C

## D



## E

## F



## G



## H

## I

## J



## K



## L



## M

## N



## O

## P

## Q



## R



## S

## T

## U



## V



## W



## Y



## Z